1+05117221

WJ 300

Hand
and t

Fifth 1

withdrawn 18/6/23

Handbook of Nutrition and the Kidney

Fifth Edition

Editors

William E. Mitch, MD
Edward Randall Distinguished Professor of Medicine
University of Texas, Galveston
Galveston, Texas

Saulo Klahr, MD
John E. and Adaline Simon Professor of Medicine
Department of Internal Medicine
Washington University School of Medicine
Barnes-Jewish Hospital
St. Louis, Missouri

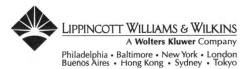

LIPPINCOTT WILLIAMS & WILKINS
A **Wolters Kluwer** Company

Philadelphia • Baltimore • New York • London
Buenos Aires • Hong Kong • Sydney • Tokyo

Acquisitions Editor: Lisa McAllister
Managing Editor: Kerry Barrett
Developmental Editor: Matthew Kory
Project Manager: Alicia Jackson
Senior Manufacturing Manager: Benjamin Rivera
Marketing Manager: Kathy Neely
Creative Director: Doug Smock
Production Service: Laserwords Private Limited
Printer: RR Donnelley-Crawfordsville

© 2005 by LIPPINCOTT WILLIAMS & WILKINS
530 Walnut Street
Philadelphia, PA 19106 USA
LWW.com

Printed in the USA

Fourth Edition, 2002 © Lippincott Williams & Wilkins

Library of Congress Cataloging-in-Publication Data

Handbook of nutrition and the kidney / editors, William E. Mitch,
    Saulo Klahr.— 5th ed. p. ; cm.
  Includes bibliographical references and index.
  ISBN 0-7817-6031-3
  1. Kidneys—Diseases—Diet therapy—Handbooks, manuals, etc. 2.
Kidneys—Diseases—Nutritional aspects—Handbooks, manuals, etc. I. Mitch,
William E. II. Klahr, Saulo. [DNLM: 1. Kidney Diseases—diet therapy—
Handbooks. 2. Kidney Diseases—metabolism—Handbooks. 3. Nutritional
Requirements—Handbooks. WJ 39 H2357 2995]
RC903.N87 2005
616.6'10654—dc22

                                                                    2005006769

To our wives, Alexandra and Carol

Contents

Contributing Authors

J. Andrew Bertolatus, MD   *Associate Professor, Department of Internal Medicine, University of Iowa College of Medicine; Staff Nephrologist, Department of Internal Medicine, University of Iowa Hospitals and Clinics, Iowa City, Iowa*

Mark C. Boxall, MRCP   *Clinical Research Associate, School of Clinical Medical Sciences, University of Newcastle upon Tyne; Specialist Registrar, Department of Nephrology, Freeman Hospital, Newcastle upon Tyne, England*

Nicole M. Daignault, RD, LD, CNSD   *Nutritionist, Nutrition and Metabolic Support Service, Emory University Hospital, Atlanta, Georgia*

Ralf Dikow, MD   *Clinical Research, Department of Nephrology, University of Heidelberg; Chief Resident, Department of Nephrology, University Hospital of Internal Medicine, Heidelberg, Germany*

Wilfred Druml, MD   *Professor of Medicine, Department of Medicine III, Medical University of Vienna; Director, Acute Nephrology Unit, Department of Nephrology, Vienna General Hospital, Vienna, Austria*

Mary E. Evans, PhD   *Postdoctoral Fellow, Departments of Medicine and Endocrinology, Emory University School of Medicine, Atlanta, Georgia*

Denis Fouque, MD, PhD   *Professor of Nephrology, Research Unit JE 2411 in Malnutrition, University Claude Bernard Lyon1; Associate Chief, Department of Nephrology, Hôpital Édouard Herriot, Lyon, France*

Jordi Goldstein-Fuchs, DSc, RD   *Assistant Clinical Professor, Department of Internal Medicine, University of Nevada School of Medicine; Kidney Nutrition Specialist, Sparks Dialysis, Sparks, Nevada*

William G. Goodman, MD   *Professor of Medicine, Department of Medicine, David Geffen School of Medicine at University of California Los Angeles, University of California Los Angeles Medical Center, Los Angeles, California*

Timothy H. J. Goodship, MD   *Professor of Renal Medicine, School of Clinical Medical Sciences, University of Newcastle upon Tyne; Consultant Nephrologist, Renal Unit, Freeman Hospital, Newcastle upon Tyne, England*

Talat Alp Ikizler, MD   *Associate Professor, Department of Medicine/Nephrology, Vanderbilt University, Vanderbilt University Medical Center, Nashville, Tennessee*

George A. Kaysen, MD. PhD   *Professor of Medicine, Chief, Division of Nephrology, Acting Chair, Department of Biochemistry, University of California Davis; Chief, Division of Nephrology, VA Northern California Health Care System, Sacramento, California*

Saulo Klahr, MD   *John E. and Adaline Simon Professor of Medicine, Department of Internal Medicine, Washington University School of Medicine, Barnes-Jewish Hospital, St. Louis, Missouri*

Vera Krane, MD   *Department of Medicine/Division of Nephrology, University Hospital, Würzburg, Germany*

Ronald M. Krauss, MD   *Adjunct Professor, Department of Nutritional Sciences, University of California, Berkeley, California; Senior Scientist and Director, Atherosclerosis Research, Children's Hospital Oakland Research Institute, Oakland, California*

Sreedhar Mandayam, MD, MPH   *Fellow in Nephrology, Department of Internal Medicine, Nephrology Division, University of Texas Medical Branch, Galveston, Texas*

Tahsin Masud, MD   *Assistant Professor, Department of Medicine, Emory University School of Medicine; Chief of Nephrology, Emory Crawford Long Hospital, Atlanta, Georgia*

Brent W. Miller, MD   *Assistant Professor of Medicine, Washington University School of Medicine; Attending Physician, Barnes-Jewish Hospital, St. Louis, Missouri*

William E. Mitch, MD   *Edward Randall Distinguished Professor of Medicine, Department of Internal Medicine, Nephrology Division, University of Texas Medical Branch, Galveston, Texas*

Eberhard Ritz, MD   *Professor of Medicine Emeritus, Department of Internal Medicine, Division of Nephrology, Ruperto Carola University, Heidelberg, Germany*

Christoph Wanner, MD   *Professor of Medicine, Head, Division of Nephrology, Department of Medicine, University of Würzburg, Würzburg, Germany*

Jane Y. Yeun, MD   *Associate Professor, Director, Nephrology Fellowship Program, Department of Medicine, Division of Nephrology, University of California Davis, Sacramento, California; Staff Nephrologist, Nephrology Section, Medical Service, Sacramento Veterans Administration Medical Center, Mather, California*

Vernon R. Young, PhD, DSc   *Professor of Nutritional Biochemistry, Department of Biochemistry, Massachusetts Institute of Technology, Cambridge, Massachusetts*

Thomas R. Ziegler, MD   *Associate Professor of Medicine, Department of Medicine, Emory University School of Medicine; Co-Director, Nutrition and Metabolic Support Service, Emory University Hospital, Atlanta, Georgia*

Preface

In the fifth edition of this book, we have again concentrated on describing the influence of diet on kidney function and vice versa. In addition, we have made important changes in the *Handbook of Nutrition and the Kidney*. First, new authors have brought new perspectives for 6 of the 14 chapters. Second, we have tried to make the *Handbook* more readily available and easily accessible to physicians, dietitians, nurses, and other professionals who provide care to patients with renal disease. This increased accessibility is reflected in extended use of figures and tables to demonstrate nutritional principles.

The role of nutrition in treating patients with kidney disease cannot be underestimated for several reasons. First, the requirements for protein, minerals, and other elements change substantially with advancing renal failure. Second, nutritional principles should be used to provide optimal care for patients with kidney disease. All the chapters in this edition have been revised and updated by authors who are experts in nephrology and clinical nutrition. Our goal is to integrate scientific foundations and clinical wisdom with the information needed to provide a rational approach to the nutritional needs of patients with acute and chronic renal failure, for patients undergoing dialysis (both hemodialysis and peritoneal dialysis) or renal transplantation, for patients with diabetes and nephropathy, and for patients with nephrotic syndrome. This goal requires that the information be of practical use, and we have emphasized this requirement.

We are grateful to all the authors for their thoughtful and excellent contributions to the *Handbook*. We especially thank Ms. Jill Hof and Ms. Rosalie Dustmann for their expert editorial help, and we thank Ms. Kerry Barrett and Mr. Matthew Kory at Lippincott Williams & Wilkins for their patience and advice.

William E. Mitch, MD
Saulo Klahr, MD

1

Nutritional Requirements of Healthy Adults

Nicole M. Daignault, Mary E. Evans,
Ronald M. Krauss, Vernon R. Young,
and Thomas R. Ziegler

THE NUTRIENTS

Six general classes of nutrients exist: carbohydrates, fats, proteins, vitamins, minerals, and water. Those nutrients that are essential components of the diet are listed in Table 1-1. Without these elements, the individual cannot function. Moreover, sufficient energy from the diet is required for growth and maintenance of the body as well as individual organs.

Fats

Fats, or lipids, are concentrated sources of dietary energy and carriers of the fat-soluble vitamins. The sensory properties of fats make a diet flavorful, varied and rich, and they are important in determining the palatability of the diet. In body tissues, they play essential roles in many enzyme reactions, in the positioning and function of cellular proteins, and in maintaining membrane structure and function. Dietary fats are also the source of the essential fatty acids, which are intimately involved in membrane structure and serve as precursors of the eicosanoids, with their diverse, local hormone-type actions involving gastric secretion, smooth muscle metabolism, and nervous system activity. The eicosanoids are a large family of oxygenated C_{20} fatty acids, consisting of three classes: the prostanoids (prostaglandins and thromboxanes), the leukotrienes, and the epoxides. Previously, the unsaturated fatty acid linoleic acid (18:2), an n-6 fatty acid commonly found in vegetable oils and many other foods, was regarded as the primary essential fatty acid, together with its derivative n-6 fatty acids, of which arachidonic acid (20:4) is the most important. However, two classes of fatty acids appear to be essential for health (Fig. 1-1). Besides the n-6 fatty acids, a second class of essential unsaturated fatty acids includes the n-3 fatty acids, including α-linolenic acid (18:3), and its longer-chain, more unsaturated, derivative docosahexanoic acid (22:6). The n-3 fatty acids are found in a wide variety of foods, including some liquid vegetable oils and green leafy vegetables, and their higher derivatives are found in shellfish, fish, and sea mammals. Finally, the n-9 fatty acid, oleic acid (18:1), is the primary dietary monosaturated fatty acid; it is not an essential dietary constituent, but at modest intakes appears to be "neutral" in terms of changing plasma cholesterol concentrations.

The requirement for n-6 fatty acids has been suggested to be from approximately 2% to 6% of total energy, and this percentage probably should include both linoleic and arachidonic acids.

Table 1-1.　The essential nutrients in human nutrition

Amino/Fatty Acids	Vitamins	Minerals/Elements
L-Threonine	Thiamine	Oxygen
L-Valine	Niacin	Water
L-Isoleucine	Riboflavin	Sodium
L-Leucine	Pyridoxine	Potassium
L-Lysine	Folic acid	Calcium
L-Tryptophan	Vitamin B_{12}	Magnesium
L-Methionine & cyst(e)ine	Ascorbic acid	Chloride
L-Phenylalanine & Tyrosine	Biotin	Phosphorus
L-Histidine	Pantothenic acid	Iron
Taurine[a]	Vitamin A	Copper
Essential fatty acids	Vitamin D	Zinc
n-6 Family	Vitamin E	Chromium
n-3 Family	Vitamin K	Manganese
		Selenium
		Molybdenum
		Fluoride

[a] Essential in non-hepatic cells, which cannot synthesize taurine in appreciable quantities.

The dietary requirement for n-3 fatty acids in adults has not been established; in infancy, the requirement is thought to be from 0.5% to 1% of total energy, with a ratio of the n-6 to n-3 fatty acid intake in the range of approximately 4:10.

Clearly, fats and their constituent fatty acids provide more than just energy. Some are essential for maintaining normal metabolism and health. Conversely, excessive intakes of certain fats, specifically saturated fats and cholesterol, increase blood levels of low-density lipoprotein (LDL) cholesterol, and hence can increase the risk for coronary artery disease. Further, a high fat intake can increase adiposity.

Unsaturated fatty acids in plants and vegetable oils typically have the *cis* configuration (two hydrogen atoms on the same side of the double bond). Commercial edible fats contain a measurable level of *trans*-fatty acids (hydrogen atoms in the opposite direction), which appears particularly during the hydrogenation process

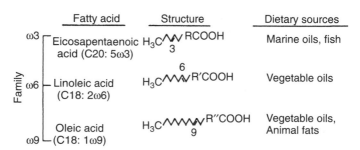

Figure 1-1.　The three families of unsaturated fatty acids and the structure of the terminal end of the fatty acid chain in each series.

that changes liquid, edible oils into solid fats. Like saturated fatty acids, *trans*-fatty acids increase blood levels of LDL cholesterol and reduce levels of protective high-density lipoprotein (HDL) cholesterol. The average intake of *trans*-fatty acids in the United States is difficult to assess accurately, because the *trans*-fatty acid content of foods is not routinely available. As of January 1, 2006, the new Food and Drug Administration (FDA) regulations will mandate that most conventional foods and some dietary supplements list the *trans*-fat content on the nutrition label.

Carbohydrates

Carbohydrates account for approximately 45% of energy intake in the United States. The nutritionally important carbohydrates can be divided into three major classes: simple sugars (monosaccharides), such as glucose, galactose, and fructose; disaccharides, such as sucrose (table sugar, consisting of glucose and fructose), maltose (starch sugar, consisting of two glucoses), and lactose (milk sugar, consisting of glucose and galactose); and polysaccharides, including starch, glycogen (animal starch), celluloses, and hemicelluloses. Celluloses and hemicelluloses are not digested or used to a major extent by humans to provide energy balance and requirements but contribute instead to the fiber component of the diet. The role these compounds play in maintaining normal gastrointestinal function, metabolism, and overall health is the focus of considerable interest. Dietary fiber can influence nutrient catabolism by (a) modulating absorption, (b) accelerating sterol metabolism, (c) increasing cecal bacterial mass and fermentation, and (d) changing intestinal transit time and stool weight. The various components of dietary fibers affect these different events in a specific manner, depending on their chemical form and physical structure.

Proteins

In addition to acting as a dietary energy source, food proteins provide the amino acids that are used as building blocks for synthesizing body proteins. Thus, proteins and their constituent amino acids are essential to life and fulfill a variety of physiologic roles, including their functions in the growth and maintenance of new tissue and in the regulation of internal water and acid–base balance, and as components of enzymes, antibodies, hormones, and peptide growth factors. In the course of carrying out their physiologic and functional roles, proteins and amino acids in the body turn over, and part of their nitrogen and carbon is lost through the excretory pathways, including the carbon dioxide in expired air and primarily urea and ammonia in urine. To maintain an adequate protein and amino acid status in the body, these losses must be balanced by a dietary supply of (a) a usable source of nitrogen to maintain function; and (b) the essential amino acids and, under specific states, the nonessential or "conditionally indispensable" amino acids, to replace those lost during the course of daily metabolic transactions, deposited during growth or repletion of tissue, or excreted with milk during lactation. The essential amino acids are valine, leucine, isoleucine, threonine, methionine, phenylalanine, lysine, tryptophan, and histidine. The nonessential amino acids are alanine, serine, cystine, aspartic acid, glutamic acid, and hydroxyproline. A third category, which can be designated "conditionally essential," is based on the existence of specific dietary or host conditions under which function is best maintained or improved when these amino acids are part of the nutrient intake. This category includes glycine, cystine, tyrosine, proline, arginine, citrulline, glutamine, and taurine.

Vitamins

Vitamins are organic compounds necessary for normal growth, health maintenance, and reproduction. Thirteen such compounds have been established as essential dietary constituents for humans. Some vitamins such as thiamine, pyridoxine, and riboflavin act as organic catalysts, or coenzymes, and a lack of or low dietary intake of these vitamins reduces the activities of enzymes responsible for promoting the conversion of food components into forms that can be used effectively by cells.

Additional functions, forms, and mechanisms of action of the vitamins have been identified. For example, retinol (vitamin A) is required for growth, vision, and reproduction, and it carries out its function, at least in part, by binding to a nuclear receptor and enhancing transcription of specific genes. The specialized functions of retinol depend on specific retinoid derivatives. For example, II-cis-retinol constitutes the chromophore of the visual pigment rhodopsin, whereas 14-hydroxy-4, 14-retro-retinol appears to mediate growth of lymphocytes and fibroblasts. The link between collagen synthesis and ascorbic acid has long been recognized, but vitamin C also is an antioxidant that maintains iron and copper ions in some enzymes in their required reduced form and neutralizes harmful oxidants and free radicals; it also influences many enzymes and physiologic processes.

Most vitamins are converted into an active form after they have been absorbed. Interactions occur between vitamins and other nutrients, affecting their bioavailability. For example, ascorbic acid increases iron bioavailability, protein intake increases calcium retention (with the exception of high protein intake); and energy intake increases the efficiency of protein (amino acid) use. As Figure 1-2 suggests, vitamin B_{12} deficiency is manifested clinically as anemia and neuropathy, because this deficiency interferes with the functioning of folate cofactors. These vitamins and vitamin B_6 are intimately involved in the metabolism of the amino acid homocysteine. Inadequate dietary intake of B vitamins, including folic acid, vitamin B_6, and vitamin B_{12}, can increase the risk for homocysteine toxicity, neuropathologies, and cognitive disturbances. Additional examples of various types of interactions among vitamins, listed in Table 1-2, indicate that changes in the amount of one vitamin could potentially affect the absorption, transport, metabolism, and excretion of another.

Minerals

The macro-inorganic elements—sodium, potassium, chloride, calcium, magnesium, and phosphorus—are all present in the body in substantial quantities, approximating a total of 3 kg in the adult body. The microelements, or trace minerals, total only 30 g in the body and are required in small amounts in the diet,

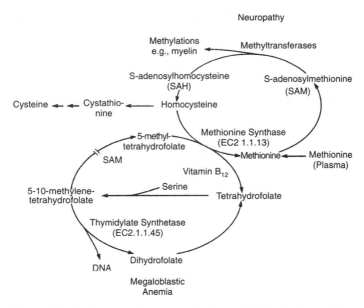

Figure 1-2. Relations between vitamin B_{12} and folate in the metabolism of one-carbon units, involving serine and DNA biosynthesis or methyl group use for synthesis of myelin and other brain structures. (From Scott JM. Folate–vitamin B_{12} interrelationships in the central nervous system. *Proc Nutr Soc* 1992;51:219, with permission.)

usually less than 30 mg per day. As in the case of vitamins, interactions occur between minerals. An example of mineral–mineral interaction is that between iron and zinc: a high iron intake often reduces the efficiency of zinc absorption. For these reasons, the total amount of mineral or of a certain vitamin in a food may not be the critical information for the nutritionist; it is more important to know what *fraction* of the total is available for absorption and for meeting the physiologic needs of the host.

The major mineral elements—sodium, potassium, calcium, magnesium, and chloride—fulfill electrochemical functions. Calcium, potassium, magnesium, copper, and zinc serve as catalysts in enzyme systems, and some minerals contribute to body structure (e.g., calcium, phosphorus, and fluorine in bone and tooth formation). Other essential mineral elements include iodine, used to form thyroid hormones, and iron, a constituent of heme, which is necessary to form hemoglobin, the pigment that transports oxygen to body tissues and organs.

An intriguing example of mineral interactions is that iodothyronine deiodinase, which is needed to convert thyroxine to triiodothyronine, the active form of the hormone, is a selenium-containing protein. Selenium plays a key role in thyroid hormone metabolism; widespread iodine-deficiency disorders, ranging from

Table 1-2.   Examples of types of vitamin–vitamin interactions

One vitamin needed for optimal absorption of another
  Vitamin B_6/vitamin B_{12}
  Folate/thiamine

A high level of one vitamin can interfere with absorption or metabolism of another
  Vitamin E/vitamin K
  Vitamin B_6/niacin
  Thiamine/riboflavin

One vitamin needed for metabolism of another
  Riboflavin/vitamin B_6 and niacin

One vitamin can protect against excess catabolism or urinary losses of another
  Vitamin C/vitamin B_6

One vitamin can protect against oxidative destruction of another
  Vitamin E/vitamin A
  Vitamin C/vitamin E

A high level of one vitamin can obscure the diagnosis of deficiency of another
  Folate/vitamin B_{12}

From Machlin L J, Langseth L. Vitamin–vitamin interactions. In: Bodwell C, Erdman JW Jr, eds. *Nutrient interactions.* New York: Marcel Dekker, 1988: 287–311, with permission.

cretinism to goiter, are frequently associated with low selenium in the soil and potentially marginal or inadequate selenium intakes. Thus, the clinical features of selenium deficiency might not be wholly attributable to the diminished activity of the selenium-requiring enzyme glutathionine peroxidase; abnormal thyroid metabolism also may be important.

THE QUANTITATIVE NEEDS FOR NUTRIENTS

The Approach

The sequence of events that leads to the appearance of symptoms of a clinical deficiency state begins with an inadequate supply of a nutrient to the body tissues (see Fig. 1-3). This state can result from a primary dietary deficiency or from factors that either reduce the absorption or availability of the nutrient or increase the need for it relative to intake. One approach used to determine nutrient requirements is to assess how much of a nutrient is consumed by people in populations free of symptoms or signs that are associated with an inadequate intake of the nutrient. This information is then compared with nutrient intakes by people in populations in which the specific nutritional deficiency occurs.

In this way, it is possible to determine an approximate range of intakes below which the disease appears and above which it is absent. This approach does not enable exact estimates of requirements, because determining precisely the amount of nutrients

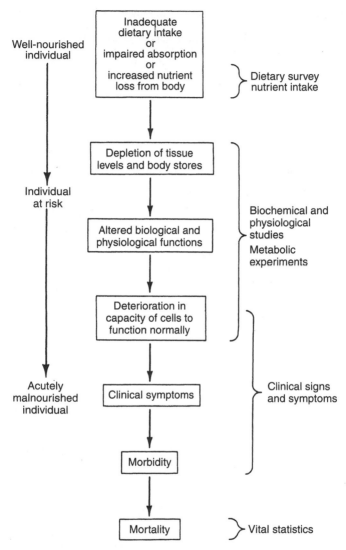

Figure 1-3. Major metabolic steps in the sequence of events leading to the precipitation of nutrition deficiency disease and associated observations. (Adapted from Beaton GH, Patwardhan VN. Physiological and practical considerations of nutrient function and requirements. In: Beaton GH, Bengoa JM, eds. *Nutrition in preventive medicine.* World Health Organization monograph series No. 62. Geneva: World Health Organization, 1976:445–481, with permission.)

that people consume is difficult. Moreover, the diagnosis of subclinical deficiency is often uncertain. Nevertheless, the procedure
helps to forecast the minimal levels of nutrient intake likely to
maintain health in normal humans.

If the dietary intake of a nutrient or its availability in body tissues continues to be low and inadequate, the content of the nutrient in body tissues and fluids decreases, a decrease often
paralleled by a diminished rate of excretion or conversion of the
nutrient to end products. If the dietary insufficiency continues,
biochemical and physiologic lesions develop. Changes can occur
in enzyme activities or in the rates at which blood proteins are
formed. The capacity to use energy-yielding nutrients can be diminished, as reflected in changes in levels of cell and blood compounds that arise during metabolism of these nutrients. These
responses are characteristic of the subclinical phase of a nutritional disease, and they are followed, eventually, by the appearance of clinical signs and symptoms of nutrient deficiency.

Dietary Reference Intakes (DRIs) comprise a set of four nutrient-based reference values that extends the *Recommended Dietary
Allowances,* published regularly since 1941 by the National
Academy of Sciences. They include the Estimated Average Requirement (EAR), Recommended Dietary Allowance (RDA), Adequate
Intake (AI), and tolerable Upper Intake Level (UL). A requirement is defined as the lowest continuing intake level of a nutrient that will maintain a defined level of nutriture in an individual.
RDAs and AIs are levels of intake recommended for healthy individuals that should reduce the risk for developing a condition
that is associated with the nutrient in question. Meeting the recommended intakes for the macronutrients would not necessarily provide enough for individuals who are already malnourished,
nor would they be adequate for certain disease states marked by
increased nutritional requirements. The RDA is the average
daily dietary intake level that is sufficient to meet the nutrient
requirement of nearly all (97% to 98%) healthy individuals in a
particular life stage and gender group. The EAR is the daily intake value that is estimated to meet the requirement, as defined
by the specified indicator of adequacy, in 50% of the apparently
healthy individuals in a life stage or gender group. A normal or
symmetric distribution (median and mean are similar) is usually assumed for nutrient requirements. At this level of intake, the
nutritional needs of the other 50% of the specified group would
not be met. If sufficient scientific evidence is not available to calculate an EAR, a reference intake called an AI is provided instead of an RDA. The AI is a value based on experimentally
derived intake levels or approximations of observed mean nutrient intakes by a group (or groups) of healthy people. The AI is
expected to meet or exceed the amount needed to maintain a defined nutritional state or criterion of adequacy in essentially all
members of a specific healthy population. Examples of defined
nutritional states include normal growth, maintenance of normal circulating nutrient values, or other aspects of nutritional
well-being or general health. The AI is set when data are considered to be insufficient or inadequate to establish an EAR on
which an RDA would be based. The UL is the highest level of
daily nutrient intake that is likely to pose no risk for adverse

health effects for almost all individuals in the specified life-stage group. As intake increases above the UL, the risk for adverse effects increases. The UL is not intended to be a recommended level of intake, and no benefit has been established in healthy individuals who consume a nutrient in amounts exceeding the recommended intake (the RDA or AI).

Current Dietary Recommended Intakes

The Food and Nutrition Board has issued reports providing DRIs for three categories of nutrients: calcium, vitamin D, phosphorus, magnesium, and fluoride; folate and other B vitamins; and antioxidants (e.g., vitamins C and E and selenium). A summary of the RDAs for these nutrients (or AI when RDA was not determined) is given in Table 1-3. Forthcoming volumes will deal with macronutrients (fats, carbohydrates, protein and amino acids, and energy balance); trace elements (e.g., iron and zinc); and other food components (e.g., fiber and phytoestrogens).

Factors Affecting Nutrient Requirements

Not everyone of the same age, body build, and sex has the same nutrient requirements. These differences may be attributable, in part, to variations in genetic background. Various environmental, physiologic, psychological, and pathologic influences affect the variability in physiologic requirements for nutrients among individuals (see Table 1-4). For example, the growing infant or child requires higher nutrient intakes per unit of body weight than does the adult. Besides energy, for which the daily requirement declines with age because of reduced lean body mass and physical activity, most nutrient needs of healthy aged subjects do not change significantly from those of young adults, with the exception of increased intakes suggested for vitamin D, vitamin B$_6$, and calcium in men and women over 50 years old. Furthermore, a characteristic of aging (especially beyond 70 years of age) is an increased incidence of disease and morbidity, which is likely to be far more important than age *per se* in determining practical differences between the nutrient requirements of younger adults and elderly people.

Numerous dietary factors determine the required intake of a particular nutrient. For example, all forms of dietary iron are not equally available, and the type of diet and composition of individual meals influence the availability of the iron consumed. Acute or chronic gastrointestinal infections can interfere with the absorption of nutrients. The result is that body nutrients are depleted, and then the physiologic requirement for nutrients increases during the recovery phase to promote recovery and to compensate for the earlier losses.

Finally, various drugs can affect nutrient requirements by decreasing nutrient absorption or by altering the use of nutrients. For example, a reduced appetite is a frequent consequence of drug therapy, and reduced appetite and food intake exaggerate the effects of drug treatment on the person's nutritional status, particularly if the diet is already marginally adequate. The diet of alcoholics is usually inadequate, and ethanol interferes with the absorption or use of various nutrients, thereby increasing nutrient needs above those required by healthy people.

Table 1-3. Dietary reference intakes: recommended intakes for individuals

Life Stage	Calcium* (mg/d)	Phosphorus (mg/d)	Magnesium (mg/d)	Vitamin A[a] (µg/d)
0–6 mo	210*	100*	30*	400*
7–12 mo	270*	275*	75*	500*
1–3 yr	500*	**460**	**80**	**300**
4–8 yr	800*	**500**	**130**	**400**
Men				
9–13 yr	1,300*	**1,250**	**240**	**600**
14–18 yr	1,300*	**1,250**	**410**	**900**
19–30 yr	1,000*	**700**	**400**	**900**
31–50 yr	1,000*	**700**	**420**	**900**
51–70 yr	1,200*	**700**	**420**	**900**
>70 yr	1,200*	**700**	**420**	**900**
Women				
9–13 yr	1,300*	**1,250**	**240**	**600**
14–18 yr	1,300*	**1,250**	**360**	**700**
19–30 yr	1,000*	**700**	**310**	**700**
31–50 yr	1,000*	**700**	**320**	**700**
51–70 yr	1,200*	**700**	**320**	**700**
>70 yr	1,200*	**700**	**320**	**700**
Pregnancy				
≤18 yr	1,300*	**1,250**	**400**	**750**
19–30 yr	1,000*	**700**	**350**	**770**
31–50 yr	1,000*	**700**	**360**	**770**
Lactating				
≤18 yr	1,300*	**1,250**	**360**	**1,200**
19–30 yr	1,000*	**700**	**310**	**1,300**
31–50 yr	1,000*	**700**	**320**	**1,300**

Recommended dietary allowance (RDAs): in **bold**.
* Adequate Intakes (AIs).
[a] As retinol activity equivalent (RAEs). 1 RAE = 1 µg retinol, 12 µg β-carotene, 24 µg α-carotene, or 24 µg β-cryptoxanthin.
[b] As cholecalciferol. 1 µg cholecalciferol = 40 IU vitamin D.
[c] In the absence of adequate exposure to sunlight.
[d] As niacin equivalents (NE). 1 mg niacin = 60 mg of tryptophan; 0–6 mo = preformed niacin (not NE).
[e] As dietary folate equivalents (DFE). 1 DFE = 1 µg food folate = 0.6 µg of folic acid from fortified food or as a supplement consumed with food = 0.5 µg of a supplement taken on an empty stomach.
[f] In view of evidence linking folate intake with neural tube defects in the fetus, all women capable of becoming pregnant should consume at least 400 µg of folate daily from supplements or fortified foods, in addition to intake of food folate from a varied diet.
[g] It is assumed that women will continue consuming 400 µg folate from supplements or fortified food until their pregnancy is confirmed and their prenatal care, which ordinary occurs after the end of the periconceptional period—the critical time for formation of the neural tube.

Vitamin D* (μg/d)[b,c]	Fluoride* (mg/d)	Thiamine (mg/d)	Riboflavin (mg/d)	Niacin[d] (mg/d)
5*	0.01*	0.2*	0.3*	2*
5*	0.5*	0.3*	0.4*	4*
5*	0.7*	0.5	0.5	6
5*	1*	0.6	0.6	8
5*	2*	0.9	0.9	12
5*	3*	1.2	1.3	16
5*	4*	1.2	1.3	16
5*	4*	1.2	1.3	16
10*	4*	1.2	1.3	16
15*	4*	1.2	1.3	16
5*	2*	0.9	0.9	12
5*	3*	1	1	14
5*	3[k]	1.1	1.1	14
5*	3*	1.1	1.1	14
10*	3*	1.1	1.1	14
15*	3*	1.1	1.1	14
5*	3*	1.4	1.4	18
5*	3*	1.4	1.4	18
5*	3*	1.4	1.4	18
5*	3*	1.4	1.6	17
5*	3*	1.4	1.6	17
5*	3*	1.4	1.6	17

continued

[h] Because 10% to 30% of older people may malabsorb food-bound B_{12}, people older than 50 years should meet their RDA mainly by consuming foods fortified with B_{12} or a supplement containing B_{12}.

[i] Although AIs have been set for choline, few data are available to assess whether a dietary supply of choline is needed at all stages of the life cycle, and it may be that the choline requirement can be met by endogenous synthesis at some of these stages.

[j] As α-tocopherol. α-tocopherol includes RRR-α-tocopherol, the only form that occurs naturally in foods, and the 2R-stereoisomeric forms of α-tocopherol (RRR-, RSR-, RRS-, and RSS-α-tocopherol) that occur in fortified foods and supplements. It does not include the 2S-stereoisomeric forms of α-tocopherol (SRR-, SSR-, SRS-, and SSS-α-tocopherol), also found in fortified foods and supplements.

Table 1-3. *Continued.*

Vitamin B_6 (mg/d)	Folate[e] (μg/d)	Vitamin B_{12} (μg/d)	Pantothenic Acid* (mg/d)
0.1*	65*	0.4*	1.7*
0.3*	80*	0.5*	1.8*
0.5	150	0.9	2*
0.6	200	1.2	3*
1.0	300	1.8	4*
1.3	400	2.4	5*
1.3	400	2.4	5*
1.3	400	2.4	5*
1.7	400	2.4[h]	5*
1.7	400	2.4[h]	5*
1.0	300	1.8	4*
1.2	400	2.4	5*
1.3	400[f,g]	2.4	5*
1.3	400[f,g]	2.4	5*
1.5	400	2.4[h]	5*
1.5	400	2.4[h]	5*
1.9	600	2.6	6*
1.9	600	2.6	6*
1.9	600	2.6	6*
2.0	500	2.8	7*
2.0	500	2.8	7*
2.0	500	2.8	7*

From *Dietary Reference Intakes for Calcium, Phosphorus, Magnesium, Vitamin D, and Fluoride (1998); Dietary Reference Intakes for Thiamine, Riboflavin, Niacin, Vitamin B₆, Folate, Vitamin B₁₂, Pantothenic Acid, Biotin, and Choline (1998); Dietary Reference Intakes for Vitamin C, Vitamin E, Selenium, and Carotenoids (2000); Dietary Reference Intakes for Vitamin A, Vitamin K, Arsenic, Boron, Chromium, Copper, Iodine, Iron, Manganese, Molybdenum, Nickel, Silicon, Vanadium, and Zinc (2001); and Dietary Reference Intakes for Water, Potassium, Sodium, Chloride, and Sulfate (2004).* Food and Nutrition Board, Institute of Medicine, National Academy of Sciences, National Academy Press, 2004, with permission.

ENERGY UTILIZATION AND REQUIREMENTS

Components of the Energy Requirement

A person's energy requirement might be described in terms of the energy-balance equation (see Table 1-5). The major components of the energy requirement include *obligatory* thermogenesis, consisting of the basal metabolic rate (BMR) and the thermic effect of food, and *facultative* thermogenesis. Facultative thermogenesis comprises the energy transformations associated with physical activity and diet-induced thermogenesis (i.e., the more variable component of energy expenditure). When considering energy needs in adults, two important questions must be asked: (a) how large are various components of the daily energy expenditure and (b) do they change during the progression of the adult years, and if so, why?

Biotin* (μg/d)	Choline[i] (mg/d)	Vitamin C (mg/d)	Vitamin E[j] (mg/d)	Selenium (μg/d)
5*	125*	40*	4*	15*
6*	150*	50*	5*	20*
8*	200*	15	6	20
12*	250*	25	7	30
20*	375*	45	11	40
25*	550*	75	15	55
30*	550*	90	15	55
30*	550*	90	15	55
30*	550*	90	15	55
30*	550*	90	15	55
20*	375*	45	11	40
25*	400*	65	15	55
30*	425*	75	15	55
30*	425*	75	15	55
30*	425*	75	15	55
30*	425*	75	15	55
30*	450*	80	15	60
30*	450*	85	15	60
30*	450*	85	15	60
35*	550*	115	19	70
35*	550*	120	19	70
35*	550*	120	19	70

An appropriate "composition" of the daily energy expenditure in a relatively sedentary adult is shown in Figure 1-4, indicating that the BMR accounts for approximately 60% or more of the daily energy flux. Various factors, including familial and genetic influences, nutritional, metabolic, and disease conditions, as well as gender and body composition, determine the BMR. The BMR is reduced in older people, largely, if not entirely, because of the age-related decrease in lean body mass, especially in muscle mass.

The other component of obligatory thermogenesis, that of the thermic effect of food, arises from the energy transformations required for ingesting, digesting, absorbing, processing, and storing the energy-yielding nutrients. The energy costs of the thermic effect of food vary according to the immediate metabolic fate of these nutrients, whereas the facultative component of dietary thermogenesis results from metabolic cycle activity and activation of the sympathetic nervous system.

Actual Energy Requirements

The energy requirement has been defined by Food and Agriculture Organization/World Health Organization/United Nations University (FAO/WHO/UNU) as follows:

The energy requirement of an individual is the level of energy intake from food that balances energy expenditure when the individual has the body size and composition and a level of physical activity that is consistent with long-term good health. The

Table 1-4.   Agent, host, and environmental factors that influence nutrient requirements and nutritional status

Agent (dietary) factors
  Chemical form of nutrient
  Energy intake
  Food processing and preparation (can increase or decrease
    dietary needs)
  Effect of other dietary constituents
Host factors
  Age
  Sex
  Genetic makeup
  Pathologic states
  Drugs
  Infection
  Physical trauma
  Chronic disease, cancer
Environmental factors
  Physical (unsuitable housing, inadequate heating)
  Biologic (poor sanitary conditions)
  Socioeconomic (poverty, dietary habits and food choices,
    physical activity)

requirement also enables the individual to maintain economically necessary and socially desirable physical activity. In children and pregnant or lactating women, the energy requirement includes the energy needs associated with the deposition of tissue or the secretion of milk.

The approach followed by FAO/WHO/UNU to set or define this level of energy intake was to estimate the energy costs of various factors, expressed in relation to multiples of the BMR. These factors are (a) the BMR; (b) growth, in the case of the young; (c) physical activity, which is divided into "occupational" and "discretionary" activities; and (d) the thermic effect of food.

The maintenance component was taken to be approximately 1.4 times BMR for both men and women; when the other components

**Table 1-5.   The energy-balance equation:
energy stored = energy intake – energy expenditure**

Energy Intake	Energy Expenditure (Thermogenesis)
Metabolic food energy	Obligatory thermogenesis
	Basal metabolic rate
	Thermic effect of food
	Facultative thermogenesis
	Physical activity
	Nonshivering thermogenesis
	Diet-induced thermogenesis

From Young VR. Energy requirements in the elderly. *Nutr Rev* 1992;50:95, with permission.

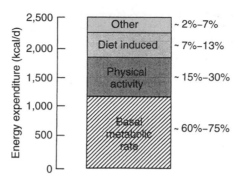

Figure 1-4. An approximate distribution of the major components of daily energy expenditure in a sedentary adult. (From Young VR. Energy requirements in the elderly. *Nutr Rev* 1992;50:95, with permission.)

were expressed as a function of BMR, the average daily energy requirement of an adult might be approximated as 1.55 to 1.75 times BMR (see Table 1-6). A more thorough estimation of the average energy needs of a group of healthy retired men, for example, is shown in Table 1-7. Likewise, estimations for energy requirements by the U.S. Food and Nutrition Board are based upon the use of regression equations for different body mass index (BMI) classifications and ranges of physical activity. As a general guide, the average energy requirement in adults appears to be approximately 1.5 times the resting energy expenditure (Table 1-6).

Source of Energy-Yielding Nutrients

It is important to determine whether the mixture of dietary energy sources is of metabolic, pathophysiologic, or nutritional significance because positive epidemiologic associations have been observed between fat intake and body composition. These associations suggest that the composition of the diet is a factor in determining body energy balance, composition, and obesity.

Macronutrient or energy balance can be achieved by fat alone for the following reasons: (a) dietary carbohydrate and fat have unequal effects on energy substrate metabolism and energy balance; (b) the conversion of carbohydrate to fat is not an important pathway of carbohydrate disposal in the person who is close to energy balance or when glycogen stores are depleted; (c) dietary carbohydrate promotes carbohydrate oxidation and reduces lipid oxidation, whereas dietary fat does not enhance fat oxidation or influence carbohydrate oxidation; and (d) imbalances between intake and oxidation are more likely to occur for fat than for carbohydrate, because carbohydrate balance is under a stricter metabolic control than is body-fat balance. From these observations, three conclusions can be drawn: (a) carbohydrate and fat balances are regulated differently; (b) appreciable storage of glycogen occurs before any important *de novo* lipogenesis occurs from dietary carbohydrate; and (c) adjustment of fat oxidation to altered dietary fat occurs only after a considerable expansion of adipose tissue. Excess body fat increases plasma fatty acid concentrations and promotes fat oxidation.

Table 1-6. Dietary reference intakes (DRIs): estimated energy requirements (EER) for men and women 30 years of age[a]

Height [m (in)]	PAL[b]	Weight for BMI[c] of 18.5 kg/m² [kg (lb)]	Weight for BMI of 24.99 kg/m² [kg (lb)]
1.50 (59)	Sedentary Low active Active Very Active	41.6 (92)	56.2 (124)
1.65 (65)	Sedentary Low active Active Very Active	50.4 (111)	68.0 (150)
1.80 (71)	Sedentary Low active Active Very Active	59.9 (132)	81.0 (178)

[a]For each year below 30, add 7 kcal per day for women and 10 kcal per day for men. For each year above 30, subtract 7 kcal per day for women and 10 kcal per day for men.
[b]PAL, physical activity level.
[c]BMI, body mass index.
[d]Derived from the following regression equations based on doubly labeled water data:
Adult man: EER = 662 − 9.53 × age (y) + PA × [15.91 × wt (kg) + 539.6 × ht (m)]
Adult woman: EER = 354 − 6.91 × age (y) + PA × [9.36 × wt (kg) + 726 × ht (m)].

It follows that voluntarily restricting fat might well be desirable simply from an energy balance and requirement standpoint, regardless of the adverse effects of a high fat intake and the risks of cardiovascular and cerebrovascular disease. Thus, appropriate consideration must be given to the *source* of the energy intake, as well as *total* energy expenditure, in determining the energy requirement and for making recommendations about energy intakes. No broad consensus exists on the "ideal" or "appropriate" mixture of the net energy from carbohydrate and lipid sources.

PROTEIN AND AMINO ACID REQUIREMENTS

The joint FAO/WHO/UNU Expert Consultation defined the protein requirement as follows:

The protein requirement of an individual is defined as the lowest level of dietary protein intake that will balance the losses of nitrogen from the body in persons who maintain energy balance at modest levels of physical activity. In children and pregnant or lactating women, the protein requirement is taken to include the needs associated with the deposition of tissues or the secretion of milk at rates consistent with good health.

Most estimates of human protein and amino acid requirements have been obtained directly, or indirectly, from measurements of nitrogen balance. The 1985 report of the FAO/WHO/UNU Expert Consultation provides an extensive discussion of the approaches used to estimate the mean requirements for protein in various

| EER, Men[d] (kcal/d) | | EER, Women[d] (kcal/d) | |
BMI of 18.5 kg/m^2	BMI of 24.99 kg/m^2	BMI of 18.5 kg/m^2	BMI of 24.99 kg/m^2
1,848	2,080	1,625	1,762
2,009	2,267	1,803	1,956
2,215	2,506	2,025	2,198
2,554	2,898	2,291	2,489
2,068	2,349	1,816	1,982
2,254	2,566	2,016	2,202
2,490	2,842	2,267	2,477
2,880	3,296	2,567	2,807
2,301	2,635	2,015	2,211
2,513	2,884	2,239	2,459
2,782	3,200	2,519	2,769
3,225	3,720	2,855	3,141

PA, coefficient for PAL.

PAL = total energy expenditure ÷ basal energy expenditure

PA = 1.0 if PAL ≥1.0<1.4 (sedentary)
PA = 1.12 if PAL ≥1.4<1.6 (low active)
PA = 1.27 if PAL ≥1.6<1.9 (active)
PA = 1.45 if PAL ≥1.9<2.5 (active).

From Food and Nutrition Board, Institute of Medicine, National Academy of Science, 2004, with permission.

age and physiologic groups. A brief summary of protein requirements for adults, including those for elderly people and women, is illustrated in Table 1-8.

The practical recommendation emerging from estimations of requirements is for a "safe protein intake" (equivalent to the RDA) that includes a factor accounting for the variation in protein requirements among apparently similar people. The interindividual variability in protein requirements among adults amounts to a coefficient of variation of 12.5%. Hence, a value of 25% (2 SD) above the *mean* minimal physiologic requirement for the adult of 0.6 g protein/kg/d, would meet the needs of all but 2.5% of people in the adult population. The mean minimal requirement should be increased to 0.75 g/kg/d to achieve a safe protein intake for healthy adults. Apparently, most people require less than this minimum to maintain an adequate state of protein nutrition. It follows that some adult subjects might require as little as 0.45 g high-quality protein/kg/d. This approach for including variability is applied to other age groups, but in the case of infants, an adjustment also is made for the interindividual and individual variations in growth rate.

Table 1-9 gives estimates for the amino acid requirements in various age groups. Indispensable amino acid needs, when expressed per unit of body weight, decrease markedly between infancy and adulthood. The requirement for indispensable amino

Table 1-7.   Average energy requirement of healthy, retired elderly men [average age, 75 years; weight, 60 kg; height, 1.6 m; body mass index (BMI), 23.5; estimated basal metabolic rate (BMR), 54 kcal (225 kJ)/h]

	H	kcal	kJ
In bed at 1.0 × BMR	8	430	1,810
Occupational activities	0	0	0
Discretionary activities			
Socially desirable (3.3 × BMR)	2	355	1,490
Household tasks (2.7 × BMR)	1	145	610
Cardiovascular and muscular maintenance (4 × BMR)	1/3	70	300
For residual time, energy needs			
12 at 1.4 × BMR	2/3	960	4,020
Total (= 1.5 × BMR)		1960	8,200

BMI, body mass index; BMR, basal metabolic rate.
From Food and Agriculture Organization/World Health Organization/United Nations University (FAO/WHO/UNU). *Energy and protein requirements: report of a joint FAO/WHO/UNU expert consultation.* Technical report series no. 724. Geneva: World Health Organization, 1985:77, with permission.

acids, expressed per unit of the total need for protein, is also lower in the adult than in the infant or preschool child. Table 1-9 compares a pattern of amino acid requirements for the adult with that proposed for the preschool child by the joint FAO/WHO/UNU Expert Consultation. These two patterns are quite similar, but the amino acid requirements for the adult are increased, on average, by a factor of 2.5.

Table 1-8.   Protein requirements in adults, in elderly persons, and women: Summary of essentials of the approach taken by Food and Agriculture Organization (FAO)/World Health Organization (WHO)/United Nations University (UNU)

1. Young men: Short-term N balance (mean, 0.63 g/kg)
      Long-term N balance (~0.58 g/kg)
      Mean, approximately 0.6 g; CV 12.5%
      Hence, safe level = 0.6 + 25% = 0.75 g/kg/d
2. Young women: Concluded to be the same as for men
3. Older people: not lower than 0.75 g/kg/d
4. Pregnancy: based on average 925-g protein increment + 30%, with 0.70 efficiency factor; therefore, 1.2 g, 6.1 g, and 10.7 g additional protein during 1st, 2nd, 3rd trimesters, respectively
5. Lactation: from protein secreted; + 0.7 efficiency factor + CV, 12.5% (birth weight); +16 g daily (0–6 mo); 12 g daily (6–12 mo)

N, nitrogen; CV, coefficient of variation.
From Young VR. Protein and amino acid requirements in humans: metabolic basis and current recommendations. *Scand J Nutr* 1992;36:47, with permission.

Table 1-9. 1985 Food and Agriculture Organization (FAO)/World Health Organization (WHO)/United Nations University (UNU) estimates of amino acid requirements at different ages

Amino Acid	Infants (3–4 mo) mg/kg/d	Children (2 yr) mg/kg/d	School Boys (10–12 yr) mg/kg/d	Adults mg/kg/d
Histidine	28	?	?	8–12
Isoleucine	70	31	28	10
Leucine	161	73	44	14
Lysine	103	64	44	12
Methionine and cystine	58	27	22	13
Phenylalanine and tyrosine	125	69	22	14
Threonine	87	37	28	7
Tryptophan	17	12.5	3.3	3.5
Valine	93	38	25	10
Total (-Histidine)	714	352	216	84
Total/g protein	434	320	222	111

From Food and Agriculture Organization/World Health Organization/United Nations University (FAO/WHO/UNU). *Energy and protein requirements: report of a joint FAO/WHO/UNU expert consultation.* Technical report series no. 724. Geneva: World Health Organization;1985:65, with permission.

These new figures emphasize the issue of dietary protein quality and the amino acid requirement, or *scoring,* pattern to be used for the purposes of assessing food protein quality. The amino acid score, corrected for digestibility, uses the amino acid requirement pattern for the 2- to 5-year-old child, as proposed in 1985 by FAO/WHO/UNU.

DIETARY GOALS AND GUIDELINES

With the growing epidemiologic evidence relating diet and its constituents to chronic diseases, such as cardiovascular disease, cancers at certain organ sites, osteoporosis, diabetes, hypertension, and obesity, concern has focused on eating appropriate amounts to maintain the specific and unique physiologic functions of that nutrient. Cardiovascular disease remains the leading cause of death in the United States and is common among patients with kidney disease. Notably, nearly 50% of deaths among patients undergoing dialysis in the United States are caused by cardiovascular disease. Nutritional management is critically important in preventing or ameliorating a number of cardiovascular disease risk factors, including those that are prevalent in patients with impaired renal function: dyslipidemia, diabetes mellitus, and hypertension. Dietary guidelines from the American Heart Association for preventing and managing cardiovascular disease in the general population have emphasized nutritional principles that can be effectively implemented and maintained on a long-term basis. For this reason, selecting types and quantities of foods that can be readily incorporated in an individual's diet places emphasis on achieving a favorable balance of nutrient intake. Some individuals may have multiple options for specific dietary practices that conform to the general population guidelines. Medical conditions other than kidney disease for which these guidelines can be modified include elevated plasma lipids, clinical cardiovascular disease, insulin resistance, diabetes mellitus, and congestive heart failure.

Core Dietary Guidelines

Core dietary guidelines are appropriate for the overall population and focus on four specific goals for maintaining overall health and reducing risk for cardiovascular disease:

1. Adhering to an overall dietary pattern containing a spectrum of foods that is not associated with cardiovascular and overall health risks
2. Preventing and managing excess body weight
3. Achieving a desirable plasma lipid and lipoprotein profile
4. Maintaining normal blood pressure

The concept of individualizing dietary approaches according to overall health status and specific risk factors also has received increased attention. This concept is particularly important for individuals at increased risk for cardiovascular disease, for whom population-based guidelines might not be sufficient to achieve optimal health status. It also satisfies the need to consider interindividual variability in dietary response as well as cultural and other factors that can limit adherence to a single type of dietary regimen.

Overall Dietary Pattern

Achieve and maintain a healthy eating pattern that includes foods from each of the major food groups. Consume fruits and vegetables (five to thirteen $1/2$ cup servings per day) and grain products, especially whole grains (six or more servings per day with half or more from whole grains). A diet rich in fruits, vegetables, and whole grains confers multiple health benefits. Fruits and vegetables are high in nutrients and relatively low in calories, so they have a high nutrient density. Dietary patterns with high intake of fruits and vegetables are associated with a lower risk for developing heart disease, stroke, and hypertension and also are associated with reduced risk for certain cancers. Grain products provide complex carbohydrates and vitamins, minerals, and fiber. Dietary patterns high in grain products have been associated with decreased risk for cardiovascular disease.

Soluble fibers (notably glucan and pectin) modestly reduce total and LDL-cholesterol levels beyond those achieved by a diet low in saturated fat and cholesterol. Additionally, dietary fiber can promote satiety by slowing gastric emptying and helping to control calorie intake and body weight. Grains, vegetables, fruits, legumes, and nuts are good sources of fiber.

Preventing and Managing Excess Body Weight

Match intake of total energy (calories) to overall energy needs; achieve a level of physical activity that matches (for weight maintenance) or exceeds (for weight loss) energy intake. The increasing incidence of overweight and obesity in the United States has a serious effect on risk for cardiovascular disease, diabetes, and hypertension. According to the U.S. Dietary Guidelines for Americans, excess body weight is defined by a BMI of more than 25 kg per m², and obesity is classified by a BMI of more than 30. In view of the limited success of dietary programs in achieving long-term weight loss, considerable emphasis should be placed on preventing weight gain, particularly in childhood and adolescence. The key principle is to balance total energy intake with energy expenditure. Although a variety of popular weight-loss programs have focused on limiting specific macronutrients, no convincing evidence suggests that such diets are more effective long-term than those in which total energy intake is limited. The most efficacious approach is to limit the intake of foods with high caloric density, such as those high in fat (9 cal per g versus 4 cal per g for protein and carbohydrate), and particularly those with low nutrient density.

Achieving and Maintaining a Desirable Plasma Cholesterol and Lipoprotein Profile

Limit intake of foods with high content of cholesterol-raising fatty acids (saturated and *trans*-fatty acids) and cholesterol by substituting with grains and unsaturated fatty acids from fish, vegetables, legumes, and nuts.

On the basis of abundant evidence for the role of LDLs in the development of coronary artery disease and the demonstrated benefits of LDL reduction for reducing coronary disease risk, LDL remains a main target for dietary intervention. For the population as a whole, both the American Heart Association and the U.S. Dietary Guidelines recommend limiting intake of cholesterol-increasing fatty acids (saturated plus *trans*-fatty acids) to no more than 10% of total calories, and dietary cholesterol to less than 300 mg per day. Anticipated labeling of *trans*-fatty acid content of foods will improve the ability to monitor intake. Further limiting intake of these substances (saturated and *trans*-fat to less than 7% of calories and cholesterol to less than 200 mg per day) is warranted for individuals above risk-based LDL-cholesterol targets put forward by Adult Treatment Panel III of the National Cholesterol Education Program (NCEP). Ancillary dietary measures for reducing elevated LDL include plant sterols and stanols, soluble fiber (e.g., oat bran and psyllium), and soy protein. Substituting whole grains and unsaturated fats for saturated fats achieves equivalent reductions in LDL cholesterol. However, diets high in carbohydrate, particularly those enriched in simple sugars, can induce an atherogenic lipoprotein profile associated with insulin resistance and increased coronary disease risk. Features of this profile include increased plasma triglycerides, reduced HDL, and smaller, denser LDL particles. In individuals with this trait, diets lower in carbohydrate and higher in unsaturated fat should be considered. Omega-3 polyunsaturated fatty acids, found in fatty fish (e.g., salmon and tuna) and in certain vegetables and nuts, may exert beneficial effects on risk for coronary heart disease, independent of their lipid-lowering effects.

Achieving and Maintaining Normal Blood Pressure

Limit salt (sodium chloride) intake; maintain a healthy body weight; limit alcohol intake; and consume a dietary pattern that emphasizes fruits, vegetables, and low-fat dairy products and is reduced in fat.

Based on abundant epidemiologic and clinical trial evidence, limitation of sodium chloride intake is recommended to avoid increased blood pressure. Current guidelines advise no more than 2,300 mg sodium (1 teaspoon or 6 g sodium chloride) per day for the general population, but further salt restriction can be of additional benefit, particularly in hypertensive individuals. Increased intake of other minerals, particularly potassium, calcium, and magnesium, can also be of benefit. Moderate or low levels of sodium intake, consumption of a diet enriched in fruits and vegetables (five to thirteen ½ cup servings per day) and low-fat dairy products (three cups per day) can achieve further substantial blood pressure reductions. In hypertensive individuals, avoiding alcohol and, when indicated, reducing weight are also advisable. Further recommendations regarding acceptable macronutrient distribution and energy, carbohydrate, fiber, fat, protein, water, and electrolyte requirements are shown in Tables 1.10, 1.11, 1.12, and 1.13.

Vitamins and Other Supplements

For most healthy individuals, currently recommended nutrient intakes can be achieved by consuming an adequate dietary pattern of foods, without supplements. Potential exceptions are calcium, and folic acid for women of childbearing age. Claims

Table 1-10. Dietary reference intakes: recommended intakes for individuals: macronutrients

	Range (percent of energy)		
Macronutrient	Children, 1–3 yr	Children, 4–18 yr	Adults
Fat	30–40	25–35	20–35
n-6 polyunsaturated fatty acids[a] (linoleic acid)	5–10	5–10	5–10
n-3 polyunsaturated fatty acids[a] (α-linolenic acid)	0.6–1.2	0.6–1.2	0.6–1.2
Carbohydrate	45–65	45–65	45–65
Protein	5–20	10–30	10–35

[a]Approximately 10% of the total can come from longer-chain n-3 or n-6 fatty acids.
From Food and Nutrition Board, Institute of Medicine. *Dietary reference intakes for energy, carbohydrate, fiber, fat, fatty acids, cholesterol, protein, and amino acids.* Washington, DC: National Academy Press, 2002, with permission.

Table 1-11. Dietary reference intakes (DRIs): recommended intakes for individuals: macronutrients

Life Stage Group	Total Water[a] (L/d)	Carbo-hydrate (g/d)	Total Fiber (g/d)	Fat (g/d)	Linoleic Acid (g/d)	α-Lino-lenic Acid (g/d)	Protein[b] (g/d)
Infants							
0–6 mo	0.7[c]	60[c]	ND	31[c]	4.4[c]	0.5[c]	9.1[c]
7–12 mo	0.8[c]	95[c]	ND	30[c]	4.6[c]	0.5[c]	**13.5**
Children							
1–3 yr	1.3[c]	**130**	19[c]	ND	7[c]	0.7[c]	**13**
4–8 yr	1.7[c]	**130**	25[c]	ND	10[c]	0.9[c]	**19**
Men							
9–13 yr	2.4[c]	**130**	31[c]	ND	12[c]	1.2[c]	**34**
14–18 yr	3.3[c]	**130**	38[c]	ND	16[c]	1.6[c]	**52**
19–30 yr	3.7[c]	**130**	38[c]	ND	17[c]	1.6[c]	**56**
31–50 yr	3.7[c]	**130**	38[c]	ND	17[c]	1.6[c]	**56**
51–70 yr	3.7[c]	**130**	30[c]	ND	14[c]	1.6[c]	**56**
>70 yr	3.7[c]	**130**	30[c]	ND	14[c]	1.6[c]	**56**
Women							
9–13 yr	2.1[c]	**130**	26[c]	ND	10[c]	1.0[c]	**34**
14–18 yr	2.3[c]	**130**	26[c]	ND	11[c]	1.1[c]	**46**
19–30 yr	2.7[c]	**130**	25[c]	ND	12[c]	1.1[c]	**46**
31–50 yr	2.7[c]	**130**	25[c]	ND	12[c]	1.1[c]	**46**
51–70 yr	2.7[c]	**130**	21[c]	ND	11[c]	1.1[c]	**46**
>70 yr	2.7[c]	**130**	21[c]	ND	11[c]	1.1[c]	**46**
Pregnancy							
14–18 yr	3.0[c]	**175**	28[c]	ND	13[c]	1.4[c]	**71**
19–30 yr	3.0[c]	**175**	28[c]	ND	13[c]	1.4[c]	**71**
31–50 yr	3.0[c]	**175**	28[c]	ND	13[c]	1.4[c]	**71**
Lactating							
14–18 yr	3.8[c]	**210**	29[c]	ND	13[c]	1.3[c]	**71**
19–30 yr	3.8[c]	**210**	29[c]	ND	13[c]	1.3[c]	**71**
31–50 yr	3.8[c]	**210**	29[c]	ND	13[c]	1.3[c]	**71**

ND, not determinable.
Recommended Dietary Allowances (RDAs) = in **bold**.
[a] Total water includes all water contained in food, beverages, and drinking water.
[b] Based on 0.8 g per kg body weight for reference body weight.
[c] Adequate intakes (AIs).
From Food and Nutrition Board, Institute of Medicine. *Dietary reference intakes for energy, carbohydrate, fiber, fat, fatty acids, cholesterol, protein, and amino acids.* Washington, DC: National Academy Press, 2002, with permission.

made for potential benefits of supplemental vitamins (particularly antioxidants), minerals, and other substances for preventing heart disease, cancer, and other diseases have not been consistently supported by experimental data. In this regard, particular attention should be paid to the upper limits for these nutrients established by the Food and Nutrition Board (see Table 1-3).

**Table 1-12.   Dietary reference intakes
(DRIs): additional macronutrient recommendations**

Macronutrient	Recommendation
Dietary cholesterol	As low as possible while consuming a nutritionally adequate diet
Trans-fatty acids	As low as possible while consuming a nutritionally adequate diet
Saturated fatty acids	As low as possible while consuming as nutritionally adequate diet
Added sugars	Limit to no more than 25% of total energy

From Food and Nutrition Board, Institute of Medicine. *Dietary reference intakes for energy, carbohydrate, fiber, fat, fatty acids, cholesterol, protein, and amino acids.* Washington, DC: National Academy Press, 2002, with permission.

**Table 1-13.   Dietary reference
intakes: electrolytes and water**

Nutrient	Life Stage Group	AI	UL[a]
Sodium		(g/d)	(g/d)
	Infants		
	0–6 mo	0.12	ND[b]
	7–12 mo	0.37	ND[b]
	Children		
	1–3 yr	1.0	1.5
	4–8 yr	1.2	1.9
	Men		
	9–13 yr	1.5	2.2
	14–18 yr	1.5	2.3
	19–30 yr	1.5	2.3
	31–50 yr	1.5	2.3
	50–70 yr	1.3	2.3
	>70 yr	1.2	2.3
	Women		
	9–13 yr	1.5	2.2
	14–18 yr	1.5	2.3
	19–30 yr	1.5	2.3
	31–50 yr	1.5	2.3
	50–70 yr	1.3	2.3
	>70 yr	1.2	2.3
	Pregnancy		
	14–18 yr	1.5	2.3
	19–50 yr	1.5	2.3
	Lactating		
	14–18 yr	1.5	2.3
	19–50 yr	1.5	2.3
Chloride	*Infants*		
	0–6 mo	0.18	ND[b]
	7–12 mo	0.57	ND[b]

continued

Table 1-13. *Continued.*

Nutrient	Life Stage Group	AI	UL[a]
	Children		
	1.3 yr	1.5	2.3
	4–8 yr	1.9	2.9
	Men		
	9–13 yr	2.3	3.4
	14–18 yr	2.3	3.6
	19–30 yr	2.3	3.6
	31–50 yr	2.3	3.6
	50–70 yr	2.0	3.6
	>70 yr	1.8	3.6
	Women		
	9–13 yr	2.3	3.4
	14–18 yr	2.3	3.6
	19–30 yr	2.3	3.6
	31–50 yr	2.3	3.6
	50–70 yr	2.0	3.6
	>70 yr	1.8	3.6
	Pregnancy		
	14–18 yr	2.3	3.6
	19–50 yr	2.3	3.6
	Lactating		
	14–18 yr	2.3	3.6
	19–50 yr	2.3	3.6
Potassium	*Infants*		
	0–6 mo	0.4	No
	7–12 mo	0.7	UL
	Children		
	1–3 yr	3.0	
	4–8 yr	3.8	
	Males		
	9–13 yr	4.5	
	14–18 yr	4.7	
	19–30 yr	4.7	
	31–50 yr	4.7	
	50–70 yr	4.7	
	>70 yr	4.7	
	Females		
	9–13 yr	4.5	
	14–18 yr	4.7	
	19–30 yr	4.7	
	31–50 yr	4.7	
	50–70 yr	4.7	
	>70 yr	4.7	
	Pregnancy		
	14–18 yr	4.7	
	19–50 yr	4.7	
	Lactating		
	14–18 yr	5.1	
	19–50 yr	5.1	

continued

Table 1-13. *Continued.*

Nutrient	Life Stage Group	AI	UL[a]
Water	*Infants*		
	0–6 mo	0.7	No
	7–12 mo	0.8	UL
	Children		
	1–3 yr	1.3	
	4–8 yr	1.7	
	Males		
	9–13 yr	2.4	
	14–18 yr	3.3	
	19–30 yr	3.7	
	31–50 yr	3.7	
	50–70 yr	3.7	
	>70 yr	3.7	
	Females		
	9–13 yr	2.1	
	14–18 yr	2.3	
	19–30 yr	2.7	
	31–50 yr	2.7	
	50–70 yr	2.7	
	>70 yr	2.7	
	Pregnancy		
	14–18 yr	3.0	
	19–50 yr	3.0	
	Lactating		
	14–18 yr	3.8	
	19–50 yr	3.8	

AI, adequate intake.

[a] UL = The maximum level of daily nutrient intake that is likely to pose no risk for adverse effects.

[b] ND = Not determinable because of lack of data on adverse effects in this age group and concern about lack of ability to handle excess amounts.

From Food and Nutrition Board, Institute of Medicine. *Dietary reference intakes for water, potassium, sodium, chloride, and sulfate.* Washington, DC: National Academy Press, 2004, with permission.

SELECTED READINGS

Austen SK, Coombes JS, Fassett RG. Homocysteine-lowering therapy in renal disease. *Clin Nephrol* 2003;60(6):375–385.

Campbell WW, Evans WJ. Protein requirements of elderly people. *Eur J Clin Nutr* 1996;50:S180–S183.

Committee on Diet and Health, Food and Nutrition Board, National Research Council. *Diet and health: implication for reducing chronic disease risk.* Washington, DC: National Academy Press, 1989.

Committee on Dietary Guidelines Implementation, Food and Nutrition Board, Institute of Medicine. *Improving America's diet and health: from recommendations to action.* Washington, DC: National Academy Press, 1991.

Department of Health. *Dietary reference values for food, energy and nutrients for the United Kingdom: report on health and social subjects, no. 41.* London: Her Majesty's Stationery Office, 1991.

Dupont C. Protein requirements during the first year of life. *Am J Clin Nutr* 2003;77(6):1544S–1549S.

Flatt JP. Importance of nutrient balance in body weight regulation. *Diabetes Metab Rev* 1998;4:571.

Food and Agriculture Organization/World Health Organization/United Nations University (FAO/WHO/UNU). *Energy and protein requirements: report of a joint FAO/WHO/UNU expert consultation.* Technical Report Series, no. 724. Geneva: World Health Organization, 1985.

Food and Drug Administration, Health and Human Services. Food labeling: trans fatty acids in nutrition labeling, nutrient content claims, and health claims. *Fed Reg* 2003;68(133):41433–41506.

Food and Nutrition Board, Institute of Medicine. *Dietary reference intakes for thiamine, riboflavin, niacin, vitamin B_6, folate, vitamin B_{12}, pantothenic acid, and choline.* Washington, DC: National Academy Press, 1998.

Food and Nutrition Board, Institute of Medicine. *Dietary reference intakes for vitamin A, vitamin K, arsenic, boron, chromium, copper, iodine, iron, manganese, molybdenum, nickel, silicon, vanadium, and zinc.* Washington, DC: National Academy Press, 2001.

Food and Nutrition Board, Institute of Medicine. *Dietary reference intakes for energy, carbohydrate, fiber, fat, fatty acids, cholesterol, protein, and amino acids.* Washington, DC: National Academy Press, 2002.

Food and Nutrition Board, Institute of Medicine. *Dietary reference intakes for water, potassium, sodium, chloride, and sulfate.* Washington, DC: National Academy Press, 2004.

Food and Nutrition Board, Institute of Medicine. *Dietary reference intakes for calcium, phosphorus, magnesium, vitamin D, and fluoride.* Washington, DC: National Academy Press, 1998.

Food and Nutrition Board, Subcommittee on Criteria for Dietary Evaluation, National Research Council. *Nutrient adequacy: assessment using food consumption surveys.* Washington, DC: National Academy Press, 1986.

Freire WB, Howson CP, Cordero JF. Recommended levels of folic acid and vitamin B12 fortification: a PAHO/MOD/CDC technical consultation. *Nutr Rev* 2004;62:6.

Grundy SM, Cleeman JI, Merz NB, et al. NCEP report: implications for recent clinical trials for the national cholesterol education program adult treatment panel III guidelines. *Circulation* 2004;110:227–239.

Hegsted DM. Point of view: defining a nutritious diet: need for new dietary standards. *J Am Coll Nutr* 1992;11:241.

Horowitz A, MacFadyen DM, Munro HN et al., eds. *Nutrition in the elderly.* Oxford: Oxford University Press, 1989.

Kinney JM, Tucker HN, eds. *Energy metabolism: tissue determinants and cellular corollaries.* New York: Raven Press, 1992.

Kromhout D. Diet and cardiovascular diseases. *J Nutr Health Aging* 2001;5:3.

Poos MI, Murphy SP. Dietary reference intakes: summary of application in dietary assessment. *Pub Health Nutr* 2002;5:843–849.

Reed PJ. Criteria and significance of dietary protein sources in humans: dispensable and indispensable amino acids for humans. *J Nutr* 2000;130:1835S–1840S.

Reeds P, Schaafsma G, Tome D, et al. Criteria and significance of dietary protein sources in humans: summary of recommendations. *J Nutr* 2000;130:1874S–1876S.

Scrimshaw NS, Young VR. Requirements of human nutrition. *Sci Am* 1976;253:51.

Solomons NW. Physiological interactions of minerals. In: Bodwell C, Erdman JW, eds. *Nutrients interactions*. New York: Marcel Dekker Inc, 1988:115–148.

Trumbo P, Schlicker S, Yates AA, et al. Dietary reference intakes for energy, carbohydrate, fiber, fat, fatty acids, cholesterol, protein, and amino acids. *J Am Diet Assoc* 2002;102:1621–1630.

Young VR. Energy requirements in the elderly. *Nutr Rev* 1992;50:95.

Young VR, Borgonha S. Nitrogen and amino acid requirements: the Massachusetts Institute of Technology amino acid requirement pattern. *J Nutr* 2000;130:1841S–1849S.

Young VR, El-Khoury AE. The notion of the nutritional essentiality of amino acids revisited with a note on the indispensable amino acid requirements in adults. In: Cynober LC, ed. *Amino acid metabolism and therapy in health and nutritional disease*. Boca Raton, FL: CRC Press, 1995:191–232.

Young VR, Pellet PL, Bier DM. A theoretical basis for increasing estimates of the amino acid requirements in adult man, with experimental support. *Am J Clin Nutr* 1989;50:80.

2

Effects of Renal Insufficiency on Endocrine Function and Nutrient Metabolism

Brent W. Miller and Saulo Klahr

PRINCIPAL FUNCTIONS OF THE KIDNEY

The kidney regulates body homeostasis not only by its excretory functions but also by a number of synthetic and degradative properties of glomerular cells and tubular epithelial cells. These properties include synthesis of hormones, degradation of peptides and low-molecular-mass proteins [less than 50 kilodaltons (kDa)], and metabolic events aimed at conserving energy and regulating the composition of body fluids. The kidney is the site of synthesis of a number of hormones [i.e., erythropoietin (EPO), 1,25-dihydroxyvitamin D_3 (1,25-dihydroxycholecalciferol), and renin] and is an important catabolic site for several polypeptide hormones [e.g., insulin, glucagon, and parathyroid hormone (PTH)] and glycoproteins (see Table 2-1).

THE CONSEQUENCES OF PROGRESSIVE KIDNEY DISEASE

Accumulation of Substances Excreted by the Kidney

A sustained decrease in glomerular filtration rate (GFR) is the hallmark of progressive kidney disease. As GFR decreases, solutes that are excreted by the kidney (creatinine and urea) accumulate in body fluids, and the concentration of solutes in the plasma increases. Other solutes also can accumulate in body fluids, including phosphates, sulfates, uric acid, and hydrogen ions. The accumulation of hydrogen ions leads to the development of metabolic acidosis. As renal insufficiency advances, other compounds that are retained in body fluids include phenols, guanidines, organic acids, indols, myoinositol and other polyols, polyamines, β_2-microglobulin, certain peptides, urofuremic acids, and trace elements, such as aluminum, zinc, copper, and iron. β_2-microglobulin and some trace elements can accumulate in and cause dysfunction of various organs. Although the most profound changes occur with severe impairment of GFR, many of these abnormalities with associated adaptive or maladaptive responses begin at GFR of 50 mL/min/1.73 m^2 or more. The accumulation of these substances can lead to hormonal deficiencies (testosterone, fetuin, etc.), inability to appropriately respond to stimuli (insulin resistance, EPO resistance, etc.), or overproduction (prolactin).

Decreased Flexibility in Responding to Changes in Intake

As kidney function decreases, patients' abilities to adapt to changes in dietary intake, particularly those involving sodium,

Table 2-1. Principal functions of the kidney

Excretion of metabolic waste products (urea, creatinine, uric acid)
Elimination and detoxification of drugs and toxins
Maintenance of volume and ionic composition of body fluids
Acid–base regulation
Regulation of systemic blood pressure (renin, angiotensin,
    prostaglandins, nitric oxide, sodium homeostasis)
Production of erythropoietin
Control of mineral metabolism through endocrine synthesis
    (1,25-dihydroxycholecalciferol and 24,25-dihydroxycholecalciferol)
Degradation and catabolism of peptide hormones (insulin,
    glucagon, parathyroid hormone) and low–molecular-weight
    proteins (β_2-microglobulin and light chains)
Regulation of metabolic processes (gluconeogenesis, lipid metabolism)

potassium, phosphorus, and water, is somewhat restricted. In chronic kidney disease (CKD), solute and water excretion per nephron increases as kidney function decreases, but the fewer number of functional nephrons leads to a more restricted range of solute or water excretion. As kidney disease progresses, the capacity to respond to changes in the intake of sodium, other solutes, and water becomes less flexible, and this loss of capacity can result in changes in the volume and composition of the extracellular fluid. Thus, dietary intake in patients with either acute renal failure or CKD must be adjusted.

Decreased Synthetic Functions of the Kidney

The loss of synthetic functions in the kidney contributes to the abnormalities seen in renal insufficiency. For example, decreased production of EPO, a hormone synthesized in the kidney that plays a key role in the maturation of erythrocyte precursors in bone marrow, is a major cause of the anemia in patients with renal disease. Decreased synthesis of 1,25-dihydroxycholecalciferol (calcitriol), the active metabolite of cholecalciferol, by the diseased kidney leads to decreased serum concentrations of calcitriol and decreased calcium absorption from the gastrointestinal tract. Decreased concentrations of calcitriol also contribute to the development of hyperparathyroidism and bone disease in patients with renal insufficiency.

Alterations in Degradation of Hormones and Other Peptides

The kidney is the main site of degradation for several peptides (β_2-microglobulin and light chains), proteins, and peptide hormones, including insulin, glucagon, growth hormone, and PTH (Table 2-1). The kidney is also involved in gluconeogenesis (the synthesis of glucose from noncarbohydrate precursors) and lipid metabolism. Kidney disease, therefore, leads to multiple abnormalities that affect intermediary metabolism, the concentrations of circulating hormones, and the absorption of certain nutrients. As renal failure progresses, anorexia, nausea, and vomiting can develop and compromise the intake of nutrients and energy.

RENAL METABOLISM OF PLASMA PROTEINS AND PEPTIDE HORMONES

General Considerations

The kidney is a major site for the catabolism of plasma proteins with a molecular mass less than 50 kDa but not for proteins with a molecular mass greater than 68 kDa (e.g., albumin and immunoglobulins). Because most polypeptide hormones have molecular masses greater than 30 kDa, they are metabolized by the kidney to some extent. Renal metabolism of polypeptide hormones often involves the binding of the hormone to specific receptors in the basolateral membrane of tubular cells or glomerular filtration and tubular reabsorption. Degradation results in the generation of amino acids, which are returned to the circulation. Removal of peptide hormones by filtration depends on the molecular mass, shape, and charge of the molecule; for example, growth hormone, with a molecular mass of 21.5 kDa, has a filtration coefficient of 0.7, whereas insulin, with a molecular mass of 6 kDa, is freely filtered. Binding of a hormone to large proteins prevents its filtration. Other factors, including impaired renal and extrarenal degradation of a hormone or abnormal secretion, are also operative in renal disease. Most filtered peptides are reabsorbed in the proximal tubule, so that less than 2% of filtered polypeptides appear in the urine. In experimental animals, nephrectomy prolongs the plasma half-life of insulin, proinsulin, glucagon, PTH, growth hormones, and others. Consequently, the circulating levels of numerous peptide hormones are elevated in advanced renal insufficiency (see Table 2-2). In most instances, successful renal transplantation rapidly returns the circulating levels of many peptide hormones to normal levels.

Table 2-2.   Circulating levels of hormones in patients with advanced renal insufficiency

Increased	Decreased
Insulin, proinsulin, C-peptide	Erythropoietin
Glucagon	1,25-dihydroxycholecalciferol
Growth hormone	Progesterone
Parathyroid hormone	Testosterone
Calcitonin	Thyroxine
Gastrin	Triiodothyronine
Endothelin	Nitric oxide
Prolactin (particularly in women)	Hepatocyte growth factor
Vasopressin	Bone morphogenic protein-7
Luteinizing hormone	
Follicle-stimulating hormone	
Luteinizing hormone–releasing hormone	
Secretin	
Cholecystokinin	
Vasoactive intestinal peptide	
Gastric inhibitory peptide	

Insulin, Proinsulin, and C-Peptide

The major sites of insulin degradation are the kidney and the liver. In humans, less than 1% of the filtered insulin is excreted in the urine, and catabolism of insulin in the kidney involves both filtration-reabsorption and peritubular uptake. The kidney also catabolizes proinsulin and C-peptide. Renal extraction of all these peptides appears to be proportional to their arterial concentrations. Ligation of the renal pedicle of experimental animals results in a 75% increase in the levels of plasma insulin and a 300% increase in the levels of proinsulin and C-peptide. The kidney accounts for most of the catabolism of the insulin precursor, proinsulin. Conversely, the kidney accounts for only one third of the metabolic clearance rate of insulin; liver and muscle account for two thirds of the disappearance of this peptide. In patients with renal insufficiency, high plasma levels of immunoreactive insulin probably represent a greater contribution of proinsulin and C-peptide rather than of the active insulin. Consequently, when renal function is decreased, dissociation can occur between the insulin level indicated by radioimmunoassay and the amount of biologically active insulin actually present.

Glucagon

The kidney accounts for about one third of the metabolic clearance of glucagon. Glomerular filtration is the major route of glucagon removal. The filtered hormone is degraded in the brush-border membrane of the proximal tubule and, to a lesser extent, by reabsorption and subsequent intracellular degradation of the intact hormone, so that glucagon excretion in the urine is less than 2% of the amount filtered (some peritubular removal of glucagon occurs). Plasma glucagon levels are increased in patients with chronic renal insufficiency, and the metabolic clearance rate of injected glucagon is markedly prolonged. Glucagon secretion in response to stimulants is exaggerated in patients with uremia, but the high plasma glucagon levels in uremia are apparently caused by decreased metabolic clearance, rather than hypersecretion of the hormone. Immunoreactive glucagon in the circulation of patients with renal insufficiency is heterogeneous: approximately 20% of the total immunoreactive hormone is the biologically active, 3.5 kDa species; another 60% is a 9 kDa species with little or no biologic activity; and the remainder is a high–molecular-mass form in excess of 40 kDa. The 9 kDa species is rarely present in the plasma of healthy subjects; thus, both biologically active and inactive forms of glucagon accumulate in patients with uremia. Patients with renal failure show an altered physiologic response to glucagon; they demonstrate a three- to fourfold increase in the hyperglycemic response to this hormone. Over the long term, hemodialysis corrects some of these abnormalities.

Growth Hormone and Insulin-like Growth Factor I

The kidney accounts for approximately 40% to 70% of the metabolic clearance rate of growth hormone in experimental animals. Growth hormone (molecular mass, 21.5 kDa) has a somewhat restricted filtration rate of approximately 70%, compared with the rate for insulin. It is reabsorbed along the nephron, and less than 1% of filtered hormone is excreted in the urine. In advanced renal insufficiency, the metabolic clearance of growth hormone is markedly decreased, and plasma levels of the immunoreactive hormone are increased; but excess growth hormone production also contributes to the high growth hormone levels observed in subjects with uremia. Some of the biologic effects of growth hormone are mediated by insulin-like growth factors I and II (IGF-I and IGF-II). Growth hormone stimulates the synthesis and release of IGFs, and circulating IGFs exert a negative effect on growth hormone secretion, thereby forming a hormonal axis.

Recent evidence indicates that IGF-I plays a role in compensatory renal hypertrophy. Administering IGF-I increases GFR and kidney weight in intact animals. After uninephrectomy, IGF-I levels increase in the contralateral kidney, even though IGF-I receptor levels are unchanged. In patients with chronic renal insufficiency, plasma levels of IGF-I are normal, but the levels of IGF-II are elevated. Interestingly, the biologic effects of IGF-I and IGF-II are blunted when assayed in the presence of uremic serum, suggesting that a uremic factor (or factors) interferes with the biologic activity of IGF-I and perhaps IGF-II. However, long-term administration of supraphysiologic amounts of growth hormone to humans increases plasma IGF-I about threefold, causes positive nitrogen balance, and can have an anabolic effect. Clinical trials, mainly in children with renal insufficiency, have shown that administering growth hormone improves both the rate of growth and the amount of growth. For this reason, growth hormone is routinely administered to children with CKD or after renal transplantation. The use of growth hormone in adults with CKD is still under investigation.

Parathyroid Hormone

In response to hypocalcemia, hyperphosphatemia, decreased levels of 1,25-dihydroxycholecalciferol, alterations in the vitamin D and calcium sensor receptors, or some combination of these factors, the circulating level of PTH (a 9.1 kDa peptide of 84 amino acids) rises. This response stems from increased secretion of PTH by the parathyroid glands and impaired degradation of this hormone in the liver and kidney. Clinical measurement of PTH must be interpreted with caution; carboxy-terminal fragments of PTH are more elevated than amino-terminal fragments in the circulation of patients with renal insufficiency, because carboxy-terminal fragments depend on filtration for their catabolism, whereas amino-terminal fragments are degraded by both filtration and peritubular uptake. The level of intact PTH depends on the balance between its production and removal by glomerular filtration and peritubular uptake. The circulating metabolic fragments of PTH are the result of enzymatic breakdown of intact PTH in the liver and, to a lesser extent, in the parathyroid glands. The kidney appears to be the only site where the carboxy-terminal fragments of the PTH molecule are degraded. Thus, the liver and the kidney are the principal sites of degradation, accounting for 60% and 30%, respectively, of intact PTH removal. A 7-84 amino acid degradation product is also present, which has no apparent biologic activity but is measured by some radioimmunoassay. In summary, assays directed against the carboxy-terminal portion of PTH or other fragments of the molecule reveal extremely high levels of immunoreactive PTH in the circulation, but these levels are out of proportion with true biologic activity.

Calcitonin

Calcitonin is a peptide with a molecular mass of 3.5 kDa. The kidney accounts for about two thirds of its metabolic clearance. Calcitonin receptors are located at both peritubular sites and the brush borders of tubular cells, and the hormone is degraded at the brush-border membrane of tubular cells and intracellularly in lysosomes. Renal failure decreases the metabolic clearance rate of calcitonin, leading to increased levels of the hormone in plasma. The calcitonin species that accumulates in the plasma of patients with renal insufficiency is a high–molecular-weight form that may or may not have biologic activity. The clinical consequences of elevated levels of calcitonin in these patients are unknown.

Gastrin

The plasma concentration of gastrin in humans is increased after nephrectomy. The hypergastrinemia seen in patients with renal failure is most likely caused by reduced degradation of this hormone by the kidney.

Endothelin

The plasma levels and urinary excretion of endothelin-1, a potent endogenous vasoconstrictor peptide, are higher in patients with renal insufficiency than in healthy subjects and correlate with the degree of renal impairment. Both the hypertension present in CKD and that occurring with EPO administration have been attributed to endothelin-1–mediated responses.

Catecholamines

Plasma levels of norepinephrine are within normal limits in patients with mild to moderate renal insufficiency, but high levels are found in patients with advanced renal insufficiency. In these patients, a threefold increase in plasma norepinephrine levels occurs when patients assume an upright position, and this response exceeds that measured in healthy subjects. Patients with renal insufficiency metabolize norepinephrine abnormally because the activity of tyrosine hydroxylase, the critical enzyme involved in the synthesis of norepinephrine in certain organs (e.g., heart and brain), is reduced. However, the norepinephrine level in patients with renal insufficiency does not appear to be caused by increased synthesis but rather by decreased degradation.

Prolactin

Approximately 16% of circulating prolactin is extracted during passage through the kidney. This hormone, which has a molecular mass of 23 kDa, is filtered to a modest extent and then is reabsorbed by the proximal tubules (less than 1% appears in the urine). Very likely, the kidney contributes to the metabolic clearance of prolactin, although adequate studies in humans are lacking. Elevated plasma prolactin levels occur in approximately 80% of women but in only 30% of men with renal insufficiency. Notably, the increase in prolactin is not modified by the administration of dopamine or bromocriptine. Patients with renal insufficiency experience a prolonged increase in prolactin levels after administration of thyroid-releasing factor, indicating that a pituitary gland disorder, plus a defect in the peripheral metabolism of the hormone, is present. The metabolic clearance of prolactin is diminished to about one third in patients with renal insufficiency. Apart from galactorrhea, other biologic effects of prolactin in patients with renal insufficiency are not clearly established.

Antidiuretic Hormone (Vasopressin)

Antidiuretic hormone (ADH) is metabolized in the liver and the kidney. The kidney accounts for approximately 60% of the total metabolic clearance of ADH, mainly through glomerular filtration, although some of it is extracted at peritubular sites. Whether vasopressin is filtered and reabsorbed in the proximal tubule with intracellular degradation, or is degraded at the brush-border membrane of proximal tubular cells, remains unclear. In patients with renal insufficiency, removal of ADH is decreased, and long-term hemodialysis usually results in high circulating levels of vasopressin.

Bone Morphogenic Protein-7

A member of the transforming growth factor-β (TGF-β) super-family, bone morphogenic protein-7 (BMP-7), is important for renal development. Numerous acute and chronic renal insults decrease the expression of BMP-7. Animal studies of urinary obstruction, diabetic nephropathy, and glomerulonephritis show that exogenous administration of BMP-7 reduces fibrosis.

Hepatocyte Growth Factor

This growth factor [hepatocyte growth factor (HGF)] was identified in 1984 and purified as a potent mitogen from primary cultures of hepatocytes. Molecular cloning revealed a heterodimeric molecule composed of a 69 kDa α chain and a 34 kDa β chain. The α chain contains an N-terminal domain and subsequent four-kringle domains, with the β chain containing a serine protease-like domain with no enzymatic activity.

Levels of HGF were observed to be higher in the urine of patients with acute renal failure than in the urine of healthy subjects or patients with chronic glomerularopathy or polycystic disease, who had low but detectable levels of HGF. Serum HGF levels are elevated in patients with CKD. Immunohistochemical analysis revealed positive staining for HGF to be 33.3% for IgA nephropathy, 66.7% for membranous glomerulonephritis, and 50% for focal glomerulosclerosis. All patients with drug-induced interstitial nephritis were positive by HGF staining, but no such staining was observed in patients with minimal change. In patients with renal cystic diseases, the HGF level in proximal cyst fluid is higher (mean 2.45 ng per mL) than that in the distal cyst fluid (0.42 ng per mL). Immunohistochemical staining showed significant positive correlations between the distribution of HGF and histologic damage, the grade of tubulointerstitial lesion, and several clinical parameters determined at biopsy in patients with IgA nephropathy (p <0.01). In transplanted human kidneys that are rejected, transcription of HGF mRNA has been observed in the urinary tubular epithelium and in mesenchymal cells (fibroblasts and smooth muscle cells in chronic vascular rejection and endothelial cells, mesangial cells, or both in transplant glomerulopathy).

RENAL METABOLISM OF GLYCOPROTEIN HORMONES

The kidney is a major site for the removal of glycoprotein hormones and their metabolites, including EPO, thyrotropin or thyroid-stimulating hormone (TSH), luteinizing hormone (LH), follicle-stimulating hormone (FSH), and human chorionic gonadotropin. Studies in animals suggest that the kidney accounts for 95%, 78%, and 32% of the metabolic clearance rate of LH, FSH, and EPO, respectively. The renal clearance of glycoprotein hormones is relatively slow compared to clearance of nonglycosylated, polypeptide hormones; the filtration of glycoproteins is apparently restricted because of their larger molecular mass (usually greater than 25 kDa), and it is unlikely that glycoprotein hormones interact with peritubular receptors and lead to degradation. Filtered glycoproteins are reabsorbed to a lesser extent than filtered polypeptides, and a large proportion of glycoproteins appear in the urine; the excretion of FSH is approximately 43% of the amount filtered by the kidney. A marked decrease in renal function results in reduced metabolic clearance of glycoprotein hormones, and the balance between hormone secretion and metabolism determines whether the plasma levels of glycoproteins are elevated in patients with renal insufficiency.

HORMONAL ABNORMALITIES IN SEXUAL DYSFUNCTION WITH CHRONIC KIDNEY DISEASE

Sexual dysfunction is a bothersome disorder for patients with renal insufficiency. Its cause is probably a dysfunction of the hypothalamic–pituitary–adrenal axis, characterized by elevated circulating levels of LH, FSH, prolactin, and LH-releasing hormone. These changes lead to lower levels of progesterone or testosterone in women and men, respectively. Although the pathogenesis of these abnormalities is unknown, contributory roles have been suggested for PTH, anemia, decreased levels of nitric oxide (NO), and zinc deficiency. Sexual dysfunction is manifested clinically by impotence, decreased libido, testicular atrophy, and reduced sperm count in men and amenorrhea, dysmenorrhea, and decreased libido in women. Androgen therapy has been used as an adjunctive therapy for anemia in CKD for many years, but androgen therapy for anabolic indications in patients with CKD remains controversial. Increased levels of prolactin can cause galactorrhea, whereas high levels of LH can cause gynecomastia. Uremia might be a cause of these abnormalities if they are reversed or markedly improved after successful renal transplantation.

HORMONAL DEFICIENCIES IN PATIENTS WITH RENAL INSUFFICIENCY

Decreased levels of two hormones synthesized by the kidney, EPO and calcitriol, contribute substantially to metabolic abnormalities in patients with renal insufficiency.

Erythropoietin

Although resistance of the bone marrow to EPO can occur, decreased synthesis of EPO by the diseased kidney is the major cause of anemia in patients with renal insufficiency. Patients with CKD have lower EPO levels than comparable anemic persons who have normal renal function. Uncomplicated anemia of kidney disease is characterized as normocytic and normochromic. Administering pharmacologic doses of recombinant human EPO to patients with renal insufficiency corrects the anemia, increases exercise tolerance, and improves subjective indices of well-being and cognitive function. If iron deficiency occurs (gastrointestinal malabsorption of iron is present in patients with advanced CKD), parenteral administration of iron is required. When adequate iron stores are restored, EPO administration corrects the anemia.

25-Hydroxycholecalciferol and 1,25-Dihydroxycholecalciferol (Calcitriol)

Vitamin D_3 is hydroxylated in the liver to 25-hydroxycholecalciferol. The enzyme 1α-hydroxylase, present in the mitochondria of proximal tubular cells, catalyzes a second hydroxylation to form the active hormonal compound, 1,25-dihydroxycholecalciferol (calcitriol). Calcitriol, in turn, has several biologic effects, including increased reabsorption of calcium and phosphorus from the gastrointestinal tract. Calcitriol also facilitates PTH-induced removal of calcium from bone. The activity of the 1α-hydroxylase in the kidney is stimulated by PTH and inhibited by high levels of calcium, organic phosphates, and calcitriol in serum. Our understanding of the pathophysiologic importance of calcitriol and other vitamin D analogues, calcium, and phosphorus on the musculoskeletal system and vascular system has become increasingly intricate (see Chapter 3). The prevalence of the deficiency is increasing because our two main sources (sun exposure and diet) of the vitamin are decreasing. The diagnosis of the deficiency is increasing when compared to historic levels. The initial recommended therapy for patients with CKD is ergocalciferol 50,000 IU orally, dosed weekly to monthly depending upon the severity of the deficiency.

Nitric Oxide

Levels of nitric oxide, a physiologically important vasodilator, are decreased in patients with CKD and in patients with end-stage renal failure, possibly because its precursor, arginine, is deficient in these patients. Other reasons for administering NO are the accumulation of inhibitors of NO synthase, increased oxidant stress, or both. Low production of NO has been found in patients with CKD and could contribute to the development of hypertension, atherosclerosis, and the progression of renal disease. NO abnormalities might also contribute to intradialytic hypotension in patients receiving hemodialysis therapy.

ABNORMALITIES IN ADRENAL HORMONES AND THYROID HORMONE IN PATIENTS WITH RENAL INSUFFICIENCY

Glucocorticoids

Plasma levels of cortisol are normal or high in patients with renal insufficiency. The response of the adrenal gland to adrenocorticotropin is decreased, but the response of adrenocorticotropin to stimulatory agents such as hypoglycemia is nearly normal. Thus, the normal or high cortisol level found might be the consequence of reduced clearance by the diseased kidney. The net effect is that adrenal function remains normal, and the expected diurnal variation remains unaltered, in patients with renal insufficiency. The presence of metabolic acidosis increases glucocorticoid production.

Aldosterone

Aldosterone is the major mineral corticoid produced by the adrenal gland and, to a lesser extent, by endothelial and vascular smooth muscle cells, so both systemic and local production of aldosterone can produce effects at the target organ. Aldosterone levels are elevated in most patients with CKD and in most animal models of renal insufficiency. Increasing evidence suggests that aldosterone might participate in the development of fibrosis and proteinuria, and these conditions may therefore respond therapeutically to aldosterone blockade.

Thyroid Abnormalities

Abnormalities of thyroid function are present in patients with CKD, because kidney disease affects the metabolism of thyroid hormones at different steps. Levels of both serum total thyroxine (TT_4) and free thyroxine index (FT_4I), measured as the product of TT_4 and the triiodothyronine (T_3) resin uptake, are frequently low. Plasma iodide levels are usually high, and the plasma level of TSH is in general within normal limits, but the response to thyroid-releasing factor is blunted, especially when metabolic acidosis is present. The prevalence of goiter in patients with renal insufficiency is high (greater than 33%) compared to that in the general population, but overt hypothyroidism is rare. Although many patients with renal insufficiency are subject to easy fatigability, lethargy, and cold intolerance, these changes are not accompanied by alterations in the basal metabolic rate or in the relaxation time for tendon reflexes (indicators of the biologic function of thyroid hormone). Low circulating levels of thyroid hormones in patients with renal failure have a protective action on protein catabolism. Thyroid supplementation is not advisable unless firm evidence of hypothyroidism exists.

Other Hormones

The levels of gastrointestinal hormones are increased in the plasma of patients with CKD because of decreased degradation. These hormones include gastrin, secretin, cholecystokinin, vasoactive intestinal peptide, and gastric inhibitory peptide. Whether changes in gastrointestinal physiology result from these increased levels is not clear.

DISORDERS OF CARBOHYDRATE METABOLISM IN RENAL INSUFFICIENCY

Patients with renal insufficiency have a certain degree of glucose intolerance. Although most patients with renal insufficiency are euglycemic when fasting, some evidence indicates that glucose intolerance occurs after oral or intravenous glucose loads.

The abnormal glucose metabolism of patients with renal insufficiency is characterized by fasting euglycemia, abnormal glucose tolerance, a delayed decrease in blood glucose in response to insulin, hyperinsulinemia, and hyperglucagonemia (see Table 2-3).

Insulin Resistance

The major mechanism underlying the development of glucose intolerance in uremia is resistance of peripheral tissues, particularly muscle, to insulin. Metabolic studies, both *in vivo* and *in vitro*, have uncovered impaired insulin-mediated glucose uptake in muscle. A circulating factor might induce insulin resistance at the level of muscle, but increased levels of growth hormone also might contribute to the resistance of peripheral tissues to insulin and impaired insulin secretion. Although the binding of insulin to its receptor is apparently normal, several studies suggest that an intracellular defect at a postreceptor step accounts for the insulin resistance. Patients with renal insufficiency demonstrate two different responses to intravenous glucose administration. In some, the decay rate of infused glucose exceeds 1, and the circulating levels of insulin are increased; in others, the decay of infused glucose is less than 1, and the plasma insulin level is either decreased or lower than predicted for the level of plasma glucose. These different responses might relate to the ability of the islets to release insulin in response to hyperglycemia.

Metabolic Acidosis

The metabolic acidosis of renal insufficiency can contribute to insulin resistance, leading to impaired glucose transport. Indeed, chronic acidosis, produced by ammonium chloride administration in healthy individuals, leads to changes in insulin-dependent glucose transport similar to those seen in patients with renal insufficiency.

The Role of β Cells

The glucose tolerance of patients with renal insufficiency can be normal if the β cells of the pancreas secrete insulin appropriately. If this condition occurs, patients have a normal fasting

**Table 2-3. Glucose metabolism
and gluconeogenic hormones
in patients with renal insufficiency**

Fasting blood glucose level is usually abnormal

Possible spontaneous hypoglycemia (because of decreased gluconeogenesis, alanine deficiency)

Fasting hyperinsulinemia, increased plasma levels of proinsulin and peptide-C

Increased plasma levels of immunoreactive glucagon and growth hormone

Decreased glucose use in response to insulin in peripheral tissues (mainly in muscle)

Impaired insulin secretion from pancreatic islets in some patients (increased intracellular calcium in islets, as a consequence of hyperparathyroidism?)

serum glucose level, but at the expense of elevated levels of insulin in plasma.

A deficiency of calcitriol (1,25-dihydroxycholecalciferol) can contribute to the resistance of peripheral tissues to insulin. Calcitriol apparently interacts with pancreatic islets to modulate the secretion of insulin. Intravenous administration of calcitriol to patients undergoing dialysis has been reported to significantly increase their secretion of insulin.

Glucose Transport in Fat Cells

Fat cells from patients with CKD exhibit decreased glucose uptake in response to insulin when compared with adipocytes obtained from healthy subjects. Lipogenesis in response to insulin is also blunted, and decreased levels of insulin or resistance to its effects can decrease the activity of lipoprotein lipase, which has an important role in removing triglycerides.

Leptin

Leptin, a 16-kDa protein, is synthesized predominately in adipocytes under the control of the *ob* gene. Leptin plays an important role in regulating food intake and energy expenditure; its main target is the hypothalamus. Levels of free leptin are generally increased (when corrected for body mass) in patients with CKD and also correlate with low EPO levels and insulin resistance. Although some renal clearance and metabolism occurs, the etiology of the increased levels remains unclear. The role of leptin in the cachexia and anorexia associated with uremia also remains controversial.

Abnormal Insulin Release

A reduced release of insulin during the initial response to hyperglycemia indicates that β cells in the pancreas have reduced sensitivity to glucose. PTH, apparently by enhancing the movement of calcium into the β cells, seems to impair insulin secretion from such cells. Thus, the secondary hyperparathyroidism present in patients with renal insufficiency can compromise the ability of the islets to secrete insulin appropriately and maintain normal glucose homeostasis. For two reasons, patients with diabetes who have progressive renal insufficiency require decreasing dosages of insulin as the disease progresses. First, they have a reduced energy intake, and second, degradation of insulin by the diseased kidney is reduced.

ENERGY NEEDS OF PATIENTS
WITH RENAL INSUFFICIENCY

The energy needs of patients with CKD and the calorie requirements of such patients are similar to those of healthy subjects. However, energy intake in patients with renal disease tends to diminish, because of the gradual onset of anorexia as the GFR decreases below 25 mL per minute. An inadequate energy intake is important, because it enhances the use of protein in patients who eat low-protein diets.

Loss of Protein Stores

Reduced protein stores can play a major role in the morbidity and mortality of patients with end-stage renal failure and are an independent risk factor for death and hospitalization. Several indicators have been used to evaluate patients with CKD (see Table 2-4), including serum albumin, transferrin, cholesterol, creatinine, and a calculated protein catabolic rate. Plasma levels of prealbumin, IGF-I, amino acid profiles in plasma and muscle, and circulating levels of PTH have also been used. Finally, changes in body composition have been analyzed by measurements of anthropometry, bioelectric impedance, and total body nitrogen. Most reports of such measurements in patients with end-stage renal disease show that the prevalence of reduced protein stores among these patients is 20% to 50%.

PROTEIN AND AMINO ACID METABOLISM
IN PATIENTS WITH RENAL INSUFFICIENCY

Six general classes of nutrients exist: carbohydrates, fats, proteins, vitamins, minerals, and water. The first three classes are organic compounds that serve as sources of energy required for the biochemical and functional activities. In addition, dietary protein provides the amino acids that are needed to synthesize body proteins and support a number of physiologic processes, including growth, repair of tissues, enzymatic activity, and ion and solute transport. Protein and amino acids also function as signaling molecules and as hormones and participate in differentiation, in immunity as antibodies, in gene expression, and so forth.

Historically, the 20 amino acids present in body proteins have been classified into two categories, essential and nonessential, depending on whether they are required in the diet to maintain

Table 2-4. Indicators of
malnutrition in patients with renal insufficiency

Dietary intake
Spontaneous low dietary intake of protein as assessed by urea nitrogen excretion in a 24-hour urine collection (values <0.7 g/kg/d)

Weight and anthropometric measures
Loss of weight or body weight <85% of ideal body weight
Decreased skin fold thickness, decreased midarm circumference or muscle strength

Laboratory findings
Low serum albumin levels (<3.5 g/dL)
Low serum creatinine levels in the presence of somewhat advanced renal insufficiency
Low serum prealbumin levels (<30 mg/dL)
Low serum transferrin levels (<200 mg/dL)
Low levels of essential amino acids in plasma or muscle
Relatively low levels of immunoreactive parathyroid hormone in patients with somewhat advanced renal insufficiency

nitrogen balance in healthy people. In 1954, the amino acids classified as essential were leucine, isoleucine, valine, threonine, methionine, phenylalanine, lysine, and tryptophan. The nonessential amino acids were glycine, alanine, serine, cystine, tyrosine, aspartic acid, glutamic acid, proline, histidine, hydroxyproline, citrulline, and arginine. Subsequent studies have suggested that this classification is not satisfactory, because histidine has been shown to be an essential amino acid, and other amino acids such as glycine, tyrosine, cystine, proline, arginine, glutamine, and taurine are now generally considered indispensable components of the normal diet in patients with various diseases.

Patients with progressive renal insufficiency are at increased risk for losing protein stores, a major factor in the excessive morbidity and mortality that occurs in patients with CKD. Metabolism of protein and amino acids is altered in patients with CKD, and as renal function decreases, nitrogenous waste products of protein metabolism accumulate, eventually resulting in symptomatic uremia (see Chapter 6). During the evolution of progressive renal insufficiency, subtle alterations occur in the concentrations of plasma proteins and in the levels of amino acids in plasma and intracellular compartments. In 25% to 50% of patients entering dialysis programs in North America albumin levels in plasma are low, and this abnormality is a good predictor of morbidity and mortality in patients undergoing dialysis. The loss of protein stores can be the result of inadequate dietary intake or of increased requirements caused by changes in intermediary metabolism that result from kidney failure. In certain instances, extravascular pools of albumin can be reduced, even though the serum albumin concentration remains normal. Serum concentrations of transferrin, considered by some to respond more rapidly to protein malnutrition, are low in many patients with moderate to advanced renal insufficiency and were also found to be low in a group of patients undergoing long-term dialysis, despite sufficient protein intake (i.e., 1 g protein per kg b.w.). Although inadequate protein or energy intake frequently can be measured, the possibility that renal failure *per se* disturbs one or several steps in the complex process of protein synthesis and degradation has not received sufficient study. Recent research indicates that increased catabolism of proteins can indeed occur in the muscle of patients with only moderate renal insufficiency. Metabolic alterations in patients with renal insufficiency that seem to cause net protein catabolism in the muscle include higher levels of circulating glucagon and PTH, accumulation of uremic toxins, and metabolic acidosis. Metabolic acidosis increases proteolysis in the muscle of experimental animals without altering protein synthesis. Correcting metabolic acidosis in patients with renal insufficiency has been shown to reduce proteolysis, and supplementing the diet of patients with renal insufficiency with bicarbonate can improve nitrogen balance.

Changes in Amino Acid Profiles in Renal Insufficiency

Patients with CKD frequently have a decreased ratio of essential to nonessential amino acids, a pattern that mimics that seen in protein–calorie malnutrition. However, the abnormalities in plasma amino acids in patients with renal insufficiency cannot be explained on the basis of malnutrition alone, because these abnormalities also occur when protein intake is optimal, suggesting that abnormal levels in plasma might be the result of changes in amino acid metabolism caused by renal insufficiency. The plasma levels of the branched-chain amino acids valine, leucine, and isoleucine, and of their respective ketoacids, are decreased, with valine being reduced to a greater extent than the others. The potential mechanism responsible for this decrease in branched-chain amino acids might be related to oxidation of such amino acids in skeletal muscle as a consequence of metabolic acidosis. Patients with renal insufficiency also exhibit decreases in the plasma concentrations of threonine and lysine, as well as low serine levels. The low serine levels might be attributable to decreased production of this amino acid from glycine in the kidney. Tyrosine levels are usually decreased, and this decrease presumably is related to defective phenylalanine hydroxylation. The plasma levels of phenylalanine are usually normal, whereas total tryptophan is decreased in patients with uremia, although free tryptophan levels are normal. The explanation for this difference is that the binding of tryptophan by plasma proteins in subjects with uremia is reduced. Levels of certain amino acids, including glycine, citrulline, cystine, aspartate, methionine, and both 1- and 3-methylhistidine, are increased in the plasma of patients with renal insufficiency. The elevated plasma concentration of citrulline is caused by a decrease in the conversion of this amino acid to arginine in the damaged kidney. Interestingly, the higher citrulline level in plasma seems to correct any arginine deficit in patients with advanced renal disease. Metabolites of sulfur-containing amino acids accumulate in blood.

Intracellular Levels of Amino Acids

Intracellular levels of amino acids in the muscle of patients with CKD also reveal abnormalities. Typically, intracellular valine levels are low, but those of other branched-chain amino acids, leucine and isoleucine, are within normal limits. The levels of intracellular taurine are decreased, despite normal plasma levels. Intracellular levels of both cystine and methionine, two precursors of taurine synthesis, are usually increased in renal insufficiency, suggesting that a low intracellular taurine level might arise from defective synthesis from these two precursors.

The abnormal concentrations of amino acids possibly might influence protein metabolism *per se*. Indeed, when predialysis patients taking 16 to 20 g of protein per day were provided with a supplement of essential amino acids, designed to modify or correct the abnormalities in amino acid levels, both nitrogen balance and the profile of intracellular amino acids improved. Decreased use of amino acids by the kidney can contribute to the accumulation in the plasma of certain amino acids, such as citrulline. The concentration of amino acids is much greater inside the cells than in plasma, however, and thus plasma levels of amino acids are not representative of intracellular amino acid levels.

VITAMINS

In patients with relatively advanced renal insufficiency who are ingesting protein-restricted diets, deficiencies of water-soluble vitamins can develop because of decreased dietary intake (see Chapter 10). Reduced concentrations of several water-soluble vitamins in serum, erythrocytes, and leukocytes have been reported, and hematologic evidence of folate deficiency was found in some patients but not in others, probably reflecting variations in dietary intake and use of vitamin supplements. In one report, patients who did not receive vitamin supplements had low plasma and leukocyte concentrations of vitamin C, and a few patients had signs suggesting mild degrees of scurvy. Plasma concentrations of other water-soluble vitamins have been reported as normal in most studies. Because the kidney is one of the routes of eliminating water-soluble vitamins and their metabolites, decreased kidney function may be a protective mechanism, especially for patients receiving hemodialysis, a treatment that can remove water-soluble vitamins. Vitamin deficiencies can be related to poor dietary intake, interference with vitamin absorption by other drugs, altered metabolism, and, in patients undergoing dialysis, loss of vitamins in the dialysate. The daily requirements of vitamins for patients with renal insufficiency are not clearly defined, but evidence suggests that supplements can prevent or correct vitamin deficiencies (see Chapter 10). Thus, patients with advanced renal insufficiency or those undergoing dialysis should take supplemental folic acid and B vitamins. Vitamin replacement may have to be increased in patients undergoing high-flux dialysis.

Plasma levels of pyridoxyl-5-phosphate are frequently low in patients with renal insufficiency. Levels of serum glutamic oxaloacetic transaminase suggest that pyridoxine deficiency is clinically relevant. Because this plasma enzyme requires pyridoxyl-5-phosphate as a cofactor, a water-soluble vitamin supplement that includes 10 to 50 mg of pyridoxine per day and 1 to 5 mg of folate per day has been suggested as a way to avoid a deficiency state. Conversely, supplementation with multivitamin preparations should be avoided or prescribed cautiously, because excessive levels of certain vitamins can develop in patients with advanced renal insufficiency. Vitamin C supplements should not exceed 150 to 200 mg per day, because higher levels can cause the accumulation of ascorbic acid metabolites such as oxalate. Oxalate can lead to complications such as calcium oxalate kidney stones plus deposits of calcium oxalate in soft tissues and organs. Levels of vitamin A are usually high in patients with advanced renal insufficiency, because decreased renal catabolism causes an increase in the serum levels of retinol-binding protein. An increase in the levels of vitamin A can cause anemia and abnormalities of lipid and calcium metabolism. Plasma levels of pyridoxyl-5-phosphate are frequently low in patients with renal insufficiency. Levels of serum glutamic oxaloacetic transaminase suggest that pyridoxine deficiency is clinically relevant.

TRACE ELEMENTS

In patients with renal insufficiency, the metabolism of many trace elements is probably deranged. The mechanisms for these alterations are not clearly established, and the contribution of trace-element deficiencies or excesses to the symptoms of advanced renal insufficiency has not been adequately studied.

Highly protein-bound substances, such as copper and zinc, are lost in excessive amounts in patients with proteinuria. No data support routine supplements of trace elements for patients with CKD, but some evidence suggests a need for additional selenium, zinc, and iron (see Chapter 10).

These supplements should be given only after the adequacy of the diet in terms of calories and protein has been evaluated. The extent of zinc deficiency in advanced renal insufficiency or in patients undergoing dialysis is debatable. Infections or steroid therapy can artificially reduce the concentration of zinc in plasma, and this condition should be taken into account before zinc supplements are prescribed. Plasma levels of selenium, which has important antioxidant properties, have been reported as low, particularly in patients undergoing dialysis, but the benefits of selenium administration in this population have not been identified. Accumulation of aluminum (such as phosphate binders) from medicines can occur, but most dialysis centers have largely eliminated the use of aluminum as a phosphate binder in treating patients with CKD. Accumulation of aluminum can cause bone disease, encephalopathy, and other clinical problems in patients with renal insufficiency.

Ideal therapy with iron supplements for the patient with CKD remains controversial. Oral iron therapy is much less successful for patients with CKD, perhaps because of gastrointestinal absorption problems. Most patients with CKD receive intravenous iron therapy for anemia, although dosages must be measured against possible organ toxicity or effects upon systemic infections.

SELECTED READINGS

Feldman HI, Jaffe M, Robinson B, et al. Administration of parenteral iron and mortality among hemodialysis patients. *J Am Soc Nephrol* 2004;15:1623–1632.

Hollenberg NK. Aldosterone in the development and progression of renal injury. *Kidney Int* 2004;66:1–9.

Klahr S. Effect of malnutrition and changes in protein intake on renal function. In: Kopple JD, Massry SG, eds. *Nutritional management of renal disease*, 2nd ed. Philadelphia: Lippincott Williams & Wilkins, 2004:213–221.

Kronenberg F, Lingenhel A, Lhotta K, et al. Lipoprotein(a) and low-density lipoprotein-derived cholesterol in nephrotic syndrome: impact on lipid-lowering therapy? *Kidney Int* 2004;66:348–354.

Lariviere R, Lebel M. Endothelin-1 in chronic renal failure and hypertension. *Can J Physiol Pharmacol* 2003;81:607–621.

Mizuno S, Nakamura T. Suppressions of chronic glomerular injuries and TGF-β1 production by HGF in attenuation of murine diabetic nephropathy. *Am J Renal Physiol* 2004;286:F134–F143.

Slatopolsky E, Brown A, Dusso A. Role of phosphorus in the pathogenesis of secondary hyperparathyroidism. *Am J Kidney Dis* 2001; 37(Suppl. 2):S54–S57.

Wang S, Chen Q, Simon TC, et al. Bone morphogenic protein-7 (BMP-7), a novel therapy for diabetic nephropathy. *Kidney Int* 2003; 63:2037–2049.

Zager RA, Johnson ACM, Hanson SY. Parenteral iron nephrotoxicity: potential mechanisms and consequences. *Kidney Int* 2004;66: 144–156.

Zoccali C, Mallamaci F, Tripepi G. Adipose tissue as a source of inflammatory cytokines in health and disease: focus on end-stage renal disease. *Kidney Int* 2003;63(Suppl. 84):S65–S68.

3

Calcium, Phosphorus, and Vitamin D

William G. Goodman

The kidneys play an essential role in regulating the metabolism of calcium and phosphorus. Excretion in the urine provides the final regulatory step for maintaining total body balance for both minerals, by accommodating variations in net intestinal calcium and phosphorus absorption and changes in net calcium and phosphorus exchange between bone and extracellular fluid. The importance of adequate renal function for maintaining mineral homeostasis is underscored by the prevalence and severity of various disturbances in calcium and phosphorus metabolism that develop in patients with chronic kidney disease.

Calcium ions are critically important for maintaining the integrity and functional properties of cell membranes, and they serve as key mediators of signal transduction within cells. Phosphorus is essential for the transfer and use of energy within cells through adenosine triphosphate (ATP), and it participates in intracellular energy storage by forming high-energy chemical bonds in organic compounds, such as creatine phosphate. Phosphorus, like calcium, is involved in a wide variety of metabolic and enzymatic processes. Calcium and phosphorus together represent the major mineral components of bone, which not only serves structural and locomotive functions but also provides a large endogenous source of calcium and phosphorus to support metabolic and homeostatic requirements. Adequate regulation of calcium and phosphorus metabolism is thus crucially important to support these and a variety of other physiologic processes.

A number of factors influence the way the renal tubule handles calcium and phosphorus. Some factors act locally within discrete nephron segments, whereas other factors act systemically to regulate renal calcium and phosphorus excretion and to modify cellular functions in other target tissues. Key among the systemic factors is parathyroid hormone (PTH), which not only affects the renal tubular transport of both calcium and phosphorus but also serves as an important modifier of bone cell metabolism. Whereas PTH is involved primarily in regulating systemic calcium homeostasis, fibroblast growth factor-23 (FGF-23) and other peptides that influence phosphorus metabolism, collectively termed phosphatonins, represent a recently recognized yet distinct set of potentially important phosphate-regulating factors whose physiologic role is not fully understood. These phosphatonins also play an important role in regulating phosphorus metabolism.

Apart from their diverse excretory functions, the kidneys play a crucial role in regulating calcium and phosphorus homeostasis by serving as the primary site for producing the most potent metabolite of vitamin D: 1,25-dihydroxyvitamin D, or calcitriol.

Cells of the proximal nephron synthesize calcitriol after the uptake of 25-hydroxyvitamin D from tubular fluid by megalin-dependent mechanisms. Calcium, phosphorus, and PTH each independently affect the level of activity of the renal 25-hydroxyvitamin D, 1α-hydroxylase. The discussion that follows offers an integrated overview of how the excretory and metabolic aspects of kidney function separately regulate calcium, phosphorus, and vitamin D metabolism.

CALCIUM

Overview of Calcium Metabolism and the Regulation of Plasma Calcium Levels

Calcium is the most abundant cation in the body. More than 99% of calcium resides in bone, whereas less than 1% is found in extracellular fluid (see Fig. 3-1). Intracellular calcium concentrations are quite low, and measurements are expressed in units of μmol per L, whereas the concentration of calcium in extracellular fluid is much higher, with measurements expressed in units of mmol per L.

In adults, the skeleton contains approximately 1.2 to 1.4 kg of elemental calcium, predominantly in the form of hydroxyapatite. Most of the calcium in the bone serves a structural need, and only a limited amount, approximately 150 to 200 mg, is exchanged daily with the extracellular fluid during the process of skeletal remodeling (Fig. 3-1). A separate, more rapidly exchangeable pool of calcium is available, however, to satisfy short-term homeostatic requirements. Calcium influx and efflux from this rapidly

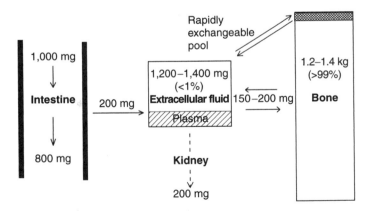

Figure 3-1. The distribution of calcium in bone and extracellular fluid and the net amounts of calcium that enter and leave the extracellular fluid each day from bone and the gastrointestinal tract. The movement of calcium between extracellular fluid and a rapidly exchangeable skeletal calcium pool serves to maintain constant levels of ionized calcium in blood and is separate from the amounts exchanged because of ongoing skeletal remodeling. Under steady conditions, calcium excretion in the urine closely approximates net intestinal calcium.

exchangeable skeletal pool is influenced by several hormones including PTH, providing a mechanism to buffer changes in blood calcium concentration that follow short-term variations in calcium entry into, or egress from, the extracellular fluid.

Calcium in extracellular fluids, specifically plasma, exists in three distinct forms (see Fig. 3-2). Approximately 40% is bound to plasma proteins, mainly albumin, whereas another 10% forms soluble complexes with various organic anions such as citrate. The physiologically most important component of calcium in extracellular fluid is the remaining ionized fraction. This fraction is the portion of calcium in blood that interacts directly with cell membranes, various membrane channels, and the calcium-sensing receptor (CaSR) (*vide infra*), and the concentration of ionized calcium in blood is regulated tightly.

Serum total calcium concentrations in humans range from a lower limit of approximately 8.4 to 8.6 mg per dL to an upper limit of approximately 10.0 to 10.2 mg per dL. Values vary somewhat among reference laboratories because of differences in the methods used for analysis. It is now apparent, however, that some of the variation in serum calcium concentrations within the general population is attributable to polymorphisms of the CaSR.

Routine measurements of serum total calcium concentration are affected most often by variations in serum albumin levels. Reductions in serum albumin concentrations diminish the binding of calcium ions to albumin by several mechanisms, thus

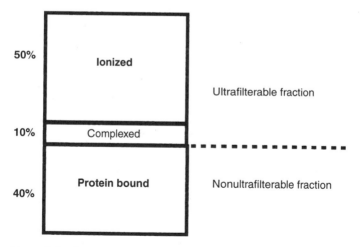

Figure 3-2. Approximately 50% of the calcium in plasma is in the ionized form. A slightly smaller portion is bound to plasma proteins, mainly albumin, whereas approximately 10% forms soluble complexes with organic and inorganic anions. The concentration of ionized calcium in blood is regulated tightly. The ionized and complexed fractions of calcium in plasma cross the filtration barrier within the glomerulus and thus represent the ultrafilterable fraction of plasma calcium. Calcium that is bound to plasma proteins does not normally traverse the glomerular filtration barrier.

lowering measured values of total serum calcium concentration. In general, reported values for serum total calcium decline by approximately 0.8 mg per dL for each 1.0 mg per dL decrement in serum albumin concentration from a reference level of 4.0 mg per dL.

Variations in systemic pH alter the net anionic charge on albumin, affect interactions between negatively charged albumin molecules and positively charged calcium ions, and thus influence measurements of serum total calcium concentration. Reductions in blood pH decrease the net anionic charge on albumin, diminish the protein-bound fraction of calcium in plasma, and lower measured values for serum total calcium concentration. Conversely, increases in plasma pH raise the net anionic charge on albumin as protons are released, leaving more anionic sites available to interact with positively charged calcium ions. The protein-bound fraction of calcium in plasma thus increases, and serum total calcium levels rise modestly. Therefore, measured values for serum total calcium should be adjusted downward by approximately 0.10 to 0.12 mg per dL for each 0.1 increment in blood pH.

The normal reference range for blood ionized calcium concentrations in healthy persons is approximately 4.4 to 5.2 mg per dL, or 1.1 to 1.3 mmol per L. Values can be measured quite accurately using calcium-specific electrodes. Such measurements are useful for assessing calcium metabolism in patients with clinical conditions that affect plasma protein concentrations and in those with various acid–base disorders.

Because of the importance of calcium in mediating a wide array of physiologic functions, the level of ionized calcium in blood is maintained within a very narrow physiologic range. This process is accomplished in subjects with normal renal and parathyroid gland function by the coordinated modulation of calcium excretion in the urine to accommodate changes in calcium entry into the extracellular fluid from the two primary sources, the gastrointestinal tract and bone (Fig. 3-1). An increase in the reclamation of calcium from tubular fluid, primarily in the distal nephron, provides an additional source of calcium input into the extracellular fluid when intestinal calcium absorption is reduced or when calcium release from bone is diminished. Conversely, calcium excretion in the urine is enhanced by reductions in calcium reabsorption in both the proximal and distal nephron when excess amounts of calcium enter the extracellular fluid from the gastrointestinal tract or from bone. PTH mediates these adaptive changes in renal calcium excretion considerably, because the minute-to-minute secretion of PTH is modulated by a CaSR located within the plasma membrane of parathyroid cells.

The CaSR is expressed abundantly in parathyroid tissue, and it represents the molecular mechanism by which parathyroid cells detect very small changes in blood ionized calcium concentration and modulate PTH secretion accordingly. Reductions in blood ionized calcium concentration inactivate the CaSR and promote PTH release (see Fig. 3-3). Because PTH enhances renal tubular calcium transport in the distal nephron, renal tubular calcium reabsorption increases, and calcium excretion in the urine falls (see Fig. 3-4). Increases in PTH secretion also promote calcium mobilization from bone, most immediately from

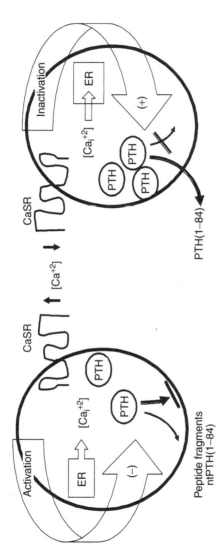

Figure 3-3. Increases in blood ionized calcium concentration activate the calcium-sensing receptor (CaSR) and inhibit parathyroid hormone (PTH) release from parathyroid cells. Such changes probably also cause the release of peptide fragments of PTH that have been truncated at their aminoterminal end (ntPTH). Conversely, decreases in blood ionized calcium concentration inactivate the CaSR and promote the secretion of full-length, biologically active PTH, or PTH (1-84).

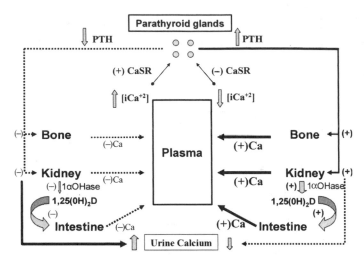

Figure 3-4. The adaptive responses to a change in plasma calcium concentration. Decreases in plasma calcium provoke parathyroid hormone (PTH) secretion, which reduces calcium excretion in the urine by enhancing calcium reabsorption in the distal nephron. PTH also mobilizes calcium from bone, and both responses increase the amount of calcium entering extracellular fluid. In contrast, increases in plasma calcium levels diminish PTH secretion leading to an increase in calcium excretion in the urine and to a reduction in calcium release from bone. The amount of calcium that enters the extracellular fluid thus decreases.

the rapidly exchangeable skeletal calcium pool. Both responses occur within minutes to hours and raise blood ionized calcium concentrations toward baseline values. When plasma PTH levels remain elevated for longer periods, 1,25-dihdroxyvitamin D synthesis by the kidney increases and intestinal calcium absorption rises, making more calcium available to support the calcium level in extracellular fluid (Fig. 3-4).

In contrast, increases in blood ionized calcium concentration activate the CaSR and inhibit PTH secretion (Fig. 3-3). As a result, renal tubular calcium reabsorption in the distal nephron diminishes, calcium excretion in the urine rises, and less calcium is released from the rapidly exchangeable skeletal calcium pool; these changes collectively lower blood ionized calcium concentration toward baseline values (Fig. 3-4). With more sustained reductions in plasma PTH levels, renal 1,25-dihdroxyvitamin D production falls, and intestinal calcium absorption decreases, reducing the amount of calcium entering extracellular fluid. The rapidity of these adaptive responses to very small changes in blood ionized calcium concentration, together with the steep reciprocal relationship between extracellular calcium concentrations and the amount of PTH released by parathyroid cells (see Fig. 3-5), provides a robust mechanism for maintaining blood ionized calcium levels within a narrow physiologic range.

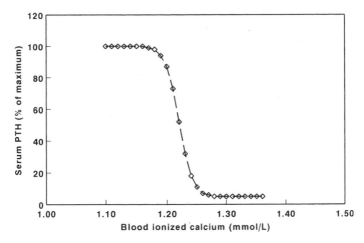

Figure 3-5. The inverse sigmoidal relationship between the concentration of ionized calcium in blood and plasma parathyroid hormone (PTH) levels. Very small changes in blood ionized calcium produce relatively large changes in plasma PTH levels within minutes, thus altering renal tubular calcium transport and calcium exchange between plasma and bone to provide a robust mechanism for maintaining the concentration of ionized calcium within a narrow physiologic range.

Calcium Metabolism and Bone

Bone is remodeled continuously throughout much of the skeleton both in adults and in children by a tightly regulated sequence of localized cellular events. Groups of osteoclasts initially remove discreet amounts of existing bone during the resorption phase of the skeletal remodeling cycle. Populations of osteoblasts subsequently replace nearly equivalent volumes of bone at each resorption site. In adults, the amounts of calcium and phosphorus mobilized during osteoclastic bone resorption approximate quite closely the amounts replaced by osteoblasts during the formation phase of bone remodeling (Fig. 3-1). Net skeletal calcium and phosphorus balance in adults is thus close to zero. Strictly speaking, however, bone resorption in the adult skeleton slightly exceeds bone formation during each remodeling cycle, and this disparity is what accounts for age-related bone loss.

Disorders that enhance the rate of skeletal remodeling, such as hyperparathyroidism and hyperthyroidism, increase the amounts of calcium and phosphorus that are exchanged daily between bone and the extracellular fluid. Conversely, the daily exchange of calcium and phosphorus between bone and extracellular fluid diminishes in clinical conditions, such as hypoparathyroidism, that are associated with reduced rates of skeletal remodeling. Despite the overall physiologic importance of these alterations, particularly with respect to long-term changes in bone mass, differences in the net exchange of calcium and phosphorus between bone and extracellular fluid caused by variations in bone remodeling have little effect on the minute-to-minute regulation of serum calcium and phosphorus levels. These changes are affected predominantly by short-term adjustments in mineral flux between plasma and the rapidly exchangeable skeletal pool.

In children and adolescents, net skeletal calcium balance is generally positive, because bones grow by endochondral bone formation. This process continues unabated until epiphyseal growth plate cartilages close at the end of adolescence, when the acquisition of peak adult bone mass is nearly complete. Net calcium retention is quite high during periods of rapid bone growth, and much of the mineral that enters the growing skeleton is retained as bones are modeled during their enlargement. The primary modeling of bones during skeletal growth occurs at sites distinct from those at which existing bone is being remodeled, and the factors that modulate these two processes differ fundamentally. As in adults, the amounts of calcium and phosphorus exchanged daily in children and adolescents between bone and extracellular fluid, because of the modeling and remodeling of bones, have little to do with the minute-to-minute regulation of serum calcium and phosphorus levels.

The fact that serum calcium levels remain unperturbed despite high rates of calcium uptake into bone in rapidly growing children underscores the fact that measurements of serum calcium concentration do not provide information about the state of total body calcium balance. This lack of association is not surprising, because blood ionized calcium levels are regulated closely by CaSR-mediated, short-term variations in PTH secretion that modulate calcium excretion in the urine, whereas the amounts of calcium entering extracellular fluid from the intestine and the amounts taken up into bone from the extracellular fluid are determined by other factors that mediate calcium transport specifically in these two tissues.

Intestinal Calcium Transport

Calcium transport occurs throughout the gastrointestinal tract. Most of the calcium is absorbed in the duodenum and upper portion of the jejunum. Although the World Health Organization recommends that the dietary intake of calcium be maintained at 1,500 mg per day to prevent age-related bone loss, the calcium content of diets in many developed countries is often considerably less, typically ranging from 800 to 1,000 mg per day. Of this amount, approximately 20% is absorbed and enters the extracellular fluid (Fig. 3-1).

The transport of calcium by intestinal epithelia occurs by two distinct mechanisms (see Fig. 3-6). One is an active, energy-dependent process that regulates the movement of calcium across intestinal epithelial cells. It is affected primarily by vitamin D and, most importantly, by calcitriol. The other is a passive, energy-independent process that traverses the paracellular pathway. This process occurs largely by diffusion, is concentration-dependent, and is unaffected by vitamin D.

The passive, or diffusional, component of intestinal calcium transport is largely unregulated. Approximately 15% to 20% of ingested calcium is absorbed by passive mechanisms across a wide spectrum of dietary calcium intakes. Net calcium absorption via passive mechanisms is small when the dietary intake of

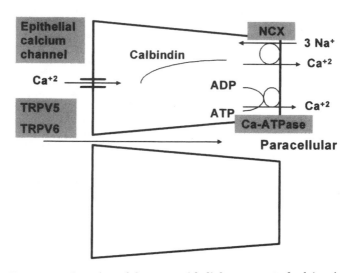

Figure 3-6.   Overview of the transepithelial movement of calcium in intestinal and renal tubular epithelial cells. Calcium entry across the apical membrane is mediated by an epithelial calcium channel, predominantly TRPV5 in kidney and TRPV6 in intestine. Calbindin D serves to buffer changes in cytosolic calcium concentration resulting from calcium entry across the apical membrane and facilitates the movement of calcium to the basolateral membrane. Calcium extrusion from the cell is mediated by a sodium–calcium exchanger (NCX) using energy provided by a calcium-ATPase. The levels of expression of calbindin D, TRPV5, and TRPV6 are affected by vitamin D. Calcium transport also occurs by diffusion through the paracellular pathway.

calcium is low, but diffusional intestinal calcium absorption increases progressively as dietary calcium intake rises. This condition accounts for the development of hypercalciuria in persons with normal renal function who ingest large amounts of calcium from either dietary or medicinal sources. It also contributes to episodes of hypercalcemia in patients with little or no residual renal function who are treated with dialysis despite the fact that the active component of intestinal calcium absorption is impaired in such individuals because of reductions in renal calcitriol production.

The active transcellular component of calcium absorption in intestinal epithelia is regulated quite tightly, predominantly by calcitriol. Vitamin D–dependent calcium transport becomes increasingly important for maintaining net intestinal calcium absorption as dietary calcium intake is reduced, and it represents a crucial adaptive response to calcium deprivation. The fractional absorption of calcium can reach 40% to 50% when dietary intake is in the range of 400 to 500 mg per day. This change is largely the result of an increase in the active, vitamin D–dependent component of intestinal calcium transport, which serves to maintain net calcium input into the extracellular fluid at approximately 200 mg per day.

The transcellular movement of calcium involves three distinct steps (Fig. 3-6). First, calcium uptake across the apical membrane of intestinal epithelial cells occurs through an epithelial calcium channel (ECaC). Second, calcium entering the cytosol binds to calbindin D_{9K}, a vitamin D–dependent protein. Calbindin D_{9K} appears to act as a transport, or shuttle, protein that facilitates the movement of calcium ions from the apical brush border to the basolateral membrane for extrusion from the cell. It also probably serves to buffer abrupt increases in cytosolic calcium concentration. Third, calcium extrusion across the basolateral membrane is mediated by a sodium–calcium exchanger (NCX) and by an ATP-dependent calcium-ATPase (Ca-ATPase).

Vitamin D has been recognized for many years as a major determinant of intestinal calbindin D_{9K} expression, providing one mechanism to account for vitamin D–mediated increases in intestinal calcium absorption. Recent work indicates, however, that vitamin D influences calcium entry into cells in calcium-transporting epithelia by modifying the level of expression of two important members of the vanilloid subfamily (TRPV) that is part of the super family of transient receptor potential (TRP) proteins. Two highly homologous members, TRPV5 and TRPV6, are expressed predominantly in calcium-transporting epithelia and play important roles in the transepithelial movement of calcium both in the kidney and in the intestine. TRPV5 is synonymous with the ECaC1 that was cloned originally from epithelial cells from rabbit kidney. TRPV6 corresponds to the ECaC2 that was cloned initially from rat duodenum.

TRPV5 and TRPV6 are constitutively activated calcium channels that mediate calcium entry across the apical membrane of renal tubular and intestinal epithelial cells, respectively (Fig. 3-6). They probably represent the rate-limiting step in the transepithelial movement of calcium in both tissues. Calcitriol, or 1,25-dihydroxyvitamin D, up-regulates the expression of both TRPV5 and TRPV6. In duodenum, TRPV6 expression and, to a lesser extent, TRPV5 expression, are also enhanced by dietary calcium supplementation through a mechanism that is vitamin D–independent.

Increases in calcitriol production by the kidney are largely responsible for the enhanced efficiency of intestinal calcium transport during dietary calcium restriction. Elevated plasma PTH levels and reductions in serum calcium concentrations both promote renal 1α-hydroxylase activity, and each probably contributes to this adaptive response. Modest elevations in serum calcitriol levels enhance the active vitamin D–dependent component of intestinal calcium absorption and optimize the efficiency of intestinal calcium transport, whereas modest elevations in plasma PTH levels serve to mobilize calcium from bone. These compensatory changes are usually sufficient to maintain serum calcium concentrations during limited periods of dietary calcium restriction, but serum calcium concentration declines when adaptive responses no longer prove adequate during extended periods of dietary calcium deficiency.

Calcium Transport within the Nephron and Renal Calcium Excretion

In adults in whom net skeletal calcium balance is neutral, the amount of calcium excreted in the urine generally reflects the amount absorbed from the gastrointestinal tract (Fig. 3-1). As described previously, net calcium absorption is approximately 200 mg in vitamin D–replete individuals who ingest diets containing adequate amounts of calcium. To maintain total body calcium balance, an equivalent amount of calcium, about 200 mg, must be excreted daily in the urine. The modulation of renal calcium excretion provides an ongoing mechanism to adapt to short-term variations in the amount of calcium entering the extracellular fluid and to maintain constant levels of calcium in plasma. Changes in the efficiency of renal tubular calcium transport, particularly in the distal nephron, mediate this adaptive response.

Renal calcium excretion begins at the glomerulus with the formation of a protein-free ultrafiltrate of plasma. Calcium that is bound to albumin does not traverse the filtration barrier within the glomerulus, whereas the ionized fraction of calcium in blood and soluble complexes of calcium in plasma are filtered freely. These two components represent the ultrafilterable fraction of calcium in plasma (Fig. 3-2). Overall, about 9,000 mg of calcium is filtered at the glomerulus each day. Approximately 70% of this amount is reabsorbed in the proximal tubule, 20% in the thick ascending limb of the loop of Henle, and the remaining 5% to 10% in the distal convoluted tubule and collecting tubule. Despite the large proportion of calcium that is reclaimed in the proximal tubule, calcium excretion in the urine is determined primarily by adjustments in calcium transport in the distal nephron.

The transcellular transport of calcium across epithelial cells in the distal nephron resembles that described previously in intestinal epithelial cells (Fig. 3-6). The entry of calcium from tubular fluid into the apical membrane is mediated by TRPV5, whereas a Ca-ATPase and the NCX accounts for calcium extrusion across the basolateral membrane. In kidney, the higher molecular weight species of calbindin D, calbindin D_{28K}, is expressed predominantly. As in the intestine, calcium transport across renal tubular epithelia also occurs via the paracellular pathway.

Because a large proportion of the filtered load of calcium is reabsorbed in the proximal nephron, variations in calcium transport in this nephron segment substantially influence net calcium excretion. The fractional reabsorption of sodium and calcium in the proximal tubule parallel one another. Increases in the filtered load of sodium caused by increases in dietary sodium intake or by extracellular volume expansion thus lower the fraction of the filtered load of sodium and calcium that is reabsorbed in the proximal convoluted tubule and increase calcium delivery to distal nephron segments. Conversely, decreases in the filtered load of sodium promote sodium and calcium reabsorption in the proximal nephron and lower net calcium excretion in the urine. Variations in the filtered load of calcium that are caused by changes in blood calcium concentration also affect proximal tubular calcium transport. Thus, increases in filtered load reduce calcium reabsorption in the proximal nephron, whereas decreases in filtered load enhance it. The level of activation of the CaSR in the thick ascending limb of the loop of Henle also serves as an important modifier of sodium, chloride, calcium, and water reabsorption, further affecting the amount of calcium delivered to more distal nephron segments and ultimately into the final urine.

PTH represents the major regulator of calcium transport in the distal tubule, promoting tubular calcium reabsorption and diminishing calcium excretion. Other calcium-regulating hormones such as vitamin D and calcitonin have less pronounced effects. The exquisite sensitivity of parathyroid cells to very small changes in blood ionized calcium concentration (Fig. 3-5) enables very rapid changes in PTH secretion to modulate distal tubular calcium transport continuously and to regulate renal calcium excretion in an ongoing fashion.

PHOSPHORUS

Overview of Phosphorus Metabolism

The total body content of phosphorus in adults is approximately 700 g. Phosphorus, like calcium, is found predominantly in mineralized skeletal tissues in the form of apatite crystals in which the molar ratio of calcium to phosphorus is 1.6:1.0 (see Fig. 3-7). Phosphorus-containing compounds are, however, important intracellular constituents, and approximately 15% of phosphorus is located in soft tissues, particularly in muscle. Less than 1% of phosphorus is found in extracellular fluid (Fig. 3-7).

The dietary intake of phosphorus in adults typically ranges from 1,000 to 1,400 mg per day and is determined largely by the ingested amounts of protein and dairy products. Total body phosphorus balance is generally neutral in healthy adults with normal renal function. As discussed previously with respect to calcium metabolism, phosphorus excretion in the urine varies primarily as a function of the amounts entering the extracellular fluid from two sources, the gastrointestinal tract and bone. The net exchange of phosphorus between soft tissue and the extracellular fluid is close to zero under basal conditions. In certain clinical disorders, however, marked changes in phosphorus exchange between plasma and soft tissues can strikingly alter renal phosphorus excretion.

Extensive damage to soft tissues arising from crush injuries to muscle, thermal burns, and massive destruction of tumor cells during chemotherapy for certain malignancies, also known as tumor lysis syndrome, can result in the release of very large amounts of phosphorus from intracellular pools. These disorders represent a unique set of clinical syndromes, in which large amounts of phosphorus enter the extracellular fluid from sources other than bone or the gastrointestinal tract. Substantial increases in serum phosphorus levels can occur even in subjects with normal renal function because the capacity of the kidney to excrete phosphorus has been overwhelmed transiently. Additional insults to renal function are often present, however, in such patients, and these disturbances further compromise the ability of

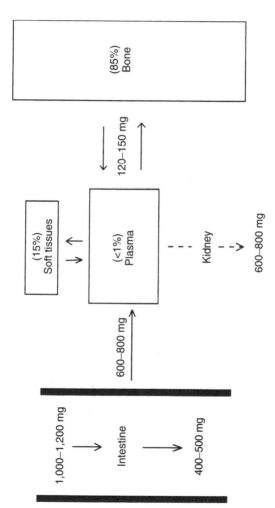

Figure 3-7. The distribution of phosphorus among bone, soft-tissues and extracellular fluid, and the net amounts of phosphorus entering and leaving the extracellular fluid each day from bone and the gastrointestinal tract. Under steady-state conditions, in adults, the amount of phosphorus excreted in the urine each day largely reflects net intestinal phosphorus absorption.

the kidney to increase phosphorus excretion, aggravating the severity of phosphorus retention.

Under basal conditions in adults, phosphorus excretion in the urine largely reflects dietary phosphorus intake because intestinal phosphorus transport is for the most part unregulated (*vide infra*). Although the capacity to increase phosphorus excretion is quite large in persons with normal renal function, phosphorus excretion in the urine becomes inadequate to accommodate the amounts absorbed daily from the gastrointestinal tract when kidney function declines from 20% to 25% of the normal. As a result, phosphorus retention develops and serum phosphorus levels rise. Dietary phosphorus intake must be restricted, therefore, in patients with moderate to advanced chronic kidney disease to prevent hyperphosphatemia from developing by limiting the intake of dairy products and protein-rich foods. Such measures are used widely to treat patients with advanced kidney disease and those who require treatment with dialysis.

Maintaining adequate nutrition, particularly adequate protein nutrition, is difficult when the dietary content of phosphorus is restricted severely. Such diets are often unpalatable, and ongoing compliance is difficult. In practical terms, the daily intake of phosphorus can be reduced to approximately 800 mg, while maintaining adequate protein nutrition, in most patients with advanced chronic kidney disease and in those undergoing long-term dialysis. More stringent dietary restrictions can contribute to inadequate protein nutrition, which has been linked to adverse clinical outcomes in such patients. Therefore, phosphate-binding medications are used commonly, together with dietary phosphorus restriction, to diminish net intestinal phosphorus absorption and to limit further the amounts of phosphorus that enter the extracellular fluid each day.

Phosphorus Metabolism and Bone

Approximately 125 to 150 mg of phosphorus enters and leaves the extracellular fluid each day as a result of ongoing skeletal remodeling (Fig. 3-7). In adults, net skeletal phosphorus balance is close to zero in the absence of overt metabolic bone disease. Because the capacity of the kidneys to modify phosphorus excretion in the urine is quite large, variations in the rate of skeletal remodeling and in the amount of phosphorus exchanged daily between bone and the extracellular fluid do not substantially affect serum phosphorus levels unless renal function is impaired markedly. High rates of phosphorus efflux from bone caused by secondary hyperparathyroidism can, however, aggravate hyperphosphatemia in patients with little of no residual renal function who require treatment with dialysis.

Several factors have been identified recently that play pivotal roles in regulating phosphorus uptake into bone by osteoblasts and in mediating skeletal mineralization. The clinical disorder of X-linked hypophosphatemia (XLH) is characterized by hypophosphatemia, growth retardation, defects in the mineralization of bone and cartilage, and abnormalities in the regulation of 1,25-dihydroxyvitamin D synthesis by the kidney. This condition is caused by inactivating mutations of the phosphate-regulating gene with homologies to endopeptidase, or PHEX. Careful assessments of humans with XLH and of mouse genetic models of the disease indicate that hypophosphatemia alone is insufficient to account fully for the severity of the defect in skeletal mineralization. Indeed, osteoblasts derived from *Hyp* mice, a murine model of XLH, do not support mineralization adequately, and they may release factors locally that interfere with matrix calcification, osteoblastic function, or both. In part, some of these disturbances are related to alterations in the expression or metabolism of matrix extracellular phosphoglycoprotein, or MEPE.

The results from these and other studies suggest quite strongly that PHEX, MEPE, and FGF-23 are components of a distinct hormonal/autocrine/paracrine network that not only affects phosphorus metabolism in bone but also regulates phosphorus homeostasis systemically. The relative importance of each, and the contribution of other phosphatonins as modifiers of phosphorus metabolism locally in skeletal tissue, has yet to be determined.

Intestinal Phosphorus Transport

Between 60% and 70% of dietary phosphorus is absorbed by the gastrointestinal tract (Fig. 3-7). Most transport occurs in the duodenum and jejunum. Although some phosphorus is lost in gastrointestinal secretions and as a result of the sloughing of intestinal epithelial cells, the net input of phosphorus into the extracellular fluid from the gastrointestinal tract is approximately 600 to 800 mg per day. This is the amount of phosphorus that is excreted in the urine each day to maintain neutral total body balance.

Intestinal phosphorus transport is, for the most part, a passive or diffusional process, occurring primarily through the paracellular pathway in a concentration-dependent manner. However, a small energy-dependent component of intestinal phosphorus transport exists, whereby the uptake of sodium and phosphorus across the apical brush-border membrane of intestinal epithelial cells is mediated by a sodium–phosphate cotransporter using energy provided by a sodium–potassium ATPase (Na/K-ATPase).

The presence of certain constituents within the intestinal lumen retards phosphorus absorption. A high dietary intake of calcium diminishes net intestinal phosphorus absorption by promoting the formation of insoluble complexes of calcium and phosphorus within the intestinal lumen. Other alkaline metals such as aluminum hydroxide, aluminum carbonate, and lanthanum carbonate also bind phosphorus in the lumen of the small intestine and diminish phosphorus absorption. These compounds and calcium-free, phosphate-binding resins such as sevelamer are used therapeutically to manage phosphorus retention and to control hyperphosphatemia in patients with chronic kidney disease.

Vitamin D sterols promote intestinal phosphorus absorption by increasing sodium–phosphate cotransport across the apical brush-border membrane. Because sustained alterations in dietary phosphorus intake affect the level of activity of the renal 25-hydroxyvitamin D, 1α-hydroxylase, changes in renal calcitriol production can provide some regulatory control over intestinal phosphorus absorption. The effect of vitamin D to enhance intestinal phosphorus absorption through sodium–phosphate cotransport-mediated mechanisms probably accounts for the worsening of hyperphosphatemia in many patients with chronic kidney disease who are given vitamin D sterols to treat secondary hyperparathyroidism.

Phosphorus Transport within the Nephron and Renal Phosphorus Excretion

Most of the inorganic phosphorus in plasma is in an ultrafilterable form. It thus readily crosses the filtration barrier within the glomerulus and is found in proximal tubular fluid at concentrations similar to those in plasma. Approximately 60% to 70% of the filtered load of phosphorus is reabsorbed in the proximal nephron, which serves as the primary site for regulating phosphorus excretion in the urine. Lesser amounts of phosphorus are reabsorbed in more distal nephron segments.

The transport of phosphorus, like calcium, across renal tubular epithelia requires the entry of phosphorus from luminal fluid across the apical brush-border membrane, vectorial movement though the cytoplasm, and extrusion from the cell across the basolateral membrane into peritubular blood. Phosphorus uptake across the apical membrane of proximal tubular cells is mediated predominantly by the type 2 sodium–phosphorus cotransporter, or Na/Pi 2 transporter, which is expressed abundantly in cells of the proximal nephron. The uptake of phosphorus across the apical brush border appears to be the rate-limiting step for the transepithelial movement of phosphorus in renal epithelia. Although other sodium–phosphorus cotransporters are expressed in the proximal tubule and in other nephron segments, the Na/Pi 2 cotransporter interacts with phosphorus specifically, and it is regulated by several key determinants of phosphorus homeostasis. The level of expression of the Na/Pi 2 cotransporter is thus thought to represent the principal molecular determinant of intestinal phosphorus transport.

Dietary phosphorus restriction leads to increased expression of the Na/Pi 2 transporter, a change that is associated with enhanced phosphorus reabsorption in the proximal tubule and decreases in phosphorus excretion in the urine. Interestingly, phosphorus excretion changes within only a few hours after the dietary intake of phosphorus is altered, and this response appears to be independent of PTH. Very short-term alterations in trafficking of the Na/Pi 2 transporter between intracellular vesicles and the apical membrane might account for this rapid adaptation.

PTH is a potent modifier of renal phosphorus excretion, and it can markedly increase renal phosphorus excretion. PTH acts primarily in the proximal nephron to diminish phosphorus reabsorption, but some evidence exists to suggest that PTH also affects phosphorus transport in the distal nephron. In the proximal tubule, PTH reduces Na/Pi 2 transporter expression by altering protein trafficking to the apical membrane and by decreasing gene expression. Changes in the level of expression of the Na/Pi 2 transporter are thus thought to be largely responsible for alterations in phosphorus transport in the proximal nephron that are mediated by PTH and by variations in dietary phosphorus intake.

Extracellular volume expansion decreases phosphorus reabsorption in the proximal nephron and promotes phosphorus excretion in the urine, independent of changes in the filtered load of phosphorus. In some studies, increases in plasma PTH levels that arise from modest reductions in blood ionized calcium concentration during rapid volume expansion might account for this change. Reductions in sodium reabsorption in the proximal tubule that arise from extracellular volume expansion probably also contribute.

Acidemia increases, whereas alkalemia decreases, phosphorus excretion in the urine. Alterations in renal tubular phosphorus transport largely account for these changes, but differences in the mobilization of calcium from bone caused by variations in plasma pH can affect the filtered load of phosphorus and modify net renal phosphorus excretion.

The effects of calcitriol on phosphorus handling by the kidney have not been defined clearly. Although administering calcitriol generally reduces phosphorus excretion in the urine, vitamin D–mediated changes in serum calcium and plasma PTH levels might be largely responsible.

Other hormones that affect renal phosphorus excretion include calcitonin, insulin, and glucagon. The effect of calcitonin on renal phosphorus excretion is relatively minor. Insulin administration generally reduces phosphorus excretion in the urine, but the anabolic effect of insulin to promote phosphorus uptake into cells can account, at least in part, for this change. Glucagon increases renal phosphorus excretion, whereas hyperglycemia increases phosphorus excretion in the urine as a result of ongoing osmotic diuresis. Diuretic agents that act in the proximal nephron, such as acetazolamide, and loop diuretics, such as furosemide, can also enhance phosphate excretion.

FGF-23 is a peptide comprised of 251 amino acid residues that markedly enhances renal phosphorus excretion. Low levels of FGF-23 can be detected in the serum of healthy persons, but levels are elevated substantially in patients with chronic kidney disease, increasing progressively as renal function declines and as serum phosphorus levels rise. FGF-23 is produced in excess amounts and released into the circulation by tumors that cause tumor-induced osteomalacia (TIO), an uncommon form of acquired hypophosphatemia and osteomalacia, which can be cured by surgically removing the offending tumor. Mutations of FGF-23 that interfere with its cleavage into inactive peptide fragments cause renal phosphorus wasting and hypophosphatemia in patients with autosomal dominant hypophosphatemic rickets (ADHR). Moreover, mice with inactivating mutations of FGF-23 exhibit hyperphosphatemia, skeletal abnormalities, and dysregulated vitamin D metabolism with markedly elevated serum calcitriol levels despite high serum phosphorus concentrations.

Recombinant FGF-23 has been shown to decrease Na/Pi 2 transporter expression in the proximal tubule and to diminish 1,25-dihydroxyvitamin D synthesis. These findings, together with observations from clinical studies of patients with selected hypophosphatemic syndromes and additional assessments of genetically modified mice, indicate that FGF-23 acts as a key determinant of phosphorus transport within the nephron.

VITAMIN D

Overview of Vitamin D Metabolism

Vitamin D is found in nature in two forms. Ergocalciferol, or vitamin D_2, originates from plant sources, whereas cholecalciferol, or vitamin D_3, comes from animal sources. The biologic actions of ergocalciferol and cholecalciferol are essentially the same, and their metabolism is quite similar (*vide infra*). Dietary sources of vitamin D_3 include fatty fishes; fish oils, such as cod liver oil; and fortified foods such as milk, cereals, and breads. Apart from dietary sources, vitamin D_3 is also produced in skin, representing an additional endogenous source of this important secosteroid. In man, previtamin D_3 is generated from 7-dehydrocholesterol in the skin during exposure to ultraviolet light. Previtamin D_3 is then converted to cholecalciferol. Cholecalciferol is released into the blood, where it circulates bound to vitamin D–binding protein (DBP).

Two important hydroxylation steps occur normally in the metabolism of vitamin D, both of which increase biologic activity (see Fig. 3-8). The carbon located at the 25-position on the side chain of native vitamin D undergoes hydroxylation in the liver to form 25-hydroxyvitamin D. This enzymatic step is not regulated tightly, is substrate-dependent, and is unaffected by chronic kidney disease. Measurements of the level of 25-hydroxyvitamin D in serum thus represent the best index of vitamin D nutrition both in the general population and in those with renal failure.

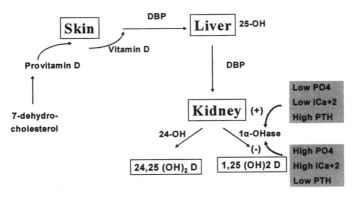

Figure 3-8.   Vitamin D metabolism. Both vitamin D_3, or cholecalciferol, and vitamin D_2, or ergocalciferol, circulate in plasma bound to vitamin D–binding protein (DBP) and undergo hydroxylation at the 25-position in the liver. The 25-hydroxylated metabolites then undergo 1α-hydroxylation in the kidney. Calcium, phosphorus, and parathyroid hormone (PTH) each modify the activity of the renal 1α-hydroxylase independently. The 24-hydroxylation of 25-hydroxyvitamin D probably represents the initial step in the degradation or inactivation of vitamin D.

Most of the 25-hydroxyvitamin D circulates in plasma bound to DBP, and only a very small fraction exists in the unbound state.

Calcitriol, or 1,25-dihydroxycholecalciferol, is biologically the most potent metabolite of vitamin D_3 and is formed by the hydroxylation of the carbon atom located at the first position of the A-ring of 25-hydroxyvitamin D. This step is mediated by a 25-hydroxyvitamin D, 1α-hydroxylase, located in the mitochondria of cells of the proximal tubule. Interestingly, substrate for the reaction comes from tubular fluid, rather than from peritubular blood. The 25-hydroxyvitamin D–DBP complex is filtered at the glomerulus, binds to megalin, and subsequently is reabsorbed across the apical membrane of proximal tubular cells. Upon entering the cytoplasm, 25-hydroxyvitamin D dissociates from DBP and is converted to calcitriol.

The renal production of calcitriol is regulated separately by calcium, phosphorus, and PTH. Low ambient levels of calcium or phosphorus and increases in PTH levels promote renal 1α-hydroxylase activity and enhance calcitriol synthesis (Fig. 3-8). Conversely, high ambient calcium or phosphorus levels and decreases in PTH diminish renal 1α-hydroxylase activity. High serum calcium levels and conditions of calcium surfeit also promote the activity of another enzyme, the renal 25-hydroxyvitamin D, 24-hydroxylase, leading to the formation 24,25-dihydroxycholecalciferol. This metabolic conversion generally represents an initial step in the degradation or inactivation of vitamin D and, together with calcium-mediated reductions in renal 1α-hydroxylase activity, diminishes calcitriol production in states of hypercalcemia.

Because renal 1α-hydroxylase activity is regulated so tightly, the serum levels of calcitriol and 25-hydroxyvitamin D are generally unrelated in healthy persons with adequate vitamin D nutrition, and measured values for the two metabolites do not correlate. The availability of substrate in the form of 25-hydroxyvitamin D has little effect on net calcitriol production, unless severe vitamin D deficiency has already developed. Renal calcitriol synthesis is maintained in less advanced states of vitamin D deficiency because of increases in renal 1α-hydroxylase activity mediated by hypocalcemia, hypophosphatemia, and elevated plasma PTH levels, either alone or together. Thus, calcitriol levels remain normal or can even be elevated despite relatively low serum levels of 25-hydroxyvitamin D, in subjects with mild or moderate vitamin D deficiency. For these reasons, serum 25-hydroxyvitamin D levels rather than serum calcitriol concentrations serve as the best biochemical index of vitamin D nutrition.

In contrast to persons with normal renal function, patients with chronic kidney disease often have levels of 25-hydroxyvitamin D and calcitriol that correlate moderately. This emergence of the relationship probably reflects disruption of the regulatory control of renal 1α-hydroxylase activity as kidney disease progresses.

Strictly speaking, calcitriol functions as a hormone. It fulfills this definition because it is produced locally in a particular tissue, circulates in plasma, and elicits biologic responses in remote target tissues. The presence of the 25-hydroxyvitamin D_3, 1α-hydroxylase in other cells such as keratinocytes, cells of the monocyte/macrophage lineage, and bone cells suggests, however, that some tissues regulate 1,25-dihydroxycholecalciferol synthesis locally.

Most of the biologic actions of calcitriol are mediated through a genomic mechanism that requires binding of the sterol to the vitamin D receptor (VDR) and subsequent translocation of the ligand-receptor complex to the cell nucleus. The ligand-bound VDR forms a heterodimer with the retinoid-X receptor (RXR), which then interacts with a vitamin D response element (VDRE) in the promoter region of various genes. These interactions enhance the expression of some genes, such as osteocalcin and the calbindins, and diminish the expression of others such as pre-pro-PTH. Because the VDR is expressed quite widely, calcitriol has effects in numerous target tissues.

Vitamin D and Calcium Metabolism

As discussed previously, vitamin D increases the expression of TRPV6, the ECaC that mediates calcium entry across the apical membrane of intestinal epithelial cells and probably represents the rate-limiting step in transcellular calcium movement. Calcitriol also up-regulates the expression of calbindin D_{9K} and other proteins such as alkaline phosphatase that are involved in the active component of intestinal calcium absorption. Calcitriol, acting through classic genomic mechanisms, thus serves as the major regulator of active intestinal calcium absorption.

Nevertheless, calcitriol also affects intestinal calcium transport through a nongenomic pathway. The addition of calcitriol to fluid in the lumen of the intestine increases the transepithelial movement of calcium within only 15 to 20 minutes, a change that is far too rapid to be explained by alterations in gene expression. This phenomenon, called "transcaltachia," can contribute to episodes of hypercalcemia in individuals treated with small oral doses of calcitriol. Data are accumulating to indicate that the nongenomic actions of vitamin D are mediated by a distinct membrane-associated, vitamin D receptor–like protein, which influences calcium transport both in the intestine and in mineralizing tissues.

Vitamin D and Phosphorus Metabolism

As mentioned previously, vitamin D promotes intestinal phosphorus absorption, but the mechanisms responsible have not been established fully. Most intestinal phosphorus absorption is passive and unregulated. Whether the effects of vitamin D on intestinal phosphorus absorption are explained solely by changes in sodium–phosphate cotransport in intestinal epithelia remains uncertain. The membrane-associated, vitamin D receptor–like protein mentioned previously as a putative mediator of the nongenomic actions of vitamin D on intestinal calcium absorption has also been reported to enhance intestinal phosphorus transport.

Disturbances in Vitamin D Metabolism Caused by Kidney Disease

Because the kidneys play such a pivotal role in the production of calcitriol, serum 1,25-dihydroxyvitamin D levels are likely to decrease progressively as kidney function declines. Results vary widely, however, among patients at any given level of renal function, whether judged by measurements of serum creatinine levels or by estimates of creatinine clearance. Technical difficulties with vitamin D assays might account for some of this variation, and differences in vitamin D nutrition can also contribute (vide infra). Nevertheless, plasma 1,25-dihydroxyvitamin D levels are normal in some patients but markedly reduced in others, who have only modest reductions in renal function. Patients whose renal function has declined from 20% to 25% of normal often have quite low serum calcitriol levels, whereas values may be only modestly reduced in others with a similar degree of renal functional impairment. The proportion of patients with subnormal serum calcitriol levels increases, however, as renal function worsens. Such changes account, at least in part, for reductions in the efficiency of intestinal calcium absorption and for modest decreases in serum calcium concentration in many patients with stage 3 and stage 4 chronic kidney disease. Indeed, hypocalciuria is a hallmark of moderate renal insufficiency, further emphasizing the importance of adequate renal calcitriol production for maintaining calcium homeostasis in those with progressive renal disease.

Other factors that can adversely affect renal calcitriol production in patients with chronic kidney disease include acidosis and interstitial renal diseases that predominantly affect the proximal renal tubular epithelial cells responsible for 1,25-dihydroxyvitamin D synthesis. Losses of DBP in the urine might account for reductions in serum vitamin D levels in some patients with proteinuria.

Vitamin D Nutrition and Renal Disease

A number of reports indicate that vitamin D nutrition is marginal or inadequate in many persons in the general population. This deficiency was demonstrated initially in studies of older persons with osteoporosis who were screened for vitamin D deficiency using measurements of 25-dihydroxyvitamin D levels in plasma. Additional epidemiologic work has documented that plasma 25-dihydroxyvitamin D levels are below recommended levels in a substantial proportion of persons in economically developed countries such as the United States and in Europe. Indeed, mild secondary hyperparathyroidism and modest elevations in plasma PTH levels are not uncommon, and repletion with vitamin D has been shown to lower plasma PTH levels in older adults with biochemical evidence of inadequate vitamin D nutrition. Such observations serve as the basis for the recent recommendation that patients with chronic kidney disease undergo biochemical screening to detect vitamin D deficiency and treatment if the disorder is identified.

Although opinions vary somewhat, plasma 25-dihydroxyvitamin D levels between 16 and 30 ng per mL reflect marginal vitamin D nutrition, or vitamin D insufficiency. Values ranging from 5 to 15 ng per mL indicate mild vitamin D deficiency, whereas values less than 5 ng per mL indicate severe vitamin D deficiency. Vitamin D repletion with ergocalciferol is recommended to restore plasma 25-dihydroxyvitamin D levels to values that exceed 30 ng per mL. Nutritional vitamin D repletion with ergocalciferol should be considered separate and distinct from the use of active vitamin D sterols to treat secondary hyperparathyroidism caused by chronic kidney disease.

A component of the secondary hyperparathyroidism that emerges as renal function declines in patients with chronic kidney disease is quite possibly caused by inadequate vitamin D nutrition and not solely by impaired calcitriol production by the diseased kidney. If present, vitamin D insufficiency, deficiency, or both are likely to aggravate the disorder. Observations from the general population show that inadequate vitamin D nutrition can contribute to the development of secondary hyperparathyroidism in individuals with adequate renal function, whereas vitamin D repletion can ameliorate the disorder in many patients or correct it fully in some patients. Additional work will be required, however, to clarify the role of vitamin D nutrition as a modifier of secondary hyperparathyroidism in patients with stage 3 or stage 4 chronic kidney disease.

Vitamin D and Bone

Vitamin D serves two critical functions in mineralizing tissues. It is an important modulator of cell differentiation and differentiated cell function both for osteoclasts and osteoblasts, and it is essential for maintaining the calcification of bone and cartilage.

Calcitriol, or 1,25-dihydroxyvitamin D_3, has major effects on the recruitment and differentiation of osteoclasts. These actions are attributable largely to calcitriol-induced up-regulation of RANK ligand (RANK-L) and its cognate receptor, RANK, that together mediate cell-to-cell interactions between marrow stromal cells and cells of the monocyte–macrophage lineage, which differentiate ultimately into fully mature osteoclasts. Although other cytokines and growth factors also influence osteoclast differentiation, calcitriol plays a critical role in the early recruitment of uncommitted precursors toward osteoclastic differentiation. Calcitriol has much less striking effects on the differentiated functions of mature osteoclasts.

Calcitriol is an important determinant of the levels of expression of selected biochemical markers of osteoblastic differentiation such as type I collagen, alkaline phosphatase, osteopontin, and osteocalcin at various stages of osteoblastic maturation. Calcitriol can, however, diminish the overall recruitment and differentiation of precursors into fully mature osteoblasts and impede differentiated functions, including collagen synthesis, in fully mature osteoblasts.

Most experimental evidence indicates that calcitriol supports skeletal mineralization primarily by maintaining adequate concentrations of calcium and phosphorus in extracellular fluid. Most compelling in this regard are data indicating that the calcification of bone and epiphyseal growth plate cartilage is normal in mice with inactivating mutations of the VDR, if serum calcium and phosphorus levels are maintained within the normal range by dietary maneuvers. Thus, calcium and phosphorus are alone sufficient to support adequate skeletal mineralization in tissues lacking a functional VDR.

ACKNOWLEDGMENTS

This work was supported in part by USPHS grant DK-60107.

SELECTED READINGS

Brown EM, MacLeod RJ. Extracellular calcium sensing and extracellular calcium signaling. *Physiol Rev* 2001;81:239–297.

Chen RA, Goodman WG. The role of the calcium-sensing receptor in parathyroid gland physiology. *Am J Physiol Renal Physiol* 2004; 286(6):F1005–F1011.

Coburn JW, Maung HM, Elangovan L, et al. Doxercalciferol safely suppresses PTH levels in patients with secondary hyperparathyroidism associated with chronic kidney disease stages 3 and 4. *Am J Kidney Dis* 2004;43(5):877–890.

den Dekker E, Hoenderop JG, Nilius B, et al. The epithelial calcium channels, TRPV5 & TRPV6: from identification towards regulation. *Cell Calcium* 2003;33(5-6):497–507.

Goodman WG. Recent developments in the management of secondary hyperparathyroidism. *Kidney Int* 2001;59:1187–1201.

Goodman WG, Coburn JW. The use of 1,25-dihydroxyvitamin D in early renal failure. *Annu Rev Med* 1992;43:227–237.

Heaney RP, Barger-Lux MJ, Dowell MS, et al. Calcium absorptive effects of vitamin D and its major metabolites. *J Clin Endocrinol Metab* 1997;82(12):4111–4116.

Hoenderop JG, Nilius B, Bindels RJ. ECaC: the gatekeeper of transepithelial Ca^{2+} transport. *Biochim Biophys Acta* 2002; 1600(1-2):6–11.

Kumar R. New insights into phosphate homeostasis: fibroblast growth factor 23 and frizzled-related protein-4 are phosphaturic factors derived from tumors associated with osteomalacia. *Curr Opin Nephrol Hypertens* 2002;11(5):547–553.

Larsson T, Nisbeth U, Ljunggren O, et al. Circulating concentration of FGF-23 increases as renal function declines in patients with chronic kidney disease, but does not change in response to variation in phosphate intake in healthy volunteers. *Kidney Int* 2003; 64(6):2272–2279.

Lips P. Vitamin D deficiency and secondary hyperparathyroidism in the elderly: consequences for bone loss and fractures and therapeutic implications. *Endocr Rev* 2001;22(4):477–501.

Lips P, Duong T, Oleksik A, et al. A global study of vitamin D status and parathyroid function in postmenopausal women with osteoporosis: baseline data from the multiple outcomes of raloxifene evaluation clinical trial. *J Clin Endocrinol Metab* 2001;86(3):1212–1221.

Malabanan A, Veronikis IE, Holick MF. Redefining vitamin D insufficiency. *Lancet* 1998;351(9105):805–806.

Quarles LD. FGF23, PHEX, and MEPE regulation of phosphate homeostasis and skeletal mineralization. *Am J Physiol Endocrinol Metab* 2003;285(1):E1–E9.

Riccardi D, Traebert M, Ward DT, et al. Dietary phosphate and parathyroid hormone alter the expression of the calcium-sensing receptor (CaR) and the Na+-dependent Pi transporter (NaPi-2) in the rat proximal tubule. *Pflugers Arch* 2000;441(2-3):379–387.

Shimada T, Mizutani S, Muto T, et al. Cloning and characterization of FGF23 as a causative factor of tumor-induced osteomalacia. *Proc Natl Acad Sci USA* 2001;98(11):6500–6505.

Shimada T, Muto T, Urakawa I, et al. Mutant FGF-23 responsible for autosomal dominant hypophosphatemic rickets is resistant to proteolytic cleavage and causes hypophosphatemia in vivo. *Endocrinology* 2002;143(8):3179–3182.

Shimada T, Urakawa I, Yamazaki Y, et al. FGF-23 transgenic mice demonstrate hypophosphatemic rickets with reduced expression of sodium phosphate cotransporter type IIa. *Biochem Biophys Res Commun* 2004;314(2):409–414.

Tenenhouse HS, Sabbagh Y. Novel phosphate-regulating genes in the pathogenesis of renal phosphate wasting disorders. *Pflugers Arch* 2002;444(3):317–326.

Tenenhouse HS, Werner A, Biber J, et al. Renal Na(+)-phosphate cotransport in murine X-linked hypophosphatemic rickets. Molecular characterization. *J Clin Invest* 1994;93:671–676.

The ADHR Consortium. Autosomal dominant hypophosphataemic rickets is associated with mutations in FGF23. *Nat Genet* 2000; 26(3):345–348.

White KE, Carn G, Lorenz-Depiereux B, et al. Autosomal-dominant hypophosphatemic rickets (ADHR) mutations stabilize FGF-23. *Kidney Int* 2001;60(6):2079–2086.

White KE, Jonsson KB, Carn G, et al. The autosomal dominant hypophosphatemic rickets (ADHR) gene is a secreted polypeptide overexpressed by tumors that cause phosphate wasting. *J Clin Endocrinol Metab* 2001;86(2):497–500.

4

Management of Lipid Abnormalities in the Patient with Renal Disease

Christoph Wanner and Vera Krane

To understand dyslipidemia in chronic kidney disease (CKD) stages 1 through 5, knowing some general aspects of lipid metabolism is useful. In general, all five major lipoproteins [chylomicrons, very–low-density lipoproteins (VLDL), intermediate-density lipoproteins (IDL), low-density lipoproteins (LDL), high-density lipoproteins (HDL)] consist of lipids (cholesterol, triglycerides, and phospholipids) and apolipoproteins. Apolipoproteins (A-I, A-II, B-48, B-100, C-I, C-II, C-III, and E) are found in different distributions among the various lipoproteins and serve as cofactors for enzymes and ligands for receptors. Levels of chylomicrons, the largest lipoprotein particle, increase after eating and are almost absent in the fasting state. These lipoproteins are formed in the intestinal epithelial cells; their main lipid content, triglycerides, is synthesized from re-esterification of dietary monoglycerides and fatty acids. Triglycerides represent 90% of chylomicrons and are hydrolyzed by lipoprotein lipase (LPL) present in adipose and vascular tissue. The residual particles, also called *chylomicron remnants*, are usually removed rapidly by the liver. In addition to dietary-derived chylomicrons, the liver has the capacity to produce endogenous lipoproteins from excess hepatocyte cholesterol and triglycerides. These lipids are synthesized and secreted as triglyceride-rich VLDL. The triglycerides present in VLDL are gradually removed by LPL (with apoC-II acting as a cofactor), resulting in IDL. IDL, also named *VLDL remnants*, represents a transition step in the lipolysis of VLDL to LDL, the main cholesterol-carrying lipoprotein, which accounts for 70% of circulating cholesterol (see Fig. 4-1). The characteristics of the various lipoproteins, and their lipid and apolipoprotein composition in healthy humans, are given in Table 4-1.

Lipoprotein(a) [Lp(a)], another apolipoprotein, should not be neglected in patients with renal disease, because high levels appear to be especially atherogenic. Lp(a) contains a structural protein called [apo(a)]. Apo(a) exhibits a high homology to plasminogen and an extreme size polymorphism, with the apo(a) isoproteins ranging in size from 420 to 840 kD. Inherited in an autosomal codominant fashion, the apo(a) isoprotein is an important factor that determines plasma Lp(a) concentrations, with an inverse correlation between the size of apo(a) isoprotein and the plasma Lp(a) concentration. The distribution of plasma Lp(a) levels is highly skewed toward lower concentrations, with more than two thirds of the population having levels lower than 20 mg per dL. High plasma concentrations of Lp(a) (more than 20 mg per dL) are associated with the risk for premature coronary

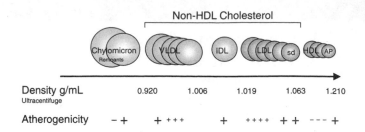

Figure 4-1. Classification of major lipoprotein particle density classes. [From Quaschning T, Krane V, Metzger T, et al. Abnormalities in urenic lipoprotein metabolism and its impact on cardiovascular disease. *Am J Kidney Dis* 2001;38(Suppl. 1):S14–S19, with permission.]

atherosclerosis, cerebrovascular atherosclerosis, and saphenous vein bypass graft stenosis.

TYPES OF DYSLIPIDEMIA IN THE DIFFERENT STAGES OF CHRONIC KIDNEY DISEASE

Qualitative characteristics of dyslipoproteinemia are the same in early renal insufficiency and in advanced renal failure. Dyslipidemia can already be detected in the early stages of CKD (stages 2 to 3) and is best characterized by abnormalities in the composition of apolipoproteins. Delayed catabolism of triglyceride-rich lipoproteins that result in increased concentrations of VLDL and IDL and reduced levels of HDL appears to be the main metabolic abnormality. A decreased apoA-I/apoC-III ratio is considered to be the hallmark of altered apolipoprotein profile. Quantitative differences might exist among patients, because the extent of dyslipidemia in patients who are non-nephrotic does not seem to depend on the urinary albumin excretion rate. The variation in urinary albumin excretion rate accounts for only 7% of the variation in non-nephrotic dyslipidemia.

Nephrotic Syndrome

Dyslipidemia is present in 70% to 90% of patients with nephrotic syndrome and can occur in several forms. Combined hyperlipidemia, with an increase in serum total cholesterol, LDL cholesterol, and serum triglycerides, is the most common form (50%). One-third of patients have elevated LDL cholesterol exclusively, whereas only 4% of patients show pure hypertriglyceridemia. Changes in the composition of lipoprotein particles also have been described, with cholesterol enrichment in IDL but not LDL. The levels of HDL cholesterol can be low, normal, or high, and the level of HDL2 is reduced. Findings of high HDL levels could be attributable to high serum levels of Lp(a) contaminating the HDL samples when cholesterol is assayed. Therefore, the inconsistent HDL results are most likely the consequence of selection criteria. HDL has been quantified in the urine in patients with nephrotic syndrome, and changes in the composition of urinary HDL have been ascribed to the effect of tubular catabolism on filtered lipoprotein. The reason that patients with nephrotic syndrome present different accumulations of triglycerides and cholesterol has not been fully elucidated but includes

Table 4-1. Lipoprotein classes of human plasma

	Density	Electrophoretic Mobility	Particle Diameter	Apolipoproteins	Composition (% mass)				
					TG	FC	CE	PL	Pr
Chylomicrons	<0.95	—	>1,000	A-I, A-IV, B-48, C, E	90	1	2	5	2
VLDL	<1.006	pre-β	55	B-100, C, E	54	7	13	16	10
IDL	1.006–1.019	pre-β-β	25	B-100, C, E	20	9	34	20	17
LDL	1.019–1.063	β	20	B-100	4	9	34	20	17
HDL	1.063–1.210	α	10	A-I, A-II, E, C	4	4	14	29	49
Lp(a)	1.080–1.100	pre-β	24	B-100, (a)	3	9	36	18	34

TG, triglyceride; FC, free cholesterol; CE, cholesteryl ester; PL, phospholipids; Pr, protein; VLDL, very–low-density lipoproteins; IDL, intermediate-density lipoproteins; LDL, low-density lipoproteins; HDL, high-density lipoproteins.

many factors, such as genetic apolipoprotein phenotypes, concomitant drug therapy, and the catabolic state of the individual. In contrast to patients with nephrotic syndrome who have normal kidney function, the presence of uremia in patients with nephrotic syndrome leads to further changes; however, diabetes mellitus does not affect the pattern of hyperlipoproteinemia. Markedly elevated Lp(a) concentrations have been found in most patients with proteinuria and nephrotic syndrome, even when compared to controls with the same apo(a) isoform. On average, Lp(a) levels are sixfold elevated in patients with severe nephrotic syndrome. Nephrotic syndrome likely results directly in elevated Lp(a) concentrations, because Lp(a) levels are substantially reduced when remission of the nephrotic syndrome is induced. Recent data suggest that the kidney per se is responsible for the metabolism of Lp(a).

Mechanisms of Hyperlipidemia in Nephrotic Syndrome

Not all patients with nephrotic syndrome show increased lipid levels, and those with elevations in VLDL have decreased fractional clearance rates (decreased catabolism) rather than increased synthesis. Two separate processes impede the removal of triglyceride-rich lipoproteins. The first defect is an abnormality in VLDL that decreases its ability to bind to endothelial surfaces in the presence of saturating LPL. This defect in VLDL function, and presumably structure, is a result of proteinuria. The second defect is the inability of LPL to bind effectively to the vascular endothelium (see Fig. 4-2).

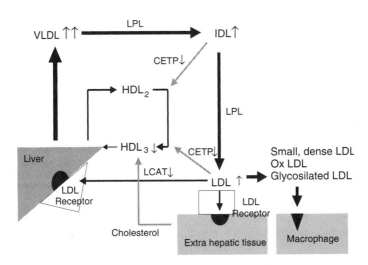

Figure 4-2. Lipoprotein metabolism in uremia is characterized by elevated VLDL, IDL, and LDL; HDL metabolism is impaired as well. The accumulation of LDL leads to its modification and consequently requires uptake via scavenger receptors. LCAT, Lecithin-cholesteryl acyltransferase; CETP, Cholesteryl ester transfer protein. [From Quaschning T, Krane V, Metzger T, et al. Abnormalities in uremic lipoprotein metabolism and its impact on cardiovascular disease. *An J Kidney Dis* 2001;38(Suppl. 1):S14–S19, with permission.]

Hemodialysis

The prevalence of dyslipidemia in end-stage renal disease (ESRD) treated with hemodialysis is greater than in the general population. Patients exhibit a characteristic dyslipidemia consisting of hypertriglyceridemia and low HDL cholesterol levels. VLDL cholesterol is typically increased. However, levels of total and LDL cholesterol are usually normal or can even be low. This profile translates into the most characteristic feature of ESRD-associated dyslipidemia: an accumulation of triglyceride-rich lipoproteins (VLDL-remnants) and IDL. In addition, qualitative changes of LDL, with the formation of small dense LDL, can be found (see Figs. 4-2 and 4-3). The overall pattern is best characterized by an accumulation of apolipoprotein B containing triglyceride-rich lipoprotein particles that contain apolipoprotein C-III and apo (a) or by lipoprotein B complex (LpBc) particles. A defect in postprandial chylomicron remnant clearance has also been described.

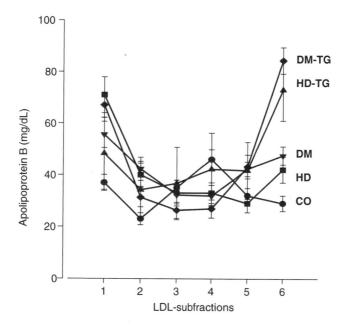

Figure 4-3. Low-density lipoprotein subfractions, obtained by density gradient ultracentrifugation in 10 healthy controls (CO) and 40 patients treated with hemodialysis (HD): 10 with type 2 diabetes (DM), 10 with hypertriglyceridemia, 10 with both type 2 diabetes and hypertriglyceridemia, and 10 who had neither diabetes nor hypertriglyceridemia. Please note the accumulation of small dense LDL in LDL subfraction 6. (From Quaschning T, Schomig M, Keller M, et al. Non-insulin-dependent diabetes mellitus and hypertriglyceridemia impair lipoprotein metabolism in chronic hemodialysis patients. *J Am Soc Nephrol* 1999;10:S332–S341, with permission.)

Continuous Ambulatory Peritoneal Dialysis

Patients treated with continuous ambulatory peritoneal dialysis (CAPD) have higher plasma cholesterol, triglyceride, and LDL cholesterol levels than patients treated with hemodialysis. In terms of atherogenic burden, CAPD patients are exposed to a higher vascular risk from dyslipidemia. This additional increase is most likely caused by two factors: (a) loss of protein (7 to 14 g per day) into the peritoneal dialysate and (b) absorption of glucose (150 to 200 g per day) from the dialysis fluid. The extent to which protein loss triggers mechanisms that are operative in the nephrotic syndrome, and whether hyperinsulinemia results in impaired receptor-mediated clearance of lipoproteins by inducing advanced glycosylation of apoB, is uncertain. The glucose load can increase triglyceride synthesis, thereby contributing to a further increase in the concentration of triglyceride-rich lipoproteins. Qualitative lipoprotein abnormalities are similar to those found in patients treated with hemodialysis, and most mechanisms that alter lipoprotein metabolism are probably also the same. An interesting study in normolipidemic patients undergoing CAPD has demonstrated less pronounced abnormalities of cholesterol transport than in patients treated with hemodialysis. This difference might be attributable to increased clearance of unknown inhibitory factors, which results in better control of uremic lipoprotein metabolism and leads to decreased concentrations of such factors. On the other hand, patients treated with CAPD also exhibit higher levels of Lp(a) than patients treated with hemodialysis, and this increase in Lp(a) levels might also outweigh other positive conditions.

Lipid Abnormalities after Kidney Transplantation

Dyslipidemia is commonly found in patients after renal transplantation and is associated with cardiovascular complications and graft atherosclerosis. Correlations have been found between dyslipidemia and renal transplantation with cyclosporine and steroids as the major causes of lipid abnormalities. Tacrolimus does not affect total cholesterol and LDL cholesterol levels, and it engenders a smaller increase in triglyceride levels (10% to 15%) compared to that caused by cyclosporine. Posttransplant dyslipidemia is qualitatively and quantitatively dependent on age, gender, body weight, and type and dose of immunosuppressive agents. Although some former studies focused mainly on elevated serum cholesterol levels as a major factor in cardiovascular disease, recent data emphasize that an increase in levels of serum triglycerides, LDL, and VLDL are major factors. Alterations in size and density contribute to configurational changes of lipoproteins. Small and dense LDL exhibits reduced receptor-specific uptake and therefore bears increased atherogenicity. This change corresponds with the finding that hypertriglyceridemia is considered to be an independent risk factor for cardiovascular disease. Because of the multiplicity of other cardiovascular risk factors, dyslipidemia might also accelerate the development of arteriosclerosis in a preinjured vascular endothelium. Immunosuppression withdrawal protocols have been used successfully to control pronounced hyperlipidemia in immunologically stable patients.

The characteristics of the various types of dyslipidemia are shown in Table 4-2.

Table 4-2. Common lipoprotein abnormalities in patients with nephrotic syndrome, patients with chronic kidney disease (CKD), and patients treated with hemodialysis and continuous ambulatory peritoneal dialysis (CAPD)

	Chylomicron Remnants	VLDL	IDL	LDL	HDL	Lp(a)
Nephrotic syndrome	—	↑	↑↑	↑↑↑	↔↓	↑↑↑
CKD	↑	↑	↑	→	→	↑
Hemodialysis	↑↑	↑↑	↑↑	→	→	↑↑
CAPD	?	↑	↑↑	↑	↔	↑↑↑
Transplantation	—	↑	—	↑	↔	↔

VLDL, very-low-density lipoproteins; IDL, intermediate-density lipoproteins; LDL, low-density lipoproteins; HDL, high-density lipoproteins; CKD, chronic kidney disease; CAPD, continuous ambulatory peritoneal dialysis.

VASCULAR RISKS ASSOCIATED WITH DYSLIPIDEMIA

Dyslipidemia should be seen not as an isolated phenomenon but in the context of cardiovascular disease. At all stages of kidney disease, the patient's cardiovascular risk should be formally assessed and documented at presentation and at 6-month intervals thereafter. Risk assessment includes modifiable risk factors such as cigarette smoking, hyperglycemia, dyslipidemia, and hypertension. Strong evidence exists from studies in the general population that cigarette smoking, glucose intolerance or poor diabetes control, hypertension, family history of vascular disease, and current or past history of vascular disease can each independently contribute to the risk for vascular disease. Including a medical record history of vascular disease as a mortality case-mix factor is recommended to quantitate the presence of vascular disease and to estimate complications and outcome.

Nephrotic Syndrome

Undoubtedly, the severe, persistent elevation of LDL, IDL, and Lp(a), regardless of cause, represents a highly atherogenic condition. But the degree to which it increases the risk for coronary heart disease (CHD) in patients with nephrotic syndrome remains uncertain. Relatively little and conflicting information has been published on the risk for atherosclerotic cardiovascular disease (ACVD). All of these studies are retrospective and flawed by small numbers, selection bias, and lack of control for other atherosclerotic risk factors (such as smoking, hypertension, and steroid therapy). Some studies include patients with minimal-change disease, who would most likely not remain nephrotic and hence not remain at risk for the long-term complications of hyperlipidemia. According to Ordonez et al., the relative risk for myocardial infarction, after adjustment for hypertension and smoking, is as high as 5.5, and the relative risk for coronary death is 2.8, which is substantial. The data were obtained in a series of patients (n = 142) matched with healthy subjects and followed prospectively for 5.6 and 1.2 years, respectively. Unfortunately, the cholesterol level data were insufficient to analyze the risk by specific lipid levels or by duration of hyperlipidemia. Until now, no study has been carried out to identify dyslipidemia as a major factor for cardiovascular complication in patients with nephrotic syndrome, nor has a regression study been performed, because of the low prevalence of the nephrotic syndrome and the large number of patients required to show a significant reduction in coronary events following lipid-lowering therapy.

Hemodialysis

The best available data are those from patients treated with dialysis documented in registries. These data show that cardiovascular disease is the leading cause of morbidity and mortality in patients treated with hemodialysis; cardiac disease accounts for 44% of overall mortality. Approximately 22% of deaths from cardiac causes are attributed to acute myocardial infarction. In patients who survive a myocardial infarction, the mortality from cardiac causes is 59% at 1 year, 73% at 2 years, and nearly 90% at 3 years. A similar abysmal long-term prognosis has been reported from the Strasbourg region (France) for patients with type 2 diabetes mellitus starting dialysis therapy. After adjusting for age, gender, race, and diagnosis of diabetes, mortality from cardiovascular disease is far greater in patients treated with hemodialysis than in the general population. The risk ranges from 500-fold in individuals 25 to 34 years old to about fivefold in individuals older than 85. The excess risk for vascular disease is caused, at least in part, by an increased prevalence of conditions that are recognized as risk factors for vascular disease in the general population ("traditional" risk factors), and further, by hemodynamic and metabolic factors characteristic of CKD ("kidney disease–related" risk factors). Most studies clearly show that dyslipidemia does not contribute to the vascular risk, and a strong confounding factor, represented by inflammation, does not allow detecting dyslipidemia as a prominent vascular risk factor in patients receiving hemodialysis therapy. The studies have also taken into account the fact that vascular damage develops during the progressive course of kidney disease and long before renal replacement therapy starts.

Atherogenicity of Dyslipidemia in Hemodialysis and Continuous Ambulatory Peritoneal Dialysis

Published data suggest that all components of dialysis or uremia-dependent dyslipidemia (elevated VLDL-remnants, IDL, small dense LDL, low HDL cholesterol) are independently atherogenic. Together, they represent a set of lipoprotein abnormalities that, in addition to elevated LDL cholesterol, promote atherosclerosis. Triglycerides are physiologically linked to small dense LDL and low HDL concentrations, and increased amounts of small dense LDL likely contribute to the atherogenic risk for hypertriglyceridemia. Atherogenic levels of small dense LDL are found in patients undergoing hemodialysis who have triglyceride levels greater than 177 mg per dL. The accumulation of these lipoprotein particles contributes to a so-called atherogenic lipoprotein phenotype. A similar type of dyslipidemia, also seen in the general population, is called *atherogenic dyslipidemia*. It frequently occurs in patients with premature coronary heart disease and appears in the absence of elevated LDL cholesterol levels. Most patients with this atherogenic lipoprotein phenotype are insulin resistant, and many also have an elevated serum apolipoprotein B. Several theories have been proposed regarding the cause of this increased atherogenicity. The primary metabolic defect is believed to be defective catabolism of triglyceride-rich lipoproteins (primarily VLDL) by the enzymes lipoprotein lipase and hepatic lipase. Lipid peroxidation products are elevated in plasma but do not seem to be generated during hemodialysis. A defect in cholesterol transport has been reported, probably caused by alterations in cholesterol ester transfer protein and lecithin cholesterol acyltransferase activities. With respect to mechanisms for small dense LDL accumulation, the suggested causes include (i) decreased affinity for the LDL receptor with increased clearance via the scavenger receptor; (ii) increased susceptibility to oxidation and glycation, partly as a result of longer residence time in the circulation; (iii) increased transcapillary permeability and filtration by the endothelium because of the smaller size of the particles; and (iv) greater affinity for binding to extracellular matrix such as arterial wall proteoglycans.

Dyslipidemia and Atherosclerotic Vascular Disease

Lipid abnormalities are a major cause of vascular disease in patients treated with hemodialysis, and reviews have focused on the subject of renal failure, dialysis, and dyslipidemia. A number of studies have examined the relationship between various lipid parameters and the presence of clinically apparent atherosclerosis in individuals receiving hemodialysis therapy. These trials have had cross-sectional designs, have included only small numbers of patients, and have failed in part to distinguish atherosclerosis-related events from other forms of cardiovascular disease. Studies also have failed to control for other risk factors and have assessed only total plasma lipid levels rather than the lipoprotein disturbances that characterize the uremic dyslipidemia. Therefore, the fact that the conclusions have been conflicting is not surprising. In the largest and longest study to date, 419 patients treated with dialysis were followed prospectively over a 21-year period. During this time, 49% died of cardiovascular disease and 23% experienced fatal or nonfatal ischemic events. Smoking, hypertension, and hypertriglyceridemia were identified as independent risk factors for ischemic cardiovascular disease. In contrast, smaller cross-sectional studies have failed to find an association between elevated triglycerides and complications that result from vascular disease. The only positive study, in a group of 196 diabetic patients receiving hemodialysis, demonstrated that elevated cholesterol levels with high LDL-to-HDL ratios were associated with an increased risk for cardiac death during a 45-month follow-up period. Hypercholesterolemia was more common in the diabetic patients than in matched dialyzed controls who did not have diabetes. Lipid measurements were done when patients commenced renal replacement therapy. Notably, serum cholesterol concentrations decline with time as treatment with dialysis continues. Most cross-sectional studies with longitudinal follow-up have also failed to demonstrate that plasma total cholesterol, LDL–cholesterol, and triglycerides are associated with increased cardiovascular mortality in patients treated with hemodialysis.

The Paradox of Cholesterol in Patients Receiving Hemodialysis Therapy

Prospective observational studies in the general population have shown that the relation between the risk for coronary artery disease and blood cholesterol is roughly loglinear. However, inverse associations were observed among patients treated with hemodialysis between blood cholesterol and all-cause or cardiovascular mortality. The relationship between serum cholesterol and mortality has been described as a U-shaped curve and, recently, as a J-shaped curve, and the risk for death is 4.3 times greater in patients treated with hemodialysis, with serum cholesterol less than 100 mg per dL (2.6 mmol per L) than in those with values between 200 and 250 mg per dL (5.2 to 6.5 mmol per L). This phenomenon is known as reverse risk factor causality and is embedded in the condition of reverse epidemiology.

Concomitant chronic illnesses that induce a compensatory decrease in cholesterol synthesis are also associated with an increased risk for death, producing artifactual negative associations between cholesterol and mortality. Indeed, Liu et al. demonstrated that hypercholesterolemia is an independent risk factor for all-cause and cardiovascular mortality in a subgroup of patients with ESRD without serologic evidence of inflammation or malnutrition but not in patients who have evidence of inflammation. This effect might limit the extent to which standard observational studies can identify the true effect of serum cholesterol on the development of vascular disease in this and other populations. The extent to which microinflammation or infections interact with dyslipidemia in the manifestation of atherosclerosis, and how lipid lowering may influence this process, is not clear.

The association between serum lipids and cardiovascular disease in patients with ESRD is shown in Table 4-3.

Kidney Transplantation

Kidney transplant recipients have high morbidity and mortality because of premature cardiovascular disease. Two studies have shown higher serum cholesterol and triglyceride values in patients with ischemic heart disease than in patients without ischemic heart disease. Vathsala et al. reported a 36-month follow-up in 500 patients treated with cyclosporine and prednisone. They found that cardiovascular or cerebrovascular episodes occurred in 9.4% of patients and were significantly more common in hyperlipidemic (15.4%) than in normolipidemic (5.2%) subjects. A recent retrospective study demonstrated

Table 4-3. Association between serum lipids and cardiovascular disease in patients with end-stage renal disease (ESRD)

Study	N	Study	TC	LDL	HDL	TG
Iseki (1996)	1,491	Prospective	↔			↔
Degoulet (1982)	1,453	Prospective	↓			↔
Kronenberg (1999)	440	Prospective	↔	↔	↓	↔
Zimmermann (1999)	280	Prospective	↔	↔	↔	↔
Cressmann (1992)	129	Prospective	↔	↔	↔	↔
Stack (2001)	4,025	Prevalence	↔	↔	↔	↔
Koch (1997)	607	Prevalence	↔	↔	↓	↔
Cheung (1992)	936	Prevalence	↔			
Overall			↔	↔	↔	↔

LDL, low-density lipoproteins; HDL, high-density lipoproteins.

significantly higher concentrations of total cholesterol, triglycerides, and apolipoproteins B, C-II, C-III, and E in 25 patients with
cardiovascular events than in 29 patients without cardiovascular
events. A significant association was found between smoking and
the proportion of patients with hypertension among those with
cardiovascular disease. Massy et al. found significantly higher
serum triglyceride concentrations, but not cholesterol levels, in patients with ischemic heart disease. Whenever studies in patients
with renal functional impairment find a significant rise in apoB—
containing, triglyceride-rich lipoprotein particles, the presence of
partially delipidized lipoproteins or so-called remnant lipoproteins
can be suspected. Indeed, Quaschning et al. demonstrated an enrichment of triglycerides in VLDL and LDL in 218 patients with
stable graft function. Triglyceride enrichment in LDL indicates an
accumulation of small dense LDL, which bears enhanced atherosclerotic risk. These lipoprotein particles are also considered to be
of particular importance in the progression of renal injury.

SCREENING FOR DYSLIPIDEMIA

For adults and adolescents with CKD stage 5 who undergo
kidney transplantation, the Kidney Disease Outcomes Quality
Initiative (K/DOQI) guidelines for managing dyslipidemias in CKD
advise assessing dyslipidemia, including a complete fasting lipid
profile with total cholesterol, LDL, HDL, and triglycerides, upon
presentation (when the patient is stable), at 2 to 3 months after a
change in treatment or when other conditions known to cause dyslipidemias become evident, and at least annually thereafter.

The same work group recommended that the Adult Treatment
panel-III (ATP III) guidelines are applicable to patients with
stage 1 to 4 CKD except to: (a) classify CKD as a CHD risk equivalent; (b) consider complications of lipid-lowering therapies that
can result from reduced kidney function; (c) consider whether indications other than preventing ACVD are present for treating
dyslipidemias; and (d) determine whether treating proteinuria
might also be an effective treatment for dyslipidemias.

LDL cholesterol should be calculated by the Friedewald formula when triglycerides are less than 400 mg per dL (4.56 mmol
per L). The Friedewald formula is valid in patients treated with
dialysis and is sufficiently accurate ($r = 0.95$ to 0.97 calculated
LDL versus measured LDL) to enable the determination of LDL
cholesterol in most patients.

[Friedewald LDL cholesterol = total cholesterol – (HDL cholesterol
+ triglyceride/5)]

Up to 20% of patients treated with hemodialysis intermittently
have total triglycerides above 400 mg per dL (4.56 mmol per L).
As in other forms of primary or secondary hyperlipoproteinemias,
LDL cholesterol should be measured by lipoprotein electrophore-
sis, or by the rarely available, analytical ultracentrifugation when
triglycerides are above 400 mg per dL (4.56 to 9.12 mmol per L).
When triglycerides are more than 800 mg per dL (9.12 mmol per
L), LDL measurement is not recommended.

Evidence suggests that each of the dyslipidemias described
above is associated with vascular disease in the general population,
and that treatment can reduce the risk for vascular disease.

Measurements are readily available in most clinical chemistry laboratories. Because of variations in extracorporal treatment methods, a complete plasma lipid profile should be ordered each time dyslipidemia assessment is recommended. Changes in therapy or other conditions that can affect dyslipidemia might require more frequent measurements.

An ongoing discussion over many years considers whether all blood collections for lipid screening should be performed on patients in the fasting state (see Fig. 4-4). The report from the Managing Dyslipidemias in Chronic Kidney Disease Work Group of the National Kidney Foundation–Kidney Disease Outcomes Quality Initiative (NKF–K/DOQI) reflects the problem and states that "whenever possible," blood should be drawn in the fasting state, immediately before, or at least 12 hours after, a regularly scheduled hemodialysis treatment. Because most studies linking dyslipidemias to vascular disease have measured lipid levels before the hemodialysis procedure, screening should be done at this time.

Patients should have a complete lipid profile measured every 6 weeks during the initiation phase of lipid-lowering intervention. When target levels have been met, the frequency can be reduced to every 4 to 6 months. Some evidence indicates that the hemodialysis procedure acutely alters lipid levels, triglyceride and free fatty acid levels in particular. Changes in therapy or other conditions that can affect dyslipidemias might make more frequent measurements necessary. Blood obtained from either fasting or nonfasting individuals can be used for total cholesterol and HDL cholesterol analysis. Any patient with elevated LDL cholesterol or other forms of dyslipidemia (elevated total cholesterol and triglycerides, low HDL cholesterol, or both) should undergo clinical or laboratory assessment to rule out other secondary causes, such as glucose intolerance, hypothyroidism, obstructive liver disease, or alcohol abuse. Other secondary disorders include progestins or anabolic steroids, drugs that increase LDL cholesterol

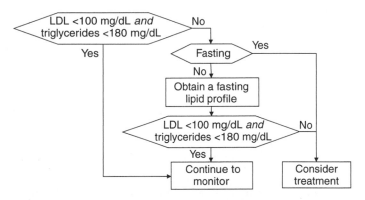

Figure 4-4. Screening for dyslipidemia in patients with renal disease and renal failure. [Modified according to National Kidney Foundation. K/DOQI clinical practice guidelines for managing dyslipidemias in chronic kidney disease. *Am J Kidney Dis* 2003;41(Suppl. 3):S23, with permission.]

and decrease HDL cholesterol. Anabolic steroids might be used to treat renal anemia in countries where erythropoietin is not widely available because of economic constraints. The use of anabolic steroids and the benefits of raising hematocrit should be weighed against the potential risk for developing several forms of dyslipidemia and possible deteriorating vascular disease. In one study, Lp(a) decreased and triglycerides increased, although most women receiving nandrolone decanoate experienced mild hirsutism and voice change. Screening for dyslipidemia should not be performed after surgery or during conditions that can acutely affect the lipid profile. Patients without any comorbid conditions and low total cholesterol levels (less than 150 mg per dL; 3.9 mmol per L) should be investigated for possible nutritional deficits. Such comorbid conditions include acute infection, diarrhea, vascular events such as myocardial infarction, or situations associated with reduced food intake. In patients admitted to the hospital for a major coronary event, LDL cholesterol levels should be measured on admission or within 24 hours. This value can be used for treatment decisions. LDL cholesterol levels begin to decline in the first few hours after a vascular event, are substantially decreased after 24 to 48 hours, and can remain low for many weeks. Thus, the initial (24-hour) LDL cholesterol level obtained in the hospital might be substantially lower than the patient's usual level. Infection is accompanied by an acute phase reaction. Activated acute phase and high levels of circulating cytokines, such as interleukin-6, lower cholesterol levels. Low or declining serum cholesterol concentrations predict increased mortality risk. Hypocholesterolemia is associated with chronic protein–energy deficits and the presence of comorbid conditions, including inflammation. Cholesterol is influenced by the same comorbid conditions, such as inflammation, that affect other nutritional markers (e.g., serum albumin).

TREATMENT GUIDELINES

General Remarks

Guidelines for detecting, evaluating, and treating high blood cholesterol in adults are available from US and European expert panels and from many national societies. These guidelines are evidence-based and were developed for the general population in a rigorous manner. Trial results from the general population might not be applicable to patients with kidney disease or those receiving kidney replacement therapy. No randomized controlled interventional trials have been conducted in patients with kidney disease or in patients receiving renal replacement therapy that show that treating dyslipidemias reduces the incidence of vascular disease. In some subpopulations of patients treated with dialysis, treating dyslipidemias might not be as safe or as effective in reducing the incidence of vascular disease as it is in the general population. Additional randomized, placebo-controlled trials are urgently needed. The use of placebo treatment arms is justified in the context of an appropriately designed trial, even when lipid levels fall within the treatment thresholds recommended by guidelines. This view, supported by current K/DOQI and European Best Practice Guidelines, allows randomizing patients into controlled clinical trials. Several of these trials are still ongoing, such as the AURORA study comparing rosuvastatin with placebo in patients treated with hemodialysis, and the SHARP trial (Study on Heart and Renal Protection) randomizing patients with CKD or those receiving dialysis treatment to either simvastatin in combination with ezetimibe or to placebo. The 4D study randomized 1,255 patients with type 2 diabetes mellitus to either atorvastatin 20 mg per dL or placebo. The study started in 1998 and was officially closed in February 2004. Data will be released at the time that this book is published. We will soon learn whether these trial results support, on a higher evidence level, the existing guidelines for using statins to prevent cardiovascular disease in patients with type 2 diabetes mellitus who are receiving hemodialysis therapy. New observations that statins affect inflammation, in addition to cholesterol–lowering, could also be evaluated on the basis of the 4D trial data.

All other patients who do not fulfill the 4D trial patients' inclusion criteria should be treated according to the recommendations of the National Cholesterol Education Program (NCEP) or other societies' guidelines. A high-risk strategy should be applied using the recommendations, targeting patients with known cardiovascular disease. Like diabetes, CKD is considered to be a coronary risk equivalent. In the absence of data from randomized trials, it can only be assumed that the interventions recommended by the various guidelines will similarly reduce vascular disease in patients with renal disease who are receiving renal replacement therapy. Although the concept of accelerated atherosclerosis has become widely accepted since it was first published by Lindner et al. in 1974, all recommended lipid-lowering treatment is done in the absence of evidence that the risk for cardiovascular death is reduced by reducing lipid levels in individuals with kidney disease or kidney failure.

Treatment Aspects

On the basis of evidence level C (= opinion), current guidelines recommend treating patients with elevated LDL cholesterol (100 to 129 mg per dL; 2.6 to 3.4 mmol per L) to achieve LDL cholesterol less than 100 mg per dL (see Fig. 4-5). Treatment beyond LDL cholesterol lowering should be initiated in patients with triglycerides greater than or equal to 180 mg per dL (2.0 mmol per L). Research on animals, laboratory investigations, epidemiology, and studies of genetic forms of hypercholesterolemia indicate that elevated LDL cholesterol is a major cause of vascular disease. In addition, recent clinical trials robustly show that LDL cholesterol-lowering therapy reduces the risk for vascular disease in the general population. For these reasons, one might decide to extrapolate, at least in part, these data to the high-risk group of patients with kidney disease and to adopt elevated LDL cholesterol as the primary target of cholesterol-lowering therapy. However, targeting LDL cholesterol alone might not be appropriate, because elevated LDL cholesterol is not the feature of lipid abnormalities complicating uremia.

Patients with CKD are automatically considered to have coronary heart disease equivalents and therefore are at the highest risk for developing vascular disease. They should have no major

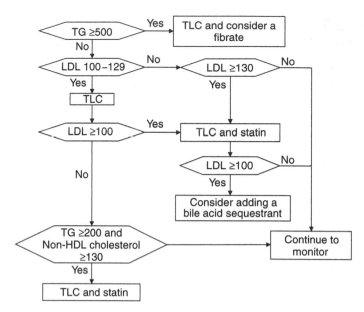

Figure 4-5.   Treatment for dyslipidemia in patients with renal disease and renal failure. [Modified according to National Kidney Foundation. K/DOQI clinical practice guidelines for managing dyslipidemias in chronic kidney disease. *Am J Kidney Dis* 2003;41(Suppl. 3):S23, with permission.]

contraindications to therapy and no illness that makes preventing or treating vascular disease unlikely to be beneficial. Lipid-lowering drugs should be administered to achieve LDL cholesterol and non-HDL cholesterol target levels, irrespective of whether ischemic heart disease symptoms are present. LDL cholesterol levels more than 100 mg per dL (2.6 mmol per L) and non-HDL cholesterol more than 130 mg per dL (3.4 mmol per L) are treatment initiation thresholds for drug therapy.

Little evidence exists to suggest that the risk attributable to LDL cholesterol is similar in patients treated with hemodialysis and in the general population, but efficacy and safety of treatment for LDL cholesterol with a statin are identical. In general, the action points for drug treatment are based primarily on risk–benefit considerations. LDL-lowering therapy greatly reduces the risk for major coronary events and stroke and yields highly favorable cost-effectiveness ratios. Patients at increased risk are likely to get greater benefit. Action points for recommended management based on therapeutic efficacy are checked against currently accepted standards for cost effectiveness. According to the current literature, hemodialysis treatment is likely to achieve cost-effectiveness ratios by reducing morbidity and subsequent hospitalizations. However, this assumption remains to be demonstrated.

Diet and Exercise

In patients with LDL cholesterol 100 to 129 mg per dL (2.6 to 3.4 mmol per L) or triglycerides more than 180 mg per dL

(2.0 mmol per L), therapeutic lifestyle changes (TLC) should be initiated, whenever possible. Patients with dyslipidemia should have dietary interviews or diaries focusing on the type and amount of fat ingested. Dietary interviews should be repeated at yearly intervals when target lipid levels are not achieved. TLC include reduced intake of saturated fat and cholesterol, increased physical activity, and weight control. However, patients undergoing hemodialysis are already subject to specific restrictions of food and fluid intake. Introducing a diet restricted in saturated fatty acids might add nutritional difficulties and can lead to protein–energy malnutrition. Some patients can benefit from replacing saturated fat with nonsaturated fat dietary sources, but these patients should be selected carefully. In patients who do not have a renal condition, diets rich in polyunsaturated fatty acids of fish-oil origin (ω-3) increase the removal of triglyceride-rich lipoprotein remnants and reduce postprandial plasma lipoprotein. Eicosapentanoic acid reduces plasma remnant lipoproteins and prevents *in vivo* peroxidation of LDL in patients undergoing dialysis. When patients are selected for dietary therapy, physicians should refer patients to qualified dietitians and nutritionists at all stages of dietary intervention.

Patients receiving hemodialysis therapy are usually less physically active than healthy sedentary controls, and this difference is pronounced in older individuals. An association exists between physical activity and nutritional status. Exercise training can, if tolerated and maintained over long periods, improve dyslipidemia and glucose tolerance in selected patients. Whether inactivity increases or exercise reduces mortality in patients receiving maintenance dialysis therapy is not known.

Weight control might be appropriate in early renal failure but is risky in advanced stages of renal failure, because it poses the danger of causing malnutrition. Optimizing body weight should best be done together with a moderate increase in physical activity. Patients receiving hemodialysis therapy normally have a reduced mean subcutaneous fat area/body mass index (SFA/BMI) and an increased visceral fat area/body mass index (VFA/BMI). Visceral fat accumulation occurs irrespective of BMI and is associated with serum triglycerides. Weight for height is a strong predictor of 12-month mortality in male and female patients receiving hemodialysis therapy. An inverse relationship between mortality rates and weight-for-height percentiles is highly significant for patients within the lower 50th percentile of body weight for height. Low BMI is associated with increased risk for hospitalization and mortality. For every unit increase in BMI more than 27.5 and up to 30, the relative risk for death is reduced by 30%. It can be important for patients to have excessive body fat and other nutrients on which they can draw in cases of inflammatory catabolic conditions. However, BMIs derived from excessive body fat should be distinguished from those derived from lean body mass or muscle mass, because the cardiovascular risk may be different.

Pharmacotherapy

Nephrotic Syndrome

The first therapeutic strategy to reduce serum lipids in nephrotic syndrome is to reduce proteinuria. Serum total and LDL cholesterol concentration and Lp(a) levels are inversely correlated with serum albumin levels and with proteinuria. Reduction in protein-uria, induced by angiotensin-converting enzyme (ACE) inhibitors, reduces serum Lp(a) and cholesterol levels and is used as an ad-juvant to standard lipid-lowering therapy. In this context, ACE in-hibitors are excellent lipid-lowering drugs in patients with proteinuria. Nevertheless, lipid-lowering therapy with statins is almost always necessary to correct excessive cholesterol eleva-tions. The bile acid–binding resins, cholestyramine and colestipol, the fibric acid gemfibrozil, and probucol have all demonstrated limited effects in short-term trials. Today the largest numbers of patients have been treated with statins, which are by far the most effective LDL cholesterol–lowering agents. Because they are well tolerated and cause few side effects, they currently represent the treatment of choice. Fish oil is a potent triglyceride-lowering agent. However, conflicting findings of increased LDL cholesterol concentrations and decreased HDL/LDL cholesterol ratios, the large number of capsules required for therapeutic effect, and the low tolerance does not make fish oil a favorite treatment. Because a considerable number of patients with nephrotic syndrome have combined hyperlipidemia, the question of combined therapy aris-es. An effective drug combination is an HMG-CoA reductase in-hibitor and a fibric acid. However, this combination increases the risk for myopathy in patients without nephrotic syndrome and has never been tested specifically in patients with nephrotic syn-drome. Therefore, combination therapy should not be used in pa-tients with nephrotic syndrome.

Treatment of Hypercholesterolemia in Patients Undergoing Hemodialysis and Peritoneal Dialysis

If after 3 months of TLC, LDL cholesterol is more than 100 mg per dL (2.6 mmol per L), treatment with a statin should be initi-ated. If the LDL cholesterol goal is not achieved after 6 weeks of treatment, the dose of the statin should stepwise be increased, and a lipid profile should be repeated after another 6 weeks. If the LDL cholesterol goal is not achieved with TLC and optimal treat-ment with a statin, additional measures should be considered.

Statins are the most effective drugs for lowering LDL cho-lesterol in patients undergoing hemodialysis and should gener-ally be the agents of first choice. If LDL cholesterol is still more than 100 mg per dL (2.6 mmol per L), despite optimal treat-ment with a statin and diet, additional LDL cholesterol–lower-ing drug classes and agents should be considered. Nicotinic acid and its derivatives lower LDL cholesterol levels by 5% to 25% but are likely to cause side effects such as flushing, hy-perglycemia, upper gastrointestinal distress, and hepatotoxici-ty. Studies investigating the effect of nicotinic acid in patients undergoing hemodialysis are sparse. Bile acid sequestrants lower LDL cholesterol levels by 15% to 30%. They cause gas-trointestinal distress and constipation when not taken with considerable amount of fluids. They are contraindicated in dysbe-talipoproteinemias, including triglyceride more than 180 mg per dL (2 mmol per L) and are likely to further increase plasma triglyc-erides. Therefore, nicotinic acid and bile acid sequestrants are not preferred treatments in patients undergoing hemodialysis. Sevelamer hydrochloride, a nonabsorbed hydrogel of cross-linked polyallylamine hydrochloride, is available as a phosphate binder. Short-term favorable effects on the lipid profile have been observed, with a 20% to 30% decrease in LDL cholesterol concentration, a 5% to 18% increase in HDL cholesterol concentration, and no change in triglyceride concentrations, presumably related to the binding of bile acids by the compound. Monitoring serum creatine kinase is mandatory only if muscle symptoms develop. Without a baseline serum value, creatine kinase values are not always conclusive in patients undergoing dialysis, so myopathy may be diagnosed clinically before laboratory assessment discovers it. The dosage of statins is usually the same as in the normal population.

Treatment for Hypertriglyceridemia and Low High-density Lipoprotein in Patients Receiving Hemodialysis and Peritoneal Dialysis Therapy

Patients with triglycerides more than 180 to 499 mg per dL (2.0 to 5.7 mmol per L) should be treated with a statin, after 3 months of TLC, to achieve a non-HDL cholesterol less than 130 mg per dL. Patients with very high triglyceride concentrations (greater than or equal to 500 mg per dL) should be treated with a fibric acid analogue, with dose adjustment according to renal function. In patients with triglyceride concentration more than 800 mg per dL (9 mmol per L), resistant to any intervention, consider administering fish oil, changing to low–molecular-weight heparin as anticoagulant during hemodialysis therapy, or both. In addition to encouraging optimized body weight, recommending abstinence from alcohol, and promoting increased physical activity, drug therapy should be initiated to achieve non-HDL cholesterol goals. The finding that elevated triglycerides are an independent cardiovascular risk factor in some studies suggests that some triglyceride-rich lipoproteins are atherogenic. These lipoproteins are partially degraded VLDL, commonly called *remnant lipoproteins*. VLDL cholesterol can be a target of cholesterol-lowering therapy. Adult treatment panel III identified the sum of LDL + VLDL cholesterol [termed non-HDL cholesterol, (total cholesterol–HDL cholesterol)] as a secondary target of therapy in patients with high triglyceride levels (180 to 499 mg per dL; 2.0 to 5.7 mmol per L). The goal for non-HDL cholesterol in patients with high triglyceride levels can be set at 30 mg per dL greater than that for LDL cholesterol, on the premise that a VLDL cholesterol level greater than or equal to 30 mg per dL is normal. Therefore, non-HDL goal should be less than 130 mg per dL (3.4 mmol per L). These target levels are more stringent and thus can have greater effect than the higher target levels suggested previously in patients receiving hemodialysis therapy. Non-HDL cholesterol has been demonstrated to remain one of the strongest predictors for intima media thickness in 897 patients receiving hemodialysis therapy, as demonstrated by multivariate Cox regression analysis. Non-HDL cholesterol has also turned out to predict aortic atherosclerosis, determined by pulse wave Doppler sonography, in a cohort of 205 patients receiving hemodialysis therapy. Therefore, non-HDL cholesterol is an independent factor affecting arterial wall thickening (intima media thickness) and stiffness (pulse wave velocity). Fibric acid analogues are effective in lowering serum triglycerides and raising HDL cholesterol levels. The most common adverse effects of drug therapy are myositis and rhabdomyolysis. These adverse effects can, however, be minimized by adjusting the dose of the drugs according to the degree of renal function. Gemfibrozil, a fibric acid analogue, is well tolerated, and the parent drug does not exhibit a tendency for accumulation and toxicity. Gemfibrozil has recently been shown to reduce cardiovascular mortality in the Veterans' Affairs High-Density Lipoprotein Intervention Trial (VA-HIT) study, a large-scale secondary prevention study, by reducing triglyceride levels and increasing HDL cholesterol without affecting LDL cholesterol levels. However, gemfibrozil is not available in all countries or, by regulation in these countries, is contraindicated in chronic renal insufficiency or if serum creatinine level is greater than 6 mg per dL, creatinine clearance is less than 15 mL per min, or if both conditions apply. Although ATP-III listed severe renal disease among the absolute contraindications for the use of fibric acids, the advice of this author, together with several other investigators, that gemfibrozil can safely be administered in a dose of 600 mg per day, is based on several reports from the literature. A pronounced lengthening of the plasma decay of fenofibric acid was observed in patients receiving both hemodialysis and peritoneal dialysis therapy. Fenofibrate should therefore be used, if at all, with great caution in patients treated with dialysis.

The ATP-III report does not specify a goal for increasing HDL levels but concedes that treatment of patients with isolated low HDL levels (less than 40 mg per dL; 1.0 mmol per L) is reserved for persons with coronary heart disease risk equivalents. Low HDL cholesterol level is a strong independent predictor of cardiovascular disease. Interesting data demonstrate that HDL, in an inflammatory milieu, can change to a proinflammatory molecule lacking effects that protect LDL from being oxidized. Similar findings were observed in patients receiving hemodialysis therapy. Apolipoprotein A-I, the major structural protein in HDL, exists in its free form in serum. Clearly, HDL composition and HDL antioxidant capacity is altered in patients receiving hemodialysis therapy. Although clinical trial results suggest that increasing HDL levels will reduce risk, the evidence is insufficient to specify a goal or therapy in the renal population. Therefore, the present working group felt that more research is needed on HDL and inflammation before recommendations for increasing HDL can be given.

Eicosapentanoic acid reduces plasma lipids and remnant lipoproteins and prevents *in vivo* peroxidation of LDL in patients receiving maintenance dialysis therapy. More importantly, *n*-3 fatty acids from fish oil do not introduce a clinically important risk for bleeding, although doubling of bleeding time is apparent. Adjuvant therapy using low–molecular-weight heparin for anticoagulation during hemodialysis or the use of polysulfone or polyamide high-flux dialysis has been shown to ameliorate hypertriglyceridemia in some but not all patients. Treating renal anemia with erythropoietin in patients receiving hemodialysis treatment lowered serum total cholesterol and triglyceride concentrations in one study but showed no effects in another one.

Combining a fibric acid analogue with a statin should be avoided, because of the high risk for rhabdomyolysis. Statins are effective and safe drugs to reduce LDL cholesterol levels and are the agents of first choice. Myositis can occur in rare cases, particularly when high dosages are used. In the 4D trial, 20 mg atorvastatin per day was administered in 1,255 patients with type 2 diabetes mellitus receiving hemodialysis therapy over a period of 4 years. There have been no major side effects reported in this cohort so far. Up to now no studies have been conducted on patients receiving hemodialysis therapy on the safety and efficacy of combination therapy.

Treating Patients After Kidney Transplantation

Statins have been proven to lower effectively serum total and LDL cholesterol concentrations in recipients of renal transplants. They are the drugs of choice in patients requiring lipid-lowering treatment. Cardiovascular complications are the most common causes of death among recipients of renal transplant, and chronic rejection is the most important cause of long-term allograft loss. Vascular lesions seen in chronic rejection and those that characterize systemic atherosclerosis share similarities. Although the Assessment of Lescol in Renal Transplantation (ALERT) trial was negative, and evidence from prospective controlled interventional studies is still lacking that statins prevent cardiovascular complications, it is reasonable to adopt the recommendations of the Joint European Societies on prevention of coronary heart disease or the National Cholesterol Education Program ATP-III guidelines. These guidelines can also be used for initial classification, risk factor assessment, treatment initiation, and to approach the target cholesterol level when drug therapy is considered.

Almost all patients receiving immunosuppressants after kidney transplantation exceed an absolute coronary artery disease risk of 20% over 10 years. They are considered to be in the highest risk group for developing a premature cardiovascular event with an even higher prevalence of lipid abnormalities. Although no event has taken place in most patients at the time of transplantation and shortly thereafter, so-called primary prevention is not routinely administered to patients. However, terms such as primary prevention are no more appropriate, because the cumulative incidence of coronary risk factors usually exceeds those that can be assessed by coronary risk charts. In addition, endothelial dependent vasodilation is impaired in nearly all patients; this finding justifies using the target cholesterol levels that are valid for patients treated for secondary prevention of cardiovascular disease. Guidelines suggest that in the presence of further risk factors for cardiovascular disease (endothelial dysfunction is already one) LDL cholesterol levels more than 100 mg per dL (2.7 mmol per L) are a treatment initiation threshold for drug therapy. In the absence of risk factors, an LDL cholesterol level up to 130 mg per dL may be acceptable.

Therefore, patients with a renal transplant are definitively considered as a high-risk population when lipid-lowering pharmacologic intervention is considered. When treatment options are evaluated with caution, most of the lipid-lowering drugs are safe and efficacious. Drug treatment is necessary in a considerable number of patients to control lipid disorders, because dyslipidemia in recipients of renal transplant is not particularly responsive to modification of dietary fat.

Cholesterol Reduction, Statins, and the Cytochrome P-450 System

Statins are the most effective drugs for reducing total and LDL cholesterol levels in recipients of transplants and should generally be the first choice among pharmacologic agents in patients requiring treatment for hypercholesterolemia. The hydrophilic statins, such as pravastatin and fluvastatin, should be distinguished from the lipophilic agents, lovastatin and simvastatin, with regard to toxicity and active metabolite accumulation. Furthermore, lovastatin, simvastatin, and the synthetic statin atorvastatin are metabolized by cytochrome P-450 3A4 (CYP3A4). Because myositis, rhabdomyolysis, or other complications can occur, maximal dosages of drugs in the latter group should be avoided, whereas pravastatin and fluvastatin have been administered at high dosages over prolonged periods without adverse effects. The ALERT study has randomized more than 2,000 patients after kidney transplantation to either fluvastatin or placebo. Recently fluvastatin, metabolized mainly via CYP2C9, was increased to 80 mg per day without adverse effects in patients who have not met target cholesterol levels. In respect to effects of statins on HDL cholesterol levels, no recommendation has been given yet.

However, drug–drug interactions are not necessarily always deleterious. Drugs with the potential to produce interactions mediated by CYP3A4 include the calcium channel blocker, diltiazem, which is used to save costs by cyclosporine immunosuppression. Some clinicians have argued that activation of this enzyme pathway (by a glass of grapefruit juice at breakfast, for example) will lead to further reductions in cholesterol and coronary heart disease. Such potential interactions should be kept in mind, and a careful approach is mandatory to avoid harmful side effects to the patients.

Use of Statins to Maintain Kidney Transplants

Two randomized controlled clinical trials have demonstrated that statins reduced the severity of angiographic coronary artery disease and improved patient survival following cardiac transplantation. The ALERT trial investigated the effects of fluvastatin on cardiac and renal endpoints in a multicenter, randomized, double-blind, placebo-controlled trial with 2,102 recipients of renal transplants. After a mean follow-up of 5.1 years, fluvastatin had lowered LDL cholesterol concentrations by 32%. Risk reduction with fluvastatin for the primary endpoint was not significant, although fewer cardiac deaths or nonfatal myocardial infarction occurred in the fluvastatin group than in the placebo group. Coronary intervention procedures and other secondary endpoints did not differ significantly between groups. If the pathogenesis of allograft vasculopathy in recipients of renal and cardiac transplants is similar, statins might hold promise for preventing and treating chronic renal allograft rejection as well. However, the mechanism whereby statins improve survival in recipients of heart transplants is still not entirely clear. Statins may have a direct, immunosuppressive effect. If so, the effect might require the presence of cyclosporine, because no evidence has demonstrated that statins are immuno-suppressive in healthy individuals. Alternatively, the reduction in lipids caused by statins might increase the immunosuppressive effect of cyclosporine. At present, the best therapeutic approach for chronic rejection might ultimately be a combination therapy of lipid lowering and appropriate immunosuppression.

Lipid Lowering with Fibrates After Kidney Transplantation

In the few patients in whom hypertriglyceridemia and low HDL cholesterol levels are the leading lipid abnormalities, fibric acid derivatives are appropriate. Combination therapy should not be administered in high doses of the various components.

Treating Patients with Elevated Lipoprotein(a) Levels

Other than hormonal therapies, such as adrenocorticotropin hormone (ACTH), D-thyroxine, and nandrolone, no effective treatments to reduce plasma Lp(a) in patients undergoing hemodialysis treatment or in the general population are currently available. Two small studies described a reduction in plasma Lp(a) with the use of nicotinic acid in patients undergoing hemodialysis treatment. Consequently, no large-scale interventional trials are available that investigate the effects of such treatments on cardiovascular disease in these patients. The use of anabolic steroids raises hematocrit but is also associated with the development of dyslipidemia. The overall effect on the cardiovascular system in subjects with normal kidney function is not beneficial, although plasma Lp(a) concentrations may be lowered. LDL apheresis is used for secondary prevention of coronary heart disease and might be considered in rare situations when primary or secondary hyperlipidemias fail to respond to maximal drug therapy. Because Lp(a) seems to have biologic consequences in patients with renal failure, and Lp(a) can effectively be removed, this therapy can be useful for selected patients with documented progressive vascular disease.

SELECTED READINGS

Attman PO, Samuelsson O, Alaupovic P. Lipoprotein metabolism and renal failure. *Am J Kidney Dis* 1993;21:573–592.

Baigent C, Burbury K, Wheeler D. Premature cardiovascular disease in chronic renal failure. *Lancet* 2000;356:147–152.

Cockcroft JR, Wilkinson IB. Cholesterol reduction, statins and the cytochrome P-450 system. *Eur Heart J* 2000;21:1555–1556.

Deighan CJ, Caslake MJ, McConnell M, et al. Atherogenic lipoprotein phenotype in end-stage renal failure: origin and extent of small dense low-density lipoprotein formation. *Am J Kidney Dis* 2000;35:852–862.

European Best Practice Guidelines for Haemodialysis (Part 1). Section VII. Vascular disease and risk factors. *Nephrol Dial Transplant* 2002;17(Suppl. 7):88–109.

Executive Summary of the Third Report of The National Cholesterol Education Program (NCEP). Expert panel on detection, evaluation, and treatment of high blood cholesterol in adults (adult treatment panel III). *JAMA* 2001;285:2486–2497.

Foley RN, Parfrey PS, Sarnak MJ. Clinical epidemiology of cardiovascular disease in chronic renal disease. *Am J Kidney Dis* 1998;32:S112–S119.

Fried LF, Orchard TJ, Kasiske BL. Effect of lipid reduction on the progression of renal disease: a meta-analysis. *Kidney Int* 2001;59: 260–269.

Holdaas H, Fellstrom B, Jardine AG, et al. Assessment of Lescol in Renal Transplantation (ALERT) study investigators: effect of fluvastatin on cardiac outcomes in renal transplant Assessment of Lescol in Renal Transplantation recipients: a multicentre, randomized, placebo-controlled trial. *Lancet* 2003;361:2024–2031.

Hulthe J, Bokemark L, Wikstrand J, et al. The metabolic syndrome, LDL particle size, and atherosclerosis: the Atherosclerosis and Insulin Resistance (AIR) study. *Arterioscler Thromb Vasc Biol* 2000;20:2140–2147.

Kalantar-Zadeh K, Block G, Humphreys MH, et al. Reverse epidemiology of cardiovascular risk factors in maintenance dialysis patients. *Kidney Int* 2003;63:793–808.

Kronenberg F, Steinmetz A, Kostner GM, et al. Lipoprotein(a) in health and disease. *Crit Rev Clin Lab Sci* 1996;33:495–543.

Liu Y, Coresh J, Eustace JA, et al. Association between cholesterol level and mortality in dialysis patients: role of inflammation and malnutrition. *JAMA* 2004;291:451–459.

Massy ZA, Chadefaux-Vekemans B, Chevalier A, et al. Hyperhomocysteinaemia; a significant risk factor for cardiovascular disease in renal transplant recipients. *Nephrol Dial Transplant* 1994;9(8):1103–1108.

Morena M, Cristol JP, Dantoine T, et al. Protective effects of highdensity lipoprotein against oxidative stress are impaired in haemodialysis patients. *Nephrol Dial Transplant* 2000;15:389–395.

National Kidney Foundation. K/DOQI clinical practice guidelines for managing dyslipidemias in chronic kidney disease. *Am J Kidney Dis* 2003;41(Suppl. 3):S1–S92.

National Heart, Lung, and Blood Institute (NHLBI). *Recommendations regarding public screening for measuring blood cholesterol*, NIH publication no. 95-3045. Bethesda, MD: National Institutes of Health, 1995.

Ordonez JD, Hiatt RA, Killebrew EJ, et al. The increased risk of caronary heart disease associated with nephrotic syndrome. *Kidney Int.* 1993;44(3);638–642.

Quaschning T, Krane V, Metzger T, et al. Abnormalities in uremic lipoprotein metabolism and its impact on cardiovascular disease. *Am J Kidney Dis* 2001;38(Suppl. 1):S14–S19.

Quaschning T, Schomig M, Keller M, et al. Non-insulin-dependent diabetes mellitus and hypertriglyceridemia impair lipoprotein metabolism in chronic hemodialysis patients. *J Am Soc Nephrol* 1999;10:S332–S341.

Shearer GC, Kaysen GA. Proteinuria and plasma compositional changes contribute to defective lipoprotein catabolism in the nephrotic syndrome by separate mechanisms. *Kidney Int* 2001;37(Suppl. 2):S119–S122.

Vathsala A, Weinberg RB, Schoenberg L, et al. Lipid abnormalities in cyclosporine-prednisone treated renal transplant recipients. *Transplantation* 1989;48(1);37–43.

Zimmermann J, Herrlinger S, Pruy A, et al. Inflammation enhances cardiovascular risk and mortality in hemodialysis patients. *Kidney Int* 1999;55:648–658.

5

Nutritional Support in Acute Renal Failure

Wilfred Druml

Adequate nutritional support is the prescription that will maintain protein stores, correct preexisting and disease-related deficits in lean body mass, and prevent "hospital-acquired" malnutrition. In patients with acute renal failure (ARF) mortality is tightly interrelated with nutritional or metabolic factors, including hypercatabolism and the induction of a proinflammatory and pro-oxidative environment. The objectives of nutritional therapy in a patient with ARF frequently exceed conventional levels of support and must be aimed at mitigating the inflammatory state, improving the oxygen-radical scavenging system, and bolstering endothelial functions. The objectives differ fundamentally from those for patients with chronic kidney disease (CKD) because diets or infusions that satisfy minimal requirements will not necessarily be sufficient for catabolic patients who have ARF.

In designing a nutritional program for patients with ARF, the metabolic consequences of functional kidney failure and the underlying disease process and associated complications must be considered. Profound alterations occur in nutrient balances that have been induced by modern replacement therapy, and these alterations must be accounted for as well. Nutritional support must, therefore, be viewed as a metabolic intervention that is coordinated with renal replacement therapy.

Patients with ARF are extremely prone to developing metabolic complications during nutritional support. The patient's tolerance to the administration of volume and electrolytes is impaired, and the metabolic processing of nutrients is altered. For these reasons, nutritional therapy for patients with ARF must be more closely monitored than it is in other disease states.

For many years, parenteral nutrition was the preferred nutritional support for patients with ARF. Recently, *enteral* nutrition has become the principal route of nutritional support for patients with ARF. Nevertheless, enteral and parenteral nutrition should not be viewed as opposed therapies but rather as complementary methods of nutritional support, because meeting requirements by the enteral route alone is often impossible, and supplementary parenteral nutrition becomes necessary.

METABOLIC ALTERATIONS CHANGE NUTRITIONAL REQUIREMENTS IN ACUTE RENAL FAILURE

The acute loss of excretory renal function in ARF not only affects water, electrolyte, and acid–base metabolism but also induces a global change in the "milieu interieur" that alters the metabolism of protein and amino acids, carbohydrates, and lipids, while exerting a proinflammatory reaction and suppressing the antioxidative system (see Table 5-1). Rarely is ARF an isolated disease process; instead, it often complicates sepsis, trauma, or multiple-organ failure so that metabolic responses are determined not only by ARF but also by the underlying disease process and complications, such as severe infections and organ dysfunction. The type and intensity of renal replacement therapy also determine metabolic response.

In summary, the optimal intake of nutrients in patients with ARF is influenced more by the nature of the illness causing ARF, the extent of catabolism, and the type and frequency of renal replacement therapy, rather than renal dysfunction *per se*. Patients with ARF present a heterogeneous group of subjects with widely differing nutrient requirements, and the nutritional requirements for an individual patient can vary during the course of disease.

Protein and Amino Acid Metabolism and their Requirements in Acute Renal Failure

The hallmark of metabolic alterations in ARF is the activation of protein catabolism, excessive release of amino acids from skeletal muscle, and sustained negative nitrogen balance. Amino acids are redistributed from muscle to the liver and extracted from the circulation to support increased hepatic gluconeogenesis and ureagenesis. Not only is protein breakdown accelerated, use of amino acids in the processes of protein synthesis is defective. In the liver, protein synthesis and secretion of acute phase proteins are stimulated.

Consequently, imbalances occur in the amino acid pools in plasma and in the intracellular fluid of muscle. In ARF, the clearance of most amino acids that support gluconeogenesis is enhanced.

The causes of hypercatabolism in ARF are complex and present a combination of nonspecific mechanisms induced by the acute disease process, the underlying illness and associated complications, the effects induced by the acute loss of renal function, and the type and intensity of renal replacement therapy (see Table 5-2). The dominating response is the stimulation of hepatic gluconeogenesis from amino acids. Hepatic glucose formation in ARF, unlike that in healthy subjects or patients with CKD, decreases but is not blocked when an excess of substrates is given.

A major stimulus of muscle protein catabolism in ARF is insulin resistance. This syndrome affects protein metabolism: the maximal rate of insulin-stimulated muscle protein synthesis is depressed, and protein degradation is increased, even in the presence of insulin.

Acidosis is another important factor that stimulates muscle protein breakdown. Metabolic acidosis activates the catabolism of protein and the oxidation of amino acids in muscle, independently of azotemia. In patients with CKD, increased muscle protein degradation can be eliminated and nitrogen balance can be improved by correcting the metabolic acidosis. Clinical experience shows that correcting acidosis also improves nitrogen balance in patients with ARF.

Additional catabolic factors operate ARF. The secretion of catabolic hormones (catecholamines, glucagon, and glucocorticoids), hyperparathyroidism, suppression of and decreased sensitivity to growth factors, and the release of proteases from

Table 5-1. Basic metabolic alterations in acute renal failure

	Main Finding	Underlying Mechanisms	Proposed Causes
Protein and amino acid metabolism	Hypercatabolism (loss of lean body mass)	activation of muscular protein catabolism depression of muscular protein synthesis augmentation of hepatic glucogneogenesis/ureagenesis/protein synthesis altered amino acid transport and metabolism decreased renal peptide catabolism	insulin resistance inflammatory mediators acidosis catabolic hormones growth factor resistance proteases substrate deficiencies loss of substrates (dialysis) increased ROS production
Carbohydrate metabolism	Hyperglycemia	peripheral insulin resistance (postreceptor defect) augmented hepatic gluconeogenesis	stress hormones cytokines (TNF) hyperparathyroidism acidosis
Lipid metabolism	Hypertriglyceridemia	inhibition of lipolysis increased hepatic triglyceride secretion?	accumulation of an inhibitor of lipoprotein—lipase, cytokines?

Table 5-2.   Protein catabolism in acute renal failure: contributing factors

Impairment of metabolic functions by uremic toxins
Endocrine factors
  Insulin resistance
  Increased secretion of catabolic hormones
    (catecholamines, glucagon, glucocorticoids)
  Hyperparathyroidism
  Suppression of release/resistance to growth factors
Acidosis
Acute phase reaction—systemic inflammatory response syndrome
    (activation of cytokine network)
Release of proteases
Inadequate supply of nutritional substrates
Renal replacement therapy
  Loss of nutritional substrates
  Activation of protein catabolism

activated leukocytes can separately (or together) stimulate protein breakdown. Release of inflammatory mediators in ARF, such as tumor necrosis factor-α (TNF-α) and interleukins, will also stimulate hypercatabolism.

Finally, the type and frequency of renal replacement therapy can affect protein balance. During hemodialysis, protein catabolism is accelerated, a process mediated in part by the loss of nutritional substrates and the activation of pathways that break down protein while inhibiting protein synthesis (see Chapter 7).

Last but not least, inadequate nutritional support contributes to the loss of lean body mass. In experimental animals, starvation aggravates the catabolic response to ARF, and clinically, indices that are compatible with a diagnosis of malnutrition have been identified as a major determinant of complications and mortality in patients with ARF.

Certain amino acids are synthesized or metabolized by the kidneys before being released into the circulation. Consequently, loss of renal function contributes to the altered amino acid pools in ARF. Several amino acids, such as arginine or tyrosine, which are conventionally termed *nonessential*, become "conditionally indispensable" in ARF because of their altered metabolism.

Potential Metabolic Interventions of Controlling Catabolism

Excessive mortality in ARF is tightly correlated with the extent of hypercatabolism. Unfortunately, no effective methods have been identified that will reduce or stop this catabolism. Hypercatabolism potentially could be modified by four types of metabolic interventions:

1. *Nutritional substrates*: Unfortunately, it is impossible to halt hypercatabolism and persisting hepatic gluconeogenesis in patients with ARF simply by providing conventional nutritional substrates; novel substrates (e.g., glutamine, leucine or its keto acid, or structured triglycerides) might exert a more pronounced anticatabolic response.

2. *Endocrine*: Experimentally, therapy with hormones [insulin, insulin-like growth factor-I (IGF-I), human growth hormone (rHGH)] or hormone antagonists (antiglucocorticoids) is at least partially effective. Available clinical results with IGF-I and rHGH (described later in this chapter) are rather disappointing, however.

3. *Mediators of inflammation*: ARF is an inflammatory state. Cytokines, such as interleukins and TNF-α, cause excessive release of amino acids from skeletal muscle and activate hepatic amino acid extraction and gluconegensis. Therapies to limit these processes are being experimentally evaluated but have not been tested clinically. Nutritional factors such as amino acids (glutamine, glycine, arginine), fatty acids, or antioxidants can modify the inflammatory response.

4. *Interventions to block catabolic pathways*: correction of acidosis is anticatabolic, because the ubiquitin–proteasome proteolytic system is blocked. Other experimental interventions that could directly inhibit catabolic pathways are under evaluation.

Amino Acid and Protein Requirements in Patients with Acute Renal Failure

Few studies have attempted to define the optimal requirements for protein or amino acids in ARF. In one study in patients who were nonhypercatabolic, a protein intake of 0.97 to 1.3 g/kg b.w./d during the polyuric phase of ARF achieved a positive nitrogen balance. However, measurement of nitrogen balance in patients experiencing rapid changes in accumulated nitrogen waste products is difficult and subject to considerable error.

In critically ill patients with ARF, who were treated with continuous renal replacement therapy (CRRT), the estimated protein catabolic rate was 1.4 to 1.75 g/kg b.w./d, with an inverse relation between protein and energy provision and protein catabolic rate. On the basis of this measurement, an amino acid/protein intake of about 1.5 g/kg b.w./d, but not exceeding 1.7 g/kg b.w./d, was recommended. However, a higher protein intake did not improve nitrogen balance. Although higher amino acid or protein intakes (e.g., 2.5 g/kg b.w./d) have been suggested, no proof exists that this intake is beneficial, and such excessive intakes increase the accumulation of unexcreted waste products. These accumulated products will aggravate uremic complications and increase the need for dialysis, which stimulates muscle protein degradation and increases nutrient losses. In short, hypercatabolism cannot be overcome by simply increasing protein or amino acid intake; even in patients with normal kidney function who have sepsis or burns, providing more than 1.5 g protein (or amino acids)/kg b.w./d does not improve catabolism.

Unless renal insufficiency is brief and no associated catabolic illness exists, we recommend that the intake of protein or amino acids should not be less than 0.8 g/kg b.w./d. Catabolic patients with ARF should receive approximately 1.2 g to 1.5 g protein (or amino acids)/kg b.w./d, which is in accordance with recommendations for critically ill patients. This recommendation will suffice even though amino acid and protein losses occur with hemodialysis, CRRT, or peritoneal dialysis.

Assessment of Protein Catabolism

In patients with renal insufficiency, urea is not excreted completely but accumulates in body fluids. Urea is distributed equally throughout total body water (about 60% of body weight), so changes in the urea pool can easily be calculated (see Table 5-3). Besides urea in urine, nitrogen losses in other body fluids, such as gastrointestinal or choledochal losses, must be added to the urinary nitrogen appearance (UNA). Excretion of nonurea nitrogen does not vary substantially with the diet and can be estimated at 0.031 g N/kg b.w./d (at nonedematous or ideal body weight). When this value is added to UNA, total waste nitrogen production can be estimated. If nitrogen intake from enteral or parenteral nutrition is known, nitrogen balance can be estimated using these principles.

Most of the nitrogen arising from amino acids liberated during protein degradation is converted to urea, so the degree of protein catabolism can be judged clinically by calculating the UNA rate. When UNA is multiplied by 6.25, it can be converted to protein equivalents. Because muscle contains approximately 20% of protein, multiplying the estimated protein loss by 5 can yield the approximate loss of muscle mass. Obviously, UNA is not a "true" rate of protein catabolism, because it does not take into account the high endogenous rate of protein turnover, 3 to 4 g protein/kg b.w./d in adults (see Chapter 7).

Energy Metabolism and Energy Requirements

In patients with uncomplicated ARF, oxygen consumption is similar to that in healthy subjects. However, in patients with sepsis or multiple-organ dysfunction syndrome plus ARF, oxygen consumption increases to 20% to 30% more than the calculated basic energy expenditure (BEE). In short, energy expenditure in patients with ARF is determined by the underlying disease, rather than by ARF.

Table 5-3.   Estimating the extent of protein catabolism

UNA (g/d) = Urinary urea nitrogen excretion
           + Change in urea nitrogen pool

$\quad = (UUN \times V) + (BUN_2 - BUN_1)\ 0.006 \times$ b.w.
$\qquad + ($b.w.$_2 -$ b.w.$_1) \times BUN_2/100$

If there are substantial GI losses, add urea nitrogen in secretions:
$\quad =$ Volume of secretions $\times BUN_2$

Net protein breakdown (g/d) = UNA $\times$ 6.25
Muscle loss (g/d) = UNA $\times$ 6.25 $\times$ 5

UNA, urea nitrogen appearance; UUN, urinary urea nitrogen concentration; V, urinary volume.
BUN_1 and BUN_2, are BUN in mg per dL on days 1 and 2; .b.w.$_1$ and b.w.$_2$, body weights in kg on days 1 and 2.

Previously, energy requirements for patients with ARF were grossly overestimated, and intakes of more than 50 kcal/kg b.w./d (i.e., approximately 100% more than BEE) were advocated. Adverse effects of exaggerated nutrient intakes are now recognized, and energy supply should not exceed actual energy requirements; complications from slightly "underfeeding" calories are less deleterious than those caused by overfeeding calories.

A direct measurement of the energy requirement of an individual patient is usually not available, but energy requirements can be calculated using a standard formula. The calculation includes the BEE from the Benedict–Harrison equation multiplied by a "stress factor" (the traditional 1.3 multiplication factor should be ignored). On an average, patients with ARF should receive 20 to 30 kcal/kg b.w./d; even in hypermetabolic conditions (sepsis or multiple-organ failure), energy expenditure is rarely higher than 130% of calculated BEE, so energy intake should not exceed 30 kcal/kg b.w./d.

Carbohydrate Metabolism

Frequently, ARF is associated with hyperglycemia because of insulin resistance. A diagnosis of insulin resistance is based on a high plasma insulin concentration, a 50% decrease in the maximal insulin-stimulated glucose uptake by skeletal muscle, and impaired glycogen synthesis in muscle. Abnormalities in glucose metabolism caused by ARF include accelerated hepatic gluconeogenesis, mainly from conversion of amino acids released during protein catabolism to glucose. Hepatic gluconeogenesis in patients with ARF, unlike that in patients with CKD or normal adults, cannot be suppressed by exogenous glucose infusion. In addition, endogenous insulin secretion is low in the basal state and during glucose infusion. Because the kidney is the main organ of insulin disposal, insulin degradation is decreased in ARF. Surprisingly, insulin catabolism in the liver is also consistently reduced in ARF.

Lipid Metabolism

Profound alterations of lipid metabolism occur in patients with ARF. The triglyceride content of plasma lipoproteins, especially very low-density lipoproteins (VLDL) and low-density lipoproteins (LDL) is increased, whereas total cholesterol, HDL-cholesterol in particular, is decreased. The major cause of lipid abnormalities in ARF is impaired lipolysis; activities of the lipolytic systems, peripheral lipoprotein lipase, and hepatic triglyceride lipase are decreased to less than 50% of normal. Metabolic acidosis can contribute to the impairment of lipolysis in ARF by inhibiting lipoprotein lipase.

Artificial lipid emulsions in parenteral nutritional solutions are degraded similar to endogenous VLDL. The nutritional consequence of the impaired lipolysis in ARF is a delay in eliminating intravenously infused lipid emulsions: the elimination half-life is doubled, and the clearance of fat emulsions is reduced by more than 50%.

Metabolism and Requirements of Micronutrients

Because of the vitamin losses that occur with renal replacement therapy, serum levels of water-soluble vitamins are low in patients with ARF, and such patients require more of these vitamins. An exception is ascorbic acid (vitamin C), a precursor of oxalic acid. Vitamin C intake should be less than 250 mg per day, to avoid secondary oxalosis and oxalate precipitates in soft tissues.

As in patients with CKD, vitamin D activation and plasma levels of 25(OH) vitamin D_3 and 1, 25-(OH) vitamin D_3 are severely depressed in patients with ARF, despite reduced rates of calcitriol degradation. Serum concentrations of vitamin A and vitamin E, unlike those in patients with CKD, are decreased in patients with ARF. Serum vitamin K levels are normal or even elevated in these patients (see Fig. 5-1). Even though fat-soluble vitamins are not lost during hemodialysis, requirements for these vitamins, with the exception of vitamin K, are increased by ARF. Most commercially available multivitamin preparations for parenteral infusions contain the recommended daily allowances (RDA) of vitamins and can be safely given to patients with ARF.

Reports about trace element metabolism in ARF include low plasma levels of iron and zinc or increased levels of copper; these findings represent "acute phase reaction" responses. Nevertheless, selenium concentrations in plasma and erythrocytes are decreased in patients with ARF. In critically ill patients, selenium replacement reduces the incidence of ARF and improves the clinical outcome. Parenteral administration of trace elements to patients with ARF should be undertaken with care, however, because

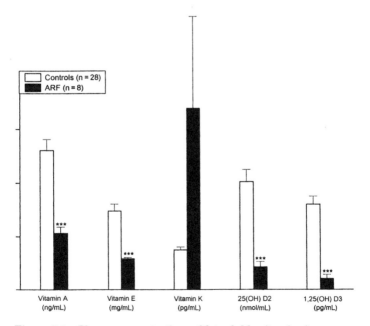

Figure 5-1.   Plasma concentrations of fat-soluble vitamins in healthy subjects and patients with acute renal failure (ARF) (***p <0.001). (Adapted from Druml W, Schwarzenhofer M, Apsner R, et al. Fat soluble vitamins in acute renal failure. *Miner Electrolyte Metab* 1998;24:220–226, with permission.)

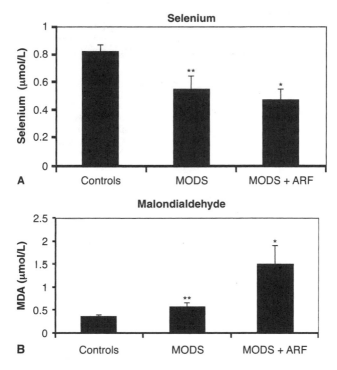

Figure 5-2. a + 2 b: Serum selenium (A) and malondialdehyde (B) concentration in healthy subjects, in patients with multiple-organ dysfunction syndrome (MODS) without acute renal failure (ARF), and with MODS and acute renal failure (MODS + ARF) (*p <0.05, **p <0.001). (From Metnitz PGH, Fischer M, Bartnes S, et al. Impact of acute renal failure on antioxidant status in patients with multiple-organ failure. *Acta Anaesthesiol Scand* 2000;44:236–240, with permission.)

gastrointestinal absorption, the main regulator of trace elements homeostasis, is bypassed, and renal excretion is impaired. The combination of these factors raises the risk of toxicity.

Micronutrients are part of the patient's defense against oxygen free radical–induced injury to cellular components. A profound depression in antioxidant status occurs in patients with ARF (see Fig. 5-2).

METABOLIC IMPACT OF EXTRACORPOREAL THERAPY

Hemodialysis therapy affects metabolism in many ways. Protein catabolism is stimulated not only by substrate losses but also by activation of protein breakdown mediated in part by release of leukocyte-derived proteases and inflammatory mediators following blood–membrane interactions, endotoxin release, or both. These responses persist for several hours after treatment. Dialysis may also inhibit muscle protein synthesis. In addition, water soluble substances, such as amino acids and vitamins, are lost during hemodialysis, and the generation of reactive oxygen species is

Table 5-4. Metabolic effects of
continuous renal replacement therapy (CRRT)

Amelioration of uremic intoxication ("renal replacement") plus

1. Heat loss
2. Excessive load of substrates (lactate, glucose, etc.)
3. Loss of nutrients (amino acids, 2 citrate, vitamins, etc.)
4. Loss of electrolytes (phosphate, magnesium)
5. Elimination of short-chain proteins (hormones, mediators?)
6. Metabolic consequences of bioincompatiblity (induction/activation of mediator-cascades, stimulation of protein catabolism?)

augmented. All of these factors can stimulate protein breakdown in muscle and other tissues.

Recently, CRRT including continuous (arteriovenous or venovenous) hemofiltration and continuous hemodialysis, have been used for patients with ARF, especially the critically ill patients. Relevant metabolic consequences of CRRT result from prolonged therapy and the high fluid turnover (see Table 5-4). One major effect of CRRT is that small- and medium-sized molecules are eliminated; for amino acids, the sieving coefficient is within the range of 0.8 to 1.0. The loss of amino acids can be estimated from the volume of the filtrate and the average plasma concentrations; usually the total loss is 5 to 15 g amino acid per day, which represents about 10% to 15% of amino acid intake. Amino acid losses during continuous hemofiltration and continuous hemodialysis are of a comparable magnitude. Water-soluble vitamins such as folic acid, vitamin B_1, vitamin B_6, and vitamin C are also eliminated during CRRT, so intake of these vitamins should be increased above the RDA to maintain plasma concentrations.

The high molecular size cut-off of the membranes used for hemofiltration means that small proteins and peptide hormones (insulin, catecholamines, and potentially cytokines and mediators) are removed. Because these elements have short half-lives, hormone losses are small and probably not of pathophysiologic importance. Depending on the type of therapy and the membrane material used, however, total protein losses can vary between 5 g and 10 g per day.

Glucose balance during CRRT depends on the glucose concentration of the substitution fluid. Peritoneal dialysis solutions should not be used for CRRT, because they lead to excessive glucose uptake. Dialysate glucose concentrations should range between 1 g to 2 g per dL in order to maintain a zero glucose balance.

Lactate is the organic base for most substitution fluids, and during CRRT, lactate uptake is substantial and close to values of endogenous lactate turnover. When lactate formation is increased (cardiogenic shock), or if lactate clearance is impaired (liver insufficiency), bicarbonate-based dialysates should be used to prevent lactate accumulation. Citrate metabolism is usually unimpaired in critically ill patients with ARF, but it is reduced in patients with liver failure.

IMPACT OF NUTRITIONAL AND ENDOCRINE INTERVENTIONS ON RENAL REGENERATION IN ACUTE RENAL FAILURE

Starvation accelerates protein breakdown and impairs protein synthesis in the kidney, whereas refeeding exerts opposite effects. In experimental animals, nutritional strategies accelerate tissue repair and recovery of renal function. In patients with ARF, however, this process has been much more difficult to prove, and only one study has reported a positive effect of parenteral nutrition on the resolution of ARF.

Amino acids (infused either before or during ischemia, or when nephrotoxicity occurs) can actually exacerbate tubular damage and accelerate the loss of renal function in rat models of ARF. This "therapeutic paradox" is related in part to the increase in metabolic work that is linked to kidney transport processes that are activated even though oxygen supply is limited. The result is aggravated ischemic injury. Similar observations can be made when excess glucose is infused during renal ischemia; however, in humans, continuous infusion of amino acids does not increase renal oxygen consumption. Infusing an amino acid solution designed to correct metabolic alterations of ARF will raise plasma amino acids levels marginally and eliminate the peaks in amino acid concentrations, possibly limiting the probability of developing untoward side effects, but this effect is not proved. During the insult phase of ARF, known as the "ebb phase," which occurs immediately after trauma, shock, major operations, and so on, excessive nutritional intake or support should be avoided, as described elsewhere in this chapter.

Certain amino acids may exert kidney protection. Glycine and, to a lesser degree, alanine and taurine, can limit tubular injury in ischemic, nephrotoxic, or both models of ARF. Arginine reportedly acts (possibly by producing nitric oxide) to preserve renal perfusion and tubular function during both nephrotoxic and ischemic injury, whereas inhibitors of nitric oxide synthase exert an opposite effect.

Parenterally infused amino acids and an enteral supply of amino acids or protein increase both renal perfusion and excretory renal function ("renal functional reserve"). Intravenous infusion of amino acids can improve renal plasma flow (approximately 25%) and glomerular filtration rate (GFR) in cirrhotic patients who have functional renal failure. Whether this effect can be used to improve renal function in patients with ARF remains unknown, but preliminary data suggest that amino acid infusions can help increase GFR and reduce the requirements for diuretics in patients with ARF. In animal experiments, enteral nutrition improves renal perfusion and function and increases survival.

In experimental models of ARF, various endocrine-metabolic interventions [e.g., thyroxine, rHGH, epidermal growth factor (EGF), IGF-1, hepatocyte growth factor (HGF)] have been shown to accelerate tubular regeneration. In clinical studies, however, these beneficial effects have not been confirmed. A multicenter study, in which IGF-I was administered to patients with ARF, was terminated early because of the lack of benefit. Administering rHGH actually increased the mortality of critically ill patients, many of whom had ARF. Administering triiodothyronine, which could potentially upregulate the EGF receptor expression, was not only ineffective in patients with ARF but also increased mortality. To date, rHGF has not been sufficiently evaluated in humans to recommend its use.

NUTRIENT ADMINISTRATION

Patient Selection

Ideally, a nutritional program should be designed for each patient with ARF. In clinical practice, however, it has proved useful to distinguish three groups of patients with ARF, on the basis of the extent of protein catabolism, leading to a suggested level of dietary requirements (see Table 5-5).

1. *Group I* includes patients without excess catabolism and a UNA of less than 6 g of nitrogen above the nitrogen intake. ARF in these patients is usually caused by nephrotoxins (aminoglycosides, contrast media). Such patients rarely present major nutritional problems and, in most cases, they can be fed orally; their prognosis is excellent.

2. *Group II* consists of patients with moderate hypercatabolism and a UNA exceeding nitrogen intake by 6 to 12 g nitrogen per day. These patients frequently suffer from complicating infections, peritonitis, or moderate injury in association with ARF. Tube feeding, intravenous nutritional support, or both are generally required, and dialysis or CRRT often becomes necessary to limit waste product accumulation.

3. *Group III* includes patients in whom ARF is associated with severe trauma, burns, or overwhelming infections in the context of multiple-organ failure syndrome. UNA is markedly elevated (more than 12 g of nitrogen above nitrogen intake). Treatment strategies are usually complex and include enteral nutrition, parenteral nutrition, or both; hemodialysis; or CRRT plus blood pressure and ventilatory support. Mortality in this group of patients exceeds 60% to 80%. The severity of the underlying illness, together with the untoward systemic consequences of ARF, accounts for the poor prognosis.

Oral Feeding

Oral feeding should be used in all patients who can tolerate it [usually, this category is restricted to patients who are non-hypercatabolic (group I)]. Energy is provided by simple carbohydrates (sugar, jellies, and other sweets) or glucose polymers, given at regular intervals. Initially, 40 g per day of high-quality protein is given (0.6 g/kg b.w./d), and protein intake is gradually increased to 0.8 g/kg b.w./d as long as the blood urea nitrogen (BUN) remains below 80 mg per dL. For patients treated with hemodialysis, protein intake should be increased to 1.0 to 1.2 g/kg b.w./d to make up for amino acids lost during dialysis and for the potential catabolic effects of the dialytic process. For patients undergoing peritoneal dialysis, protein intake should be raised to 1.4 g/kg b.w./d to counteract losses of both amino acids and protein. A supplement of water-soluble vitamins is recommended.

Enteral Nutrition (Tube Feeding)

During the last decade, enteral nutrition has become the standard method of providing nutritional support for critically

Table 5-5. Patient classification and nutrient requirements in patients with acute renal failure (ARF)

	Extent of Catabolism		
	Mild	Moderate	Severe
Excess urea appearance (above N intake)	>5 g	5–10 g	>10 g
Clinical setting (examples)	Drug toxicity	Elective surgery +/– infection	Severe injury or sepsis
Mortality	20%	60%	>80%
Dialysis/hemofiltration frequency	Rare	As needed	Frequent
Route of nutrient administration	Oral	Enteral and/or parenteral	Enteral and/or parenteral
Energy recommendations (kcal/kg b.w./d)	25	20–30	25–35
Energy substrates	Glucose	Glucose + fat	Glucose + fat
Glucose (g/kg b.w./d)	3.0–5.0	3.0–5.0	3.0–5.0
Fat (g/kg b.w./d)		0.5–1.0	0.8–1.2
Amino acids/protein (g/kg/d)	0.6–1.0 EAA(+ NEAA)	0.8–1.2 EAA + NEAA	1.2–1.5 EAA + NEAA
Nutrients used (oral/enteral/parenteral)	Food EAA + specific NEAA (general or "nephro" solutions) multivitamin and multitrace element preparations	Enteral formulas glucose 50%–70% + fat emulsions 10% or 20% EAA + specific NEAA (general or "nephro" solutions) multivitamin and multitrace element preparations	Enteral formulas glucose 50%–70% + fat emulsions 10% or 20% EAA + specific NEAA (general or "nephro" solutions) multivitamin and multitrace element preparations

EAA, essential amino acids; NEAA, nonessential amino acids.

ill patients, including those with ARF. Among the well-documented advantages of enteral nutrition, the most important is that even small amounts of luminal nutrients will maintain gastrointestinal functions and will support the barrier function of the intestinal mucosa. Enteral nutrition helps to preserve the structural integrity of the mucosal layer and prevent the development of mucosal ulcerations that lead to translocation of bacteria and systemic infections. In experimental ARF, enteral nutrition augments renal plasma flow and can improve renal function. Moreover, in two clinical studies, enteral nutrition was a factor associated with an improved prognosis in patients with ARF.

Unfortunately, few systematic studies of enteral nutrition have been conducted in patients with ARF. In the largest study to date, the feasibility and tolerance of enteral nutrition, using either a conventional diet or a preparation adapted to the metabolic needs of patients undergoing hemodialysis, was examined in 182 patients with ARF. Side effects of enteral feeding were more common in patients with ARF than in those with normal renal function but, in general, enteral nutrition was safe and effective in both groups.

In critically ill patients with ARF, providing adequate amounts of nutrients exclusively by the enteral route is frequently impossible, and supplementary or even total parenteral nutrition becomes necessary. However, enteral and parenteral nutrition should be viewed as complementary types of nutritional support, because even small amounts of enteral diets given regularly (i.e., 50 to 100 mL of polymeric diets given six times each day) can help maintain intestinal functions.

Enteral Formulas

Three types of enteral formulas have been used to treat patients with ARF, but none of these formulas was specifically developed to counteract metabolic and nutritional abnormalities (see Table 5-6).

1. *Elemental powder diets:* The concept of a low-protein diet supplemented with essential amino acids (EAA) in the oral nutrition of patients with CKD was extended to enteral nutrition in patients with ARF. Some of these diets contain the eighth EAA only and histidine, and thus, must be supplemented with energy substrates, vitamins, and trace elements.

Table 5-6.   Enteral diets for patients with acute renal failure (ARF)

1. Elemental powder diets
     designed as low-protein diets for patients with CKD
2. Standard polymeric diets designed for patients who are nonuremic
     including "immunonutrition"
     caution: high electrolyte concentrations
3. Specific polymeric ready-to-use diets
     a. adapted for predialysis patients (reduced protein and electrolyte content)
     b. adapted for patients undergoing dialysis (moderate protein content, low electrolyte concentrations, variable additions such as histidine, carnitine)

Major disadvantages are the limited spectrum of nutrients and the high osmolality of the nutrient solution, with its potential problems. These formulations should be replaced by "ready-to-use" liquid products.

2. *(Polymeric) Enteral formulas designed for patients who are nonuremic*: Many critically ill patients with ARF receive standard enteral formulas. Disadvantages with these diets are the amount and type of protein and the high content of electrolytes (e.g., potassium and phosphate). Whether diets enriched in specific substrates such as glutamine, arginine, nucleotides, or ω-3-fatty acids ("immunonutrition") might exert beneficial effects in patients with ARF is not known.

3. *Specific enteral polymeric liquid formulas adapted to correct metabolic alterations of uremia*: One of these relatively new, ready-to-use liquid diets was designed for patients with compensated CKD. These diets consist of a reduced protein and electrolyte content. A second type of preparation was created to meet the nutrient requirements of patients undergoing hemodialysis: Such preparations contain a higher protein and a reduced electrolyte content, plus a high specific energy content of 1.5 to 2.0 kcal per mL. This category of formulas represents the most reasonable approach to enteral nutrition of hypercatabolic patients with ARF in intensive care.

Parenteral Nutrition

If nutrient requirements cannot be met by the enteral route, or if the enteral route cannot be used, supplementary or total parenteral nutrition should be used. Fluids are restricted in patients with ARF; so parenteral nutritional solutions are hyperosmolar and, therefore, must be infused through central venous catheters to avoid peripheral vein damage.

Components of Parenteral Nutrition

CARBOHYDRATES. Glucose should be used as the major energy substrate, because it is metabolized by all organs, even under hypoxic conditions. Glucose intake must be restricted to less than 3 to 5 g/kg b.w./d, because higher intakes are not metabolized but promote hyperglycemia and lipogenesis (including fatty infiltration of the liver and excessive carbon dioxide production). Impaired glucose tolerance in ARF frequently requires insulin. But, because of the well-known side effects of even short-term hyperglycemia, blood glucose levels must be maintained within the physiologic range to reduce complications and improve survival.

Because of the dangers of a high glucose intake, a portion of the energy requirement should be supplied with lipid emulsions. The most suitable means of providing the energy requirements in critically ill patients is not glucose *or* lipids but glucose *and* lipids. Other carbohydrates, including fructose, sorbitol, or xylitol, which are available in some countries, should be avoided because of potential adverse metabolic effects.

FAT EMULSIONS. Advantages of intravenous lipids include their high specific energy content, a low osmolality, provision of essential fatty acids to prevent deficiency syndromes, a lower rate of hepatic lipid accumulation, a lower risk of inducing hyperglycemia, and reduced carbon dioxide production (especially relevant in patients with respiratory failure). Lipids become structural components of cell membranes and are precursors of regulatory molecules, such as hormones, prostanoids, and leukotrienes. Moreover, because oxidation of fatty acids covers a large portion of the energy metabolism of critically ill patients, lipids are directly used and present an ideal energy substrate.

Because of ARF-induced changes in lipid metabolism, the amount infused should be adjusted to meet the patient's capacity to use lipids. Usually, 1 g fat/kg b.w./d does not increase plasma triglycerides, and approximately 20% to 30% of energy requirements can be met.

Parenteral lipid emulsions usually contain long-chain triglycerides that are mostly derived from soybean oil, but fat emulsions containing a mixture of long- and medium-chain triglycerides derived from olive oil or fish oil are available. Whether a lower content of polyunsaturated fatty acids will yield the proposed advantages and reduce proinflammatory side effects is unknown. Administering medium-chain triglycerides, however, does not increase their use, because ARF retards the elimination of both types of fat emulsions equally.

Lipids should not be given to patients with hyperlipidemia (plasma triglycerides >350 mg/dL), with activated intravascular coagulation, with acidosis (pH <7.20), or with impaired circulation or hypoxemia.

AMINO ACID SOLUTIONS. Three types of amino acid solutions have been used for parenteral nutrition in patients with ARF: (a) EAA alone; (b) EAA plus nonessential amino acids (NEAA); or (c) specifically designed "nephro" solutions of different proportions of EAA plus specific NEAA that might become "conditionally essential," and hence required, for patients with ARF (see Table 5-7).

The use of solutions of EAA alone was based on principles established for treating patients with CKD using a low-protein diet plus an EAA supplement. These solutions should no longer be used, because they are incomplete and do not contain several amino acids that become conditionally essential in patients with uremia (e.g., histidine, arginine, tyrosine, serine, and cysteine). Absence of these amino acids creates imbalances, resulting in serious derangements of plasma amino acid concentrations.

Solutions including both EAA and NEAA in standard proportions or in special proportions designed to counteract the metabolic changes of renal failure ("nephro" solutions) should be used in nutritional support for patients with ARF. Tyrosine has low

Table 5-7.   Amino acid solutions used for the treatment of acute renal failure (ARF)

1. Solutions of essential amino acids only
   (should no longer be used)
2. Standard amino acid solutions
   (designed for patients with normal renal function)
3. Solutions adapted to specific metabolic situation of renal failure
   [including conditionally indispensable amino acids (arinine, histidine, tyrosine)]

water solubility, so dipeptides containing tyrosine (such as gly-cyltyrosine) are used in modern "nephro" solutions. The amino acid analogue N-acetyl tyrosine, which was used frequently as tyrosine source, cannot be converted to tyrosine in humans and should not be given.

As for other amino acid solutions, a parenteral supplement of branched-chain amino acids (BCAA) given to patients with ARF failed to exert any benefits. In a study comparing a BCAA-enriched amino acid solution and a standard amino acid solution in critically ill patients with ARF treated with CRRT, no improvement using BCAA was seen in nitrogen balance or plasma protein concentrations.

Recently, it was suggested that glutamine, an amino acid that is traditionally termed as nonessential, exerts important metabolic functions to improve nitrogen metabolism, support immunocompetence, and preserve gastrointestinal barrier function and potentially also renal function. These potential benefits would make glutamine conditionally indispensable in a catabolic illness. In a study of critically ill patients, a standard parenteral nutrition was compared to a nutrition solution enriched with glutamine; long-term survival was improved in patients who received glutamine. In a *post hoc* analysis, the improvement in prognosis was most pronounced in patients with ARF (4/24 survivors without glutamine, 14/23 with glutamine, $p < 0.02$). Because free glutamine is not stable in aqueous solutions, glutamine-containing dipeptides are administered in parenteral nutritional solutions.

ELECTROLYTES. Electrolytes should be added to the nutrition solution as required. Glucose infusion with or without insulin, amino acids, or both causes a shift of potassium and phosphate into the cells, increasing the risk of developing of hypokalemia, hypophosphatemia ("refeeding syndrome"), or both. If phosphate or calcium is added to "all-in-one" solutions containing lipid emulsions, organic salts such as glycerophosphate, glucose-1-phosphate, and calcium gluconate must be used to avoid incompatibilities with other ions and impaired stability of the fat emulsion.

Parenteral Solutions

Standard solutions with amino acids, glucose, and fat emulsions contained in a single bag are commercially available. Because required vitamins, trace elements, and electrolytes can be added to these solutions, they are known as total nutritional admixtures or "all-in-one" solutions (see Table 5-8). The stability of fat emulsions in such mixtures may not persist in the long term and should be tested. If the patient has hyperglycemia, insulin should be added to the solution or administered separately.

To ensure maximal nutrient use and to avoid metabolic derangements, the parenteral nutrition infusion should be started at a low rate (providing about 50% of requirements) and gradually increased over several days. Optimally, the solution should be infused continuously over 24 hours to avoid marked changes in substrate concentrations.

COMPLICATIONS AND MONITORING OF NUTRITIONAL SUPPORT

Technical problems and infectious complications that originate from the central venous catheter or the enteral feeding tube, as

Table 5-8.   "Renal failure fluid"—"all-in-one solution"

Component	Quantity	Remarks
Glucose 40%–70%	500 mL	In the presence of severe insulin resistance switch to D30W
Fat emulsion 10%–20%	500 mL	Start with 10%, switch to 20% if TG are <350 mg/dL
Amino acids 6.5%–10%	500 mL	General or special "nephro" amino acid solutions including EAA and NEAA
Water-soluble vitamins[a]	2 × RDA	Limit vitamin C intake <250 mg/d
Fat-soluble vitamins[a]	RDA	
Trace elements[a]	RDA	Caution: toxic effects
Electrolytes	As required	Caution: hypophosphatemia or hypokalemia after initiation of TPN
Insulin	As required	Added directly to the solution or given separately

EAA, essential amino acids; NEAA, nonessential amino acids.
"All-in-one solution" with all components contained in a single bag.
Infusion rate initially 50% of requirements, to be increased over a period of 3 days to satisfy requirements.
[a] Combination products containing the recommended daily allowances (RDA).

Table 5-9.   A minimal suggested
schedule for monitoring of nutritional support

	Patient Metabolically	
Variables	Unstable	Stable
Blood glucose, potassium	1–6 × daily	Daily
Osmolality	Daily	1 × weekly
Electrolytes (sodium, chloride)	Daily	3 × weekly
Calcium, phosphate, magnesium	Daily	3 × weekly
BUN/BUN rise/d	Daily	Daily
UNA	Daily	1 × weekly
Triglycerides	Daily	2 × weekly
Blood gas analysis/pH	Daily	1 × weekly
Ammonia	2 × weekly	1 × weekly
Transaminases + bilirubin	2 × weekly	1 × weekly

well as the metabolic complications of artificial nutrition and gastrointestinal side effects of enteral nutrition, are similar in patients with ARF to those in subjects who are nonuremic. Metabolic complications frequently occur in patients with ARF, because nutrient use is impaired and because of intolerance to administering excessive volumes of nutrients and electrolytes. Moreover, an exaggerated protein or amino acid intake results in a high BUN (and waste product) level. Glucose intolerance and decreased fat clearance can cause hyperglycemia and hypertriglyceridemia, respectively. One reason for gradually increasing the infusion rate is to avoid many side effects associated with nutritional support.

Because of the high prevalence of metabolic complications, nutritional therapy in ARF requires a tighter schedule of monitoring than in other patient groups. Table 5-9 summarizes laboratory tests used to monitor nutritional support to avoid developing metabolic complications. The frequency of testing will depend on the metabolic stability of the patient, but levels of plasma glucose, potassium, and phosphate should be monitored repeatedly after initiating nutritional therapy.

CONCLUSIONS

In patients with ARF, the impairment of renal function per se does not determine the decision to initiate nutritional support; the patient's nutritional status, the type and severity of underlying disease, and the degree of associated hypercatabolism determines this decision. For any patient with ARF who needs nutritional support, the regimen must address the complex metabolic sequels of impaired renal function, of the underlying disease process, and of renal replacement therapies.

Enteral nutrition has become the preferred type of nutrition in patients with ARF. Even small amounts of a diet entering the intestines can support gastrointestinal functions. Moreover, enteral nutrition might exert specific beneficial effects on renal function and recovery. Unfortunately, reduced morbidity and mortality as a consequence of nutritional support has not been convincingly demonstrated in patients with ARF.

The poor prognosis is related not only to the severity of the underlying illness but also to profound effects exerted by ARF per se on various metabolic functions and organ systems. Nutritional therapy, like renal replacement therapy, should be viewed as a means of supporting the patient until the underlying illness is controlled.

Future advances in nutritional therapy must leave a merely quantitatively oriented approach that meets nitrogen and energy requirements and move toward a more qualitative type of metabolic support, integrating interventions aimed at modulating the inflammatory state, the oxygen radical scavenger system, and immunocompetence and taking advantage of specific pharmacologic effects of various nutrients. Reducing the distressingly high mortality of patients with ARF will largely depend on further improvements in metabolic care.

SELECTED READINGS

Chima CS, Meyer L, Hummell AC, et al. Protein catabolic rate in patients with acute renal failure on continuous arteriovenous hemofiltration and total parenteral nutrition. *J Am Soc Nephrol* 1993;3:1516–1521.

Cianciaruso B, Bellizzi V, Napoli R, et al. Hepatic uptake and release of glucose, lactate and amino acids in acutely uremic dogs. *Metabolism* 1991;40:261–290.

Druml W. Protein metabolism in acute renal failure. *Miner Elect Metab* 1998;24:47–54.

Druml W. Metabolic aspects of continuous renal replacement therapies. *Kidney Int* 1999;56(Suppl. 72):S56–S61.

Druml W, Fischer M, Liebisch B, et al. Elimination of amino acids in renal failure. *Am J Clin Nutr* 1994;60:418–423.

Druml W, Fischer M, Sertl S, et al. Fat elimination in acute renal failure: long chain versus medium chain triglycerides. *Am J Clin Nutr* 1992;55:468–472.

Druml W, Mitch WE. Metabolic abnormalities in acute renal failure. *Semin Dial* 1996;9:484–490.

Druml W, Mitch WE. Enteral nutrition in renal disease. In: Rolandelli RH, ed. *Enteral and tube feeding*. Philadelphia: WB Saunders, 2004.

Druml W, Schwarzenhofer M, Apsner R, et al. Fat soluble vitamins in acute renal failure. *Miner Electrolyte Metab* 1998;24:220–226.

Fiaccadori E, Lombardi M, Leonardi S, et al. Prevalence and clinical outcome of malnutrition in acute renal failure. *J Am Soc Nephrol* 1999;10:581–593.

Fiaccadori E, Maggiore U, Giacosa R, et al. Enteral nutrition in patients with acute renal failure. *Kidney Int* 2004;65(3):999–1008.

May RC, Clark AS, Goheer MA, et al. Specific defects in insulin-mediated muscle metabolism in acute uremia. *Kidney Int* 1985;28:490–497.

Metnitz PGH, Fischer M, Bartnes S, et al. Impact of acute renal failure on antioxidant status in patients with multiple organ failure. *Acta Anaesthesiol Scand* 2000;44:236–240.

Metnitz PG, Krenn CG, Steltzer H, et al. Effect of acute renal failure requiring renal replacement therapy on outcome in critically ill patients. *Crit Care Med* 2002;30(9):2051–2058.

Mitch WE, Robert H. Herman Memorial Award in Clinical Nutrition Lecture, 1997. Mechanisms causing loss of lean body mass in kidney disease. *Am J Clin Nutr* 1998;67(3):359–366.

Mouser JF, Hak EB, Kuhl DA, et al. Recovery from ischemic acute renal failure is improved with enteral compared with parenteral nutrition. *Crit Care Med* 1997;25(10):1748–1754.

Price SR, Reaich D, Marinovic AC, et al. Mechanisms contributing to muscle wasting in acute uremia: activation of amino acid catabolism. *J Am Soc Nephrol* 1998;9:438–443.

Scheinkestel CD, Kar L, Marshall K, et al. Prospective randomized trial to assess caloric and protein needs of critically ill, anuric, ventilated patients requiring continuous renal replacement therapy. *Nutrition* 2003;19(11-12):909–916.

Schneeweiss B, Graninger W, Stockenhuber F, et al. Energy metabolism in acute and chronic renal failure. *Am J Clin Nutr* 1990;52:596–601.

Toback FG. Regeneration after acute tubular necrosis. *Kidney Int* 1992;41:226–246.

Van den Berghe G, Wouters PJ, Bouillon R, et al. Outcome benefit of intensive insulin therapy in the critically ill: insulin dose versus glycemic control. *Crit Care Med* 2003;31(2):359–366.

Requirements for Protein, Calories, and Fat in the Predialysis Patient

Sreedhar Mandayam and William E. Mitch

GOALS OF NUTRITIONAL THERAPY

When the diet exceeds the daily protein requirement, the excess protein is degraded to urea and other nitrogenous wastes, and these products accumulate. Foods rich in protein also contain hydrogen ions, phosphates, and other inorganic ions, and these substances must be excreted by the kidney (see Fig. 6-1). Because the severity of uremic symptoms is proportionate to the accumulation of these waste products and ions, it follows that the diet of a patient with chronic kidney disease (CKD) should not contain more than the dietary protein requirement. These considerations are the basis for the 135-year-old practice of restricting dietary protein and phosphorus: dietary modification will ameliorate symptoms of uremia and many of its metabolic complications (e.g., metabolic acidosis, insulin resistance, and secondary hyperparathyroidism). However, a diet that does not meet a patient's needs stimulates breakdown of protein stored in muscle and other organs. This process also causes accumulation of unexcreted waste products. The goals of designing a diet for a patient with CKD are (a) to diminish the accumulation of nitrogenous waste products and the metabolic disturbances of uremia; (b) to ensure that the diet will prevent malnutrition; and (c) to attempt to retard the progression of kidney disease (Quality of Evidence: Class B). Note that we have assigned levels for the "Quality of Evidence" as proposed by the Cochrane Collaborating Group.

ASSESSING PROTEIN REQUIREMENTS

Nitrogen Balance and Protein Requirements

Nitrogen balance (Bn) is the "gold standard" for assessing dietary protein requirements, because a neutral or positive Bn indicates that the body's protein stores are being maintained or increased. Although measuring Bn is time consuming and technically demanding, no readily acceptable alternative methods are available for assessing amino acid or protein requirements.

On the basis of Bn measurements, the average protein requirement for healthy adults who perform a moderate amount of physical activity and consume sufficient (but not excessive) calories is approximately 0.6 g protein/kg b.w./d. This level of dietary protein was based on Bn results from subjects who had been fed variable amounts of protein. By an extrapolation process, the World Health Organization determined that the average protein intake required to maintain neutral Bn was 0.6 g protein/kg b.w./d, and this value plus 2 standard deviations (approximately 0.75 g protein/kg b.w./d) was designated as the "safe level of intake." This amount meets the protein requirements of 97.5% or more healthy adults. Dietary protein above these levels is converted to waste products that must be excreted by the kidney.

For patients with CKD, the recommended protein intake is based on the same measurements: the average protein intake necessary to achieve neutral Bn and maintain protein stores is approximately 0.6 g protein/kg b.w./d. This recommendation is supported by long-term follow-up of patients with CKD who have maintained nutritional status at this level of intake (Quality of Evidence: Class A).

MECHANISMS RESPONSIBLE FOR NEUTRAL NITROGEN BALANCE

Healthy Subjects

For adults in Western societies, the protein intake usually exceeds the requirement; however, consuming more protein does not increase muscle mass. Instead, the body adapts by oxidizing any excess amino acids from the protein in the diet. The nitrogen liberated by amino acid oxidation is converted to waste nitrogen (principally urea) and excreted by the kidney. When the intake of protein decreases, amino acid oxidation is reduced, allowing amino acids to be recycled and yielding more efficient use of dietary essential amino acids (EAA) (see Chapter 1). In summary, when protein intake is at the minimum daily requirement, the

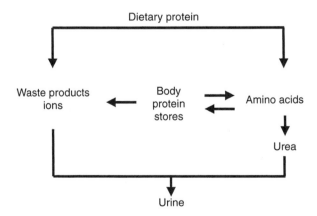

Figure 6-1. A flow diagram illustrating the use of foods rich in protein by healthy adults and by patients with chronic kidney disease (CKD). The scheme indicates that dietary protein is converted to amino acids, which can be used to build new stores of body protein. Any excess is converted to urea, which must be excreted by the kidney and, hence, will accumulate with renal insufficiency. Foods rich in protein also contain inorganic ions (e.g., H+, Na+, K+, and phosphates), and the amino acids are converted to a variety of nitrogen-containing products. These ions and waste products accumulate in patients with CKD.

production of urea and other types of waste nitrogen compounds falls, resulting in neutral Bn and a lower level of serum urea nitrogen (SUN). But, if protein intake is below the minimum daily requirement, amino acid catabolism does not decline enough to produce neutral Bn, and a loss of lean body mass occurs.

Besides amino acid oxidation, protein synthesis and degradation determine Bn. The daily rates of protein synthesis and oxidation are much larger than the rate of amino acid oxidation (see Fig. 6-2), and approximately 280 g of body protein are synthesized and degraded in a 70-kg adult each day. With fasting, body protein stores (principally skeletal muscle) are degraded to amino acids, which are used in the liver for gluconeogenesis. With feeding, protein degradation declines sharply, and protein synthesis repletes body protein stores. The net daily result is a neutral (or positive) Bn, and protein stores are preserved as long as the diet is nutritionally adequate. A principal modulator of these changes in protein turnover is insulin, the principal anabolic hormone. Insulin mainly suppresses protein degradation. In summary, healthy adults successfully adapt to dietary protein restriction by (a) suppressing catabolism of EAA and (b) inhibiting protein degradation and increasing protein synthesis with feeding.

Patients with Chronic Kidney Disease

Fortunately, even patients with advanced but uncomplicated CKD [glomerular filtration rate (GFR) approximately 5 to 10 mL per minute] can maintain protein stores and muscle mass during long-term therapy with a properly designed low-protein diet (LPD), because these patients activate the same adaptive responses to dietary protein restriction as healthy adults: by inhibiting amino acid oxidation and by suppressing whole-body

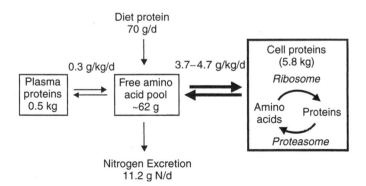

Figure 6-2.   Results illustrated in this figure are the amounts of protein in the cellular pool and in plasma as well as the amount of free amino acids in the body of an adult weighing approximately 70 kg. A very large turnover of cellular proteins (3.7 to 4.7 g protein/kg b.w./d) occurs, amounting to the protein contained in 1 to 1.5 kg of muscle. This rate is 10-fold higher than the turnover of protein in the plasma pool.

protein degradation with feeding (see Fig. 6-3). When these adaptive responses were measured in patients with advanced CKD before and after at least 1 year of therapy with an LPD, the adaptive responses were intact, and Bn was neutral. This sustained ability to adapt successfully also led to normal values of serum proteins, anthropometrics, and neutral Bn during long-term therapy with the LPD (Quality of Evidence: Class A). Additional evidence exists from the NIH (National Institute of Health) Modification of Diet in Renal Disease (MDRD) study for the nutritional adequacy and safety of LPDs in patients with CKD. Patients in this prospective trial of the effect of dietary protein restriction on nutritional status and the progression of renal failure (see Chapter 9) were followed for an average of 2.2 years. During the study, small, albeit statistically significant changes were evident in some nutritional parameters in patients prescribed different types of LPD. These nutritional signs included an *increase* in serum albumin levels and a decrease in serum transferrin levels and some anthropometric indices (see Fig. 6-4). Interestingly, the abnormal values appeared early in the trial but stabilized after the first few months of therapy.

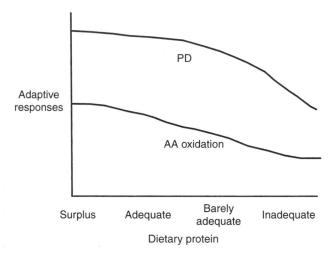

Figure 6-3.   A chart illustrating the adaptive metabolic changes that occur when healthy adults or patients with chronic kidney disease (CKD) change the amount of protein they eat. As a patient decreases dietary protein from a surplus (i.e., 1 g/kg b.w./d) to an adequate amount of 0.8 g protein/kg b.w./d, a sharp decrease occurs in amino acid (AA) oxidation. This decrease permits more efficient use of essential amino acids (EAA) in the diet. When dietary protein is reduced to a barely adequate amount (0.6 g protein/kg b.w./d), the removal of amino acids further declines, and protein degradation decreases. These responses help promote neutral nitrogen balance. However, when dietary protein decreases below the minimal value, the adaptive response cannot achieve neutral nitrogen balance, even though it limits the amount of protein being lost by the body. PD, protein degradation.

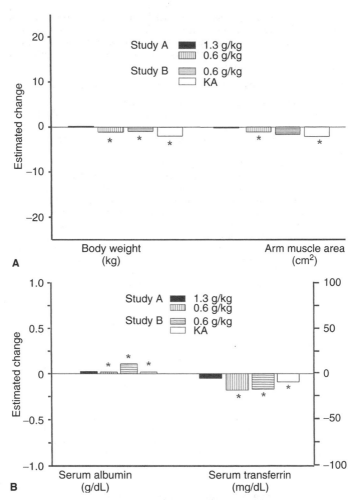

Figure 6-4.   Panel A: the average changes in body weight and arm-muscle area of patients participating in the Modification of Diet in Renal Disease (MDRD) study. Study A patients with glomerular filtration rate (GFR) values between 25 and 60 mL/min/1.73 m^2 were prescribed a diet containing either 1.3 or 0.6 g protein/kg b.w./d, whereas Study B patients with GFR values between 13 and 24 mL/min/1.73 m^2 were prescribed diets containing 0.6 or 0.3 g protein/kg b.w./d [the latter diet was supplemented with keto acids (KA) to provide essential amino acid requirements]. Although the changes in body weight and arm muscle area were significantly smaller ($p < 0.05$) in patients prescribed the low-protein diets (LPD), the changes are not biologically important, and only two patients had to stop the study because of nutritional abnormalities. Panel B: The average changes in serum albumin and transferrin in the same groups of patients. As in panel A, the changes were statistically significant ($p < 0.05$) but are not biologically important.

Nutritional status indices in the LPD groups remained within the normal range on average and, most importantly, only two patients had to drop out of the trial because of nutritional inadequacy; the LPDs were not associated with higher rates of hospitalizations or death.

Dietary Protein Restriction and Nephrotic Syndrome

Patients with nephrotic syndrome (i.e., more than 3 g proteinuria per day) could have an increased risk for malnutrition. This issue is very important, because patients who are given a well-designed LPD have decreased proteinuria and increased serum albumin concentrations compared to patients fed excessive amounts of protein. Because the severity of proteinuria is closely related to the risk for progressive kidney and cardiovascular diseases, an LPD could help prevent these problems. Fortunately, restricting dietary protein activates adaptive responses that maintain the body protein stores in patients with nephrotic syndrome. Maroni et al. measured Bn and the components of protein turnover in patients with nephrotic syndrome who consume a diet containing 0.8 or 1.6 g protein (plus 1 g dietary protein for each g proteinuria) and 35 kcal/kg b.w./d. In nephrotic and normal, age-matched adults, the low-protein diet suppressed amino acid oxidation, and protein degradation decreased while protein synthesis increased during feeding. These responses resulted in neutral or positive Bn. The increase in amino acid oxidation induced by feeding was also blunted, and evidence suggested that urinary protein losses suppressed amino acid oxidation. Thus, proteinuria in CKD does not block the adaptive responses that are required to maintain protein nutrition (see Fig. 6-5). Evidence also suggests that diets that contain less protein do not increase the risk for protein malnutrition in patients with nephrotic syndrome, including a very–low-protein diet (VLPD) that provides approximately 0.3 g protein/kg b.w./d along with a mixture of EAA.

In summary, patients with uncomplicated CKD, regardless of nephrosis, activate normal compensatory responses to an LPD, suppress EAA oxidation, and reduce feeding-induced protein degradation. The result is neutral Bn and maintenance of lean body mass during long-term dietary therapy.

Complications that Impair Adaptive Responses in Protein Turnover

Metabolic acidosis and insufficient insulin are complications of CKD, and both conditions oppose the adaptive nutritional responses to an LPD. Acidosis and acute diabetes stimulate the oxidation of EAA in muscle and accelerate the degradation of protein. Metabolic acidosis, in addition to causing negative Bn in adults and impaired growth in children and infants, also causes insulin resistance in healthy adults. Fortunately, the risks for metabolic acidosis and insulin resistance are substantially reduced with an LPD.

Acidosis-associated mechanisms have been identified that cause the degradation of EAA and protein in muscle. The branched-chain amino acids, valine, leucine, and isoleucine, are catabolized by branched-chain keto acid dehydrogenase (BCKAD), and acidosis increases the activity of this enzyme in skeletal muscle. This

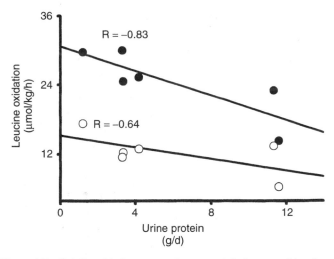

Figure 6-5. Relationship between urinary protein losses and leucine oxidation rates measured during fasting (open circles) and feeding (closed circles) when subjects with nephrotic syndrome consumed a diet providing 0.8 g protein/kg b.w./d (plus 1 g protein per g of protein-uria). By linear regression, a significant correlation was observed during feeding ($p = 0.04$). (From Maroni BJ, Staffeld C, Young VR, et al. Mechanisms permitting nephrotic patients to achieve nitrogen equilibrium with a protein-restricted diet. *J Clin Invest* 1997;99:2479–2487, with permission.)

activation includes an increase in the muscle levels of mRNAs that encode BCKAD enzyme complex, which suggests that capacity to degrade these amino acids is increased. Regarding protein degradation, acidosis accelerates the activity of the ATP-dependent, ubiquitin–proteasome proteolytic pathway and, as with BCKAD, the mRNAs that encode components of the pathway are increased.

These cellular responses explain why metabolic acidosis counteracts the adaptive responses that should occur with an LPD; acidosis accelerates the degradation of EAA and protein. Clinically, the urinary excretion of 3-methyl histidine (an index of skeletal muscle protein degradation) and urea nitrogen both increased when patients with CKD who were consuming an LPD became acidotic. These abnormalities disappeared when their acidosis was corrected by giving sodium bicarbonate. As a general rule, the serum HCO_3 should be kept at 24 mmol per L or more to prevent the loss of muscle mass (and to treat the bone, hormonal, and other complications of acidosis). Usually, two or three 650 mg sodium bicarbonate tablets (approximately 8 mEq of sodium and bicarbonate per tablet), given two to three times daily, are well tolerated and effective.

PROTEIN INTAKE DURING THE COURSE OF PROGRESSIVE CHRONIC RENAL FAILURE

Two observations have raised concerns about using LPDs. First, an association was observed in patients receiving hemodialysis therapy between hypoalbuminemia and increased mortality; second, when patients with CKD eat an unregulated diet, some patients spontaneously limit their protein intake and, therefore, certain indices of nutritional status worsen. A number of problems arise if LPDs are assumed to cause an abnormal nutritional status. First, evidence indicates (as described above) that a properly implemented LPD maintains normal serum proteins values, normal anthropometrics, and neutral Bn during long-term therapy. Second, hypoalbuminemia in patients undergoing hemodialysis is most closely related to an inflammatory response, whereas the diet plays a small role. Third, evidence suggests that proper use of an LPD in the predialysis period actually improves survival of patients with CRF during the years after hemodialysis therapy is initiated (Quality of evidence: Class A).

Emphasis must be placed on dietary education for patients with CKD, to ensure that the diet is adequate and to avoid consumption of foods that lead to the accumulation of nitrogenous wastes and aggravation of uremic symptoms. When a patient with CKD spontaneously reduces dietary protein, an educational program should be started to plan and implement an LPD.

ENERGY METABOLISM IN PATIENTS WITH CHRONIC RENAL FAILURE

Influence of Energy Metabolism on Protein Turnover

Energy intake influences protein turnover; for example, when the energy intake of patients with CKD was varied from 15 to 45 kcal/kg b.w./d while their protein intake remained constant at 0.60 g protein/kg b.w./d, Bn was more positive with higher levels of energy intake, and the urea nitrogen appearance rate was inversely correlated with energy intake (see Fig. 6-6). Because protein intake was constant, a decrease in urea appearance means that dietary protein was being used to build body protein stores. If a patient consumes too little energy, the opposite can occur, yielding a loss of body protein.

Evidence suggests that abnormalities in carbohydrate metabolism can accelerate protein degradation in muscle: the rate of lactate production in muscle of uremic rats was highly correlated with the rate of protein degradation. Metabolic acidosis also impairs energy metabolism by inducing insulin resistance and impairing triglyceride use. Finally, abnormalities occur in the plasma lipids of patients with CKD; plasma triglyceride and cholesterol levels are high, and this condition may be related to insulin insensitivity. In summary, abnormalities in the metabolism of fat and carbohydrates are related to loss of muscle mass. This effect also stresses the importance of ensuring an adequate caloric intake and correcting metabolic acidosis in patients with CKD.

Energy Requirements of Patients with Chronic Renal Insufficiency

The rates of energy expenditure (and hence, energy requirements) at rest and with exercise by patients with uncomplicated CKD are similar to those of healthy subjects. With an energy intake of approximately 35 kcal/kg b.w./d, the levels of serum proteins, anthropometric values, and Bn are maintained in patients

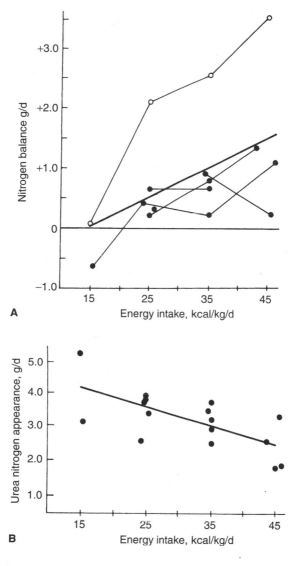

Figure 6-6. The correlation between energy intake and (A) nitrogen balance or (B) urea nitrogen appearance in six nondialyzed patients with chronic kidney disease (CKD). (A) The heavy diagonal line in both figures represents the least squares regression equation. As energy intake is increased, nitrogen balance becomes more positive. (B) Energy intake is inversely correlated with urea nitrogen appearance. (From Kopple JD, Monteon FJ, Shaib JK. Effect of energy intake on nitrogen metabolism in nondialyzed patients with chronic renal failure. *Kidney Int* 1986;29:734–742, with permission.)

consuming protein-restricted diets. Note that this recommended level of energy is commonly calculated using the patient's *ideal* body weight (IBW), because *actual* body weight may over- or underestimate energy requirements if the subject is edematous or obese, or malnourished, respectively. In elderly or obese subjects, a lower energy intake (e.g., approximately 30 kcal/kg b.w./d) may be adequate, and exercise will increase energy requirements. Clearly, the first step in achieving a sufficient energy intake is to schedule counseling sessions with a renal dietician. If changing the intake of conventional foods is unsuccessful in increasing energy intake, then high-energy or low-protein products can be used (as described above and in Chapter 14).

ABNORMALITIES IN GLUCOSE AND LIPID METABOLISM IN CHRONIC RENAL INSUFFICIENCY

Glucose Metabolism

Subjects with uremia exhibit glucose intolerance, with fasting hyperglycemia and hyperinsulinemia, especially when metabolic acidosis complicates CKD. The major metabolic abnormality resides in peripheral tissues, with decreased glucose uptake by skeletal muscle and adipose tissue, both without and with insulin. In contrast, hepatic glucose production is normal and becomes appropriately suppressed in response to insulin. This abnormality occurs after insulin interacts with its receptor (i.e., it is a postreceptor defect) and appears to reside in suppression of phosphatidyl-inositol 3 kinase activity. This glucose intolerance may be caused by a circulating substance, because dietary protein restriction improves glucose use. Evidence also suggests that insulin secretion is impaired in CKD because chronic administration of the calcium channel blocker, verapamil, normalizes intracellular calcium, insulin secretion, and glucose tolerance. Finally, exercise benefits glucose intolerance in rats with moderately severe CKD as well as in patients with uremia.

Lipid Metabolism

Hyperlipidemia is found in 20% to 70% of patients with uremia. The predominant abnormality in patients with CRF who are nonnephrotic and patients receiving hemodialysis therapy is hypertriglyceridemia, with an increase in very–low-density lipoprotein (VLDLs) levels, a decrease in high-density lipoprotein (HDL) cholesterol levels, and normal to below-normal levels of LDLs. This pattern is consistent with a type IV hyperlipoproteinemia. Besides advanced renal insufficiency, this abnormal lipoprotein pattern can be aggravated by genetic predisposition, male gender, steroid therapy, and proteinuria.

The mechanism of hypertriglyceridemia in patients with CKD is mainly defective catabolism of triglyceride-rich lipoproteins, which, in turn, is linked to decreased activity of lipoprotein lipase and hepatic triglyceride lipase. The levels of apoprotein C-II, the main activator of lipoprotein lipase, is reportedly decreased in patients with CKD, but metabolic acidosis and hyperinsulinemia in CKD can also depress lipoprotein lipase activity. Secondary hyperparathyroidism might also contribute to hypertriglyceridemia in CKD, because parathyroidectomized dogs with CKD exhibit normal serum levels of triglycerides, postheparin lipolytic activity, and intravenous fat tolerance. Another factor that aggravates hypertriglyceridemia is increased triglyceride production, which probably reflects insulin resistance. The importance of these abnormalities is that conversion of triglyceride-rich VLDL to LDL is defective, causing accumulation of potentially atherogenic IDL (intermediate density lipoproteins).

Patients with the nephrotic syndrome generally have high plasma levels of total cholesterol consisting of LDL and VLDL cholesterol, normal or low levels of HDL cholesterol, and normal or elevated triglycerides; that is, types IIa, IIb, or V hyperlipoproteinemia pattern. Early in the course of the nephrotic syndrome, VLDL is overproduced and is rapidly catabolized to LDL. However, LDL clearance is often impaired, especially in patients with severe proteinuria. The major factors that increase the risk for atherosclerosis in patients with nephrotic syndrome seem to be hypoalbuminemia and hyperlipidemia, which lead to dysregulation of HMG CoA reductase and 7α-hydroxylase expression.

ASSESSING DIETARY ADEQUACY AND COMPLIANCE

Dietary Adequacy

A key component in designing a successful plan of dietary therapy is a regular assessment of dietary adequacy and compliance. This assessment should not rely solely on indirect measures of dietary adequacy such as changes in serum albumin or transferrin, because inflammation is frequently present, leading to low values of these serum proteins. Anthropometrics are insensitive to an early decrease in nutritional status. In short, several indices should be monitored to obtain the most reliable information about nutritional status. Our approach is to monitor serum albumin, serum transferrin, and anthropometric indices of muscle mass *serially* and to interpret the values in comparison with the patient's dietary compliance.

Monitoring Compliance with the Diet Prescription

Protein Intake

For inpatients, the protein–calorie content of meals can be defined by the dietician; but for outpatients, the amount of protein ingested must be estimated. Fortunately, compliance with a dietary protein prescription can be estimated using a method based on the concept that the waste nitrogen arising from degraded protein is excreted as either urea or nonurea nitrogen (NUN). Because urea is the principal end product of amino acid degradation, the urea appearance rate (or net urea production rate) parallels protein intake. The urea nitrogen appearance rate is measured from the amount of urea excreted in urine plus the urea accumulated in body water. NUN excretion (i.e., nitrogen in feces and urinary creatinine, uric acid, amino acids, peptides, and ammonia) does not require measurement, because it does not vary with dietary protein. NUN averages 0.031 g N/kg b.w./d (see Fig. 6-7). Thus, if nitrogen balance is assumed to be neutral (i.e., when nitrogen intake equals output and no loss or gain of protein occurs), then nitrogen intake (I_N) equals urea nitrogen

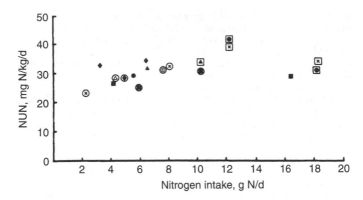

Figure 6-7. Nonurea nitrogen (NUN) losses measured in healthy
subjects (solid triangles, circles, and squares) and patients with
chronic kidney disease (CKD) being treated with low-protein diets
(LPD) (solid diamonds, open circles with cross, and open triangle),
by hemodialysis (open circle with solid square and open square with
solid triangle) or continuous ambulatory peritoneal dialysis (CAPD)
(open square with cross and open square with solid circle). These
results indicate that NUN losses (i.e., nonurea urinary nitrogen plus
fecal nitrogen) are relatively constant despite large variations in nitrogen intake and renal function. (From Maroni BJ, Steinman TI,
Mitch WE. A method for estimating nitrogen intake in patients with
chronic renal failure. *Kidney Int* 1985;27:58–65, with permission.)

appearance (U) plus the estimate of NUN losses or 0.031 g nitrogen per kg b.w. (see Table 6-1, formula 2). Nitrogen intake is converted to protein intake by multiplying I_N by 6.25, because
protein is 16% nitrogen. In the steady state [i.e., when blood urea
nitrogen (BUN) and weight are constant], the urea nitrogen appearance (U) rate is measured as the urea nitrogen in a 24-hour
urine collection [urinary urea nitrogen (UUN)]. In this case, I_N
equals UUN plus 0.031 g nitrogen per kg b.w. when nitrogen balance is zero (Table 6-1, formula 4). If weight is changing because of
an increase or decrease in body water, or if SUN is changing, the
accumulation of urea should be calculated as shown in Table 6-1.

When the calculated and prescribed values of protein intake
are similar, the patient is adhering to the amount of dietary protein prescribed. However, if the estimated protein intake is less
than prescribed, patients should be sent to the dietician to determine how to increase their protein intake. On the other hand,
if the estimated intake exceeds that prescribed by more than
25%, the difference might be caused by a superimposed catabolic illness or condition (e.g., gastrointestinal bleeding and metabolic acidosis) that is increasing waste nitrogen production by
degrading body protein stores. Alternately, the patient might
need more training to adhere to the dietary prescription. The patient should be evaluated for a catabolic condition and referred
to the dietician for counseling.

Table 6-1. Estimating compliance with the dietary protein prescription from the 24-hour urinary urea nitrogen excretion

Formulas

1. $B_N = I_N - U - NUN$, where
   $NUN = 0.031$ g N/kg b.w.
2. if $B_N = 0$, then $I_N = U + 0.031$ g N/kg b.w.
3. when BUN is unchanging, then $U = UUN$, and
4. $I_N = UUN + 0.031$ g N/kg b.w.

Example

A 40-year-old woman is seen 1 month after instruction in a diet providing 0.6 protein/kg b.w./d (i.e., 60 kg $\times$ 0.6 protein/kg = 36 g protein)

Weight: 60 kg; UUN = 4.1 g/d; NUN = 0.031 g N $\times$ 60 kg
= 1.86 g N/d

if $B_N = 0$, then $I_N = UUN + NUN$
= 4.1 + 1.86 = 5.96 g N
= 5.96 g N $\times$ 6.25 g protein/g N
= 37.3 g protein/d

N, nitrogen; B_N, nitrogen balance (g N/d); I_N, nitrogen intake (g N/d); BUN, blood urea nitrogen; U, urea nitrogen appearance (g N/d); UUN, 24-h urinary urea nitrogen (g N/d); NUN, nonurea nitrogen (g N/d).

The formula for estimating protein intake can be used for other clinical tasks; for example, if the urea clearance has been measured, the steady state SUN for any prescribed protein intake can be calculated (see Table 6-2). This formula is important, because a SUN below 60 to 70 mg per dL causes normal uremic symptoms, and the amount of dietary protein that will achieve this level of SUN can be calculated.

Energy Intake

Unlike dietary protein, no simple method is available to estimate the intake of calories (or other components of the diet), and dietary diaries or recall are the only practical methods to assess energy intake of outpatients with CKD. The accuracy of these methods depends upon accurately estimating all foods consumed, the portion size, and the number of days when each food was eaten. A skilled dietician can derive considerable information using these techniques, but another problem exists. When diets are prescribed, the patients learn what foods they should eat and often report that these foods comprise the bulk of their diet (i.e., they underestimate their actual diet). For this reason, the energy intake derived from dietary records must be interpreted cautiously; we use a 3-day food diary obtained every 3 to 4 months to monitor the energy intake of patients with CKD. If protein intake is calculated, and diet records provide a value for the percentage of calories from protein to be calculated, the total amount of dietary calories can be calculated.

The critical issue is to provide both the patient and the family with enough information so that they can be responsible for achieving compliance. Both the patient and the individual responsible for

Table 6-2. Relationship between nitrogen
balance, urea nitrogen appearance
rate, and steady state blood urea nitrogen[a]

Dietary Protein (g/d)	I_N-NUN (g N/d)	Steady State BUN (mg/dL)
80	10.6	123
60	7.4	86
40	3.9	49

where

$$BUN = \frac{I_N - 0.031 \text{ g N/kg body weight}}{C_{UREA}} \times 100$$

N, nitrogen; I_N, nitrogen intake (16% of protein intake); BUN, blood urea nitrogen; NUN, nonurea nitrogen, which averages 0.031 g N/kg b.w./d; C_{UREA}, urea clearance (L/d).
[a] Calculated for a 70-kg person with a urea clearance of 6 mL per min (8.6 L per d).

preparing the meals must have a clear understanding of the principles of dietary therapy and be trained in meal planning, knowledgeable about possible choices when the patient eats at a restaurant, and familiar with the protein contents of various foods. With this type of education, the likelihood of achieving adherence and maintaining an adequate nutritional state will be maximized. Skilled dieticians are an essential part of the treatment; they educate the patient and family in meal planning so the patient's food preferences are included. In addition, dieticians provide sample menus to enhance patient satisfaction and assist with monitoring the patient's nutritional status and dietary compliance. When patients feel comfortable with the diet, we typically examine them every 3 months. At each visit, we (a) calculate protein intake (and hence compliance) from the 24-hour UUN excretion (Table 6-1); (b) estimate caloric intake from food recall or diaries; (c) monitor serum albumin, transferrin, and anthropometrics; and, (d) use these parameters to provide a patient with feedback regarding dietary adequacy and compliance. In each case, the dietician plays a critical role.

PROTEIN REQUIREMENTS OF PREDIALYSIS PATIENTS

Two dietary regimens have been used to treat patients with progressive CKD: (a) a conventional diet that provides approximately 0.6 g protein/kg b.w./d, or (b) a VLPD that contains approximately 0.3 g protein/kg b.w./d, supplemented with a mixture of EAA or their nitrogen-free ketoanalogs (i.e., keto acids or KA) to meet EAA requirements. Because energy expenditure (and hence, energy requirements) of patients with CKD are comparable to those of healthy subjects, 35 kcal/kg b.w./d is usually recommended to achieve maximal use of the dietary protein, as described later in this chapter.

Conventional Low Protein Diet

Measurements of Bn in the early 1970s showed that some patients could achieve neutral Bn with only approximately 0.3 g protein/kg b.w./d, a value approximately 4 SDs below the average requirement for healthy subjects. This surprising finding was attributed to an ability that patients with CKD have to reuse nitrogen derived from urea degradation to make amino acids and ultimately, synthesize protein. That this finding is incorrect has now been recognized; nitrogen derived from urea does not contribute substantially to protein nutrition in patients with CKD. With LPDs, most investigators believe that approximately two thirds of the protein should be of "high biologic value" (e.g., eggs and lean meat) to ensure the EAA supply.

Essential Amino Acid Supplemented Diet Regimens

Several long-term studies have been conducted concerning the efficacy and acceptability of a VLPD that contains 25 g per day (approximately 0.3 g protein/kg b.w./d) of unrestricted quality protein (a largely vegetarian diet), plus a supplement of EAA or KA. In general, this diet regimen promptly corrects uremic symptoms while maintaining serum protein levels, muscle strength, and Bn. Generally, the EAA or KA supplement provides amino acids or KA in the proportions recommended for healthy adults, but this formulation may not be optimal because: (a) defects in amino acid metabolism have been identified in patients with uremia; (b) the plasma and intracellular concentrations of amino acids differ markedly from those in healthy adults; and, (c) with dietary protein restriction, plasma amino acid levels change differently from the pattern observed in healthy adults. For example, tyrosine synthesis from phenylalanine is impaired in uremia, and this effect can make tyrosine a "conditionally" essential amino acid, suggesting that supplemental tyrosine should be included in the mixture. Secondly, a diet that is lacking in histidine leads to a rapid decline in plasma levels of this amino acid in patients with CKD, along with a syndrome characterized by malaise, an erythematous scaling rash, and negative Bn. Supplemental histidine rapidly corrects these abnormalities, making histidine essential for patients with uremia. Serine levels are low in patients with chronic renal insufficiency (CRI), presumably because it is synthesized primarily in the kidney. Perhaps serine should be included in supplements for patients with CRI. Finally, changes in the proportions of branched-chain amino acids led to normal levels of these amino acids in muscle biopsies of patients with CKD, and during long-term therapy, Bn improved.

Keto Acid Supplemented Diet Regimens

Keto acids (the nitrogen-free analogues of EAA) are not available in the United States but are used in Europe, Asia, and Latin America. Several mixtures of KA have been evaluated. In the formulation containing the KA of branched-chain amino acids as salts of basic amino acids (lysine, ornithine, and histidine), tyrosine and a small amount of threonine and the hydroxy-analogue of methionine were provided, but the remaining EAA, tryptophan, and phenylalanine were omitted. When this mixture was given to patients with advanced CKD (average GFR of 4.8 mL per min) while they were consuming 20 to 25 g of mixed-quality protein, the patients' urea nitrogen appearance decreased; Bn remained neutral; and body weight, serum albumin, and transferrin were maintained in the normal range for 4 to 19 months. A direct comparison of a VLPD that provides 0.28 g protein/kg/d plus either an isomolar mixture of EAA or KA revealed that both diets yielded a neutral Bn but that the KA-based regimen contained approximately 15% less nitrogen; the neutral Bn with the VLPD/KA regimen was attributed to a greater decrease in urea nitrogen appearance.

Other responses to the VLPD/KA regimen in which KA were given as calcium salts showed that clinical and biochemical evidence of secondary hyperparathyroidism improved, serum phosphorus and values of alkaline phosphatase and parathyroid hormone were lower, and serum calcium and 1,25-dihydroxy cholecalciferol levels increased. These improvements are likely related to the lower intake of phosphates, because the calcium salts of KA inhibit gastrointestinal phosphate absorption. Other benefits of the regimen include an improved response to erythropoietin.

Because dietary protein is limited, the tendency for acidosis is sharply reduced, and this effect may contribute to the benefits of protein-restricted diets in patients with CKD. Finally, a KA-based regimen can improve glucose intolerance in uremia by increasing tissue sensitivity to insulin in both adults and children, leading to improvements in both fasting hyperglycemia and insulin resistance.

In summary, the nutritional status of patients treated for prolonged periods with the VLPD/KA regimen is maintained or improved, and uremic symptoms and metabolic complications of CRF (e.g., metabolic acidosis, insulin resistance, and secondary hyperparathyroidism) are reduced. A randomized trial from India also found that the VLPD/KA regimen slowed the loss of kidney function while maintaining an adequate nutritional status. The mechanism of this type of benefit is unknown, but it may be linked to suppression of proteinuria, which decreases the risk for progressive kidney failure and cardiovascular disease.

DIETARY PROTEIN PRESCRIPTION

Several reasons exist to limit the dietary protein of patients with CKD: (a) the accumulation of unexcreted waste products is reduced, and uremic symptoms are improved; (b) the severity of acidosis, secondary hyperparathyroidism, and insulin resistance is reduced; (c) proteinuria is reduced; and (d) no evidence exists that feeding an excess of protein increases body protein stores. The effect of reducing dietary protein on the progression of CKD is discussed in Chapter 9. Generally, we begin dietary protein restriction for patients with symptoms or complications of uremia, for patients with edema or poorly controlled hypertension related to salt intake, and for patients who continue to exhibit progressive renal insufficiency despite control of blood pressure and the use of angiotensin-converting enzyme inhibitors (ACEI). After discussing diet goals and methods with the patient, we use the guidelines outlined below and in Table 6-3. Dietary modification does require a substantial commitment, but when properly implemented and monitored, the dietary regimens are safe and nutritionally sound.

Moderate Chronic Renal Failure (Glomerular Filtration Rate 25 to 60 mL per minute)

Typically, dietary therapy for patients with moderate chronic renal failure begins with an LPD that provides approximately 0.6 g protein/kg b.w./d, of which approximately two thirds is provided as high–biologic value protein (meat, fish, eggs, etc.) (Table 6-3). The advantage of this strategy is that the protein limitation can be achieved using traditional foods. For patients that develop additional symptoms or problems with this dietary regimen, we begin an essentially vegetarian diet that contains approximately 0.3 g protein/kg b.w./d (approximately 15 to 25 g protein per day) supplemented with a mixture of EAA or KA. These regimens provide the daily requirement of EAA, and a variety of low-protein, high-calorie food products are available to achieve calorie requirements. Examples of these products include glucose polymers (Polycose) that can be added to beverages, high-density oral supplements (Suplena), and low-protein breads, pastas, and cookies (see Chapter 14).

Fortunately, the use of an LPD invariably limits dietary phosphates, at least if the patient limits milk intake. A low-phosphate diet is critical for preventing secondary hyperparathyroidism; generally, a patient's requirement for phosphate binders decreases sharply after the diet is begun. The rationale for dietary phosphorus restriction is discussed in Chapter 3.

Table 6-3. Managing dyslipidemia in patients with chronic kidney disease

Dyslipidemia	Target	Initial Therapy	Alternative Therapy
Triglyceride >500 mg/dL	TG <500 mg/dL	TLC + fibrate/niacin	Fibrate or niacin
LDL = 100–129 mg/dL	LDL <100 mg/dL	TLC + low-dose statin	Bile acid seq or niacin
LDL ≥130 mg/dL	LDL <100 mg/dL	TLC + max dose statin	Bile acid seq or niacin
Triglycerides >200 mg/dL and non-HDL >130 mg/dL	Non-HDL <130 mg/dL	TLC + max dose statin	Fibrate or niacin

LDL, low-density lipoproteins; HDL, high-density lipoproteins; TLC, Therapeutic Lifestyle Change; TG, Triglyceride.
Dietary component for instituting the Therapeutic Lifestyle Change includes:
Total fat: 25%–30% of calorie intake (saturated fat less than 7%, polyunsaturated 10%, mono-unsaturated 20%, total cholesterol 200 mg per day).
Carbohydrate: 50%–60% of total calories.
Fiber: 20%–30% g per day of which 10 g must be viscous fiber.
Consider plant sterols or stanols: 2 g per day.
Match calorie intake to overall energy (calorie) needs.

Table 6-4. A sample diet for patients with stage 5 chronic kidney disease (CKD) is included

Sample Menu and Nutrient Analysis

Food Items	Serving	kcal	Protein (g)	Phos (mg)	Chol (mg)	Fat (g)
Breakfast						
Oatmeal	1/2 cup	72	3	54	0	2
Toasted bagel	1/2 cup	197	3.5	60	17	1.5
Soft margarine	2 tsp	74				7.56
Honey	2 tbsp	138				
Banana	1	109	1	24		
Coffee	1 cup					
Cream powder substitute	2 tsp	22		16	0	1.5
Sugar	2 tsp	32				
Lunch						
Roast beef sandwich						
Whole wheat bread	2 slices	130	4	72	0	2
Lean roast beef	2 oz	195	15	207	46	9
Soft margarine/mustard	2 tsp	74				7.56
Lettuce and tomato				10		
Apple	1	81				
Fruit punch	1 cup	117				

Dinner

	Amount					
Baked salmon	2 oz	122	15	150		5
Noodles	1/2 cup	106	3.8	55	48	
String beans	1/2 cup	22		10		27
Olive oil	2 tbsp	243				0.78
French bread	1 slice	76	2.2	26	0	3.78
Soft margarine/mustard	1 tsp	74				9.83
Lemon meringue pie	1 slice	303	1.7	60		
Ice tea	1 cup					
Sugar/lemon	2 tsp	32				
Snack						
Graham crackers	4 squares	120	2	30		2.8
Fruit cocktail	2/3 cup	136		20		
Total		2,475	51.2	794	111	80.31

Percent calories from fat   30%

Weight (kg)	70
Calories (kcal/kg b.w./d)	2,450
Protein 0.6–0.75 g/kg b.w./d	42–52.5
Phosphorus (mg/d)	800
Cholesterol (mg/d)	<200 mg
Percent calories from fat	<35%

Advanced Chronic Renal Failure (Glomerular Filtration Rate 5 to 25 mL per minute)

The dietary regimens outlined in Table 6-3 are also appropriate for patients with advanced CKD. At this level of renal insufficiency, an LPD invariably reduces both uremic symptoms and the metabolic complications of CRI; hence, such a diet will delay the time until dialysis or transplantation is required. Albeit controversial, these diets may also slow the rate at which renal function is lost (Chapter 9).

When CKD is advanced, using the VLPD/EAA or KA regimens has potential advantages. These regimens have a lower nitrogen content, so less waste nitrogen accumulates, and dietary phosphates are reduced, while the requirement for phosphate binders is lowered. These patients also should be closely monitored to ensure an adequate intake and nutritional status.

Nephrotic Syndrome (Glomerular Filtration Rate less than 60 mL per minute)

An LPD reduces proteinuria and can ameliorate hypercholesterolemia in patients with nephrotic syndrome. Because proteinuria is considered an important risk factor for progressive renal insufficiency and for cardiovascular complications, dietary protein restriction should be used as adjunctive therapy to influence proteinuria in patients with nephrotic syndrome. Fortunately, LPD can be used safely even in patients with nephrotic syndrome: a diet providing 0.8 g protein (plus 1 g protein per g proteinuria) and 35 kcal/kg b.w./d yields neutral Bn in patients with nephrotic syndrome, regardless of the level of renal function (i.e., GFR; 19 to 120 mL per minute). Long-term studies of LPD (0.45 to 0.8 g protein/kg b.w./d) have been conducted in patients with nephrotic syndrome, and the results indicate that serum albumin levels either remain stable or increase. Although these studies emphasize the safety of dietary protein restriction in patients with nephrotic syndrome, we cannot recommend using them for patients with nephrotic syndrome who have extremely high levels of proteinuria (more than 15 g per day), in patients with catabolic illnesses (e.g., vasculitis and systemic lupus erythematosis), or those receiving catabolic medications (e.g., glucocorticoids). Evidence is insufficient for safety of dietary protein restriction in these patients.

Until the appropriate measurements are available, we recommend that patients with CKD who have infections or are receiving treatment with prednisone should increase dietary protein to the "safe" level of intake (0.75 g protein/kg b.w./d) and that the urea appearance rate (see subsequent text) be carefully monitored. If the urea appearance rate declines, the conclusion is that the patient is using amino acids to augment protein stores rather than catabolizing them to waste products. If urea appearance rises, then the patient is not using the dietary protein to increase protein stores; in this case, no reason exists to raise dietary protein.

Terminal Renal Failure (Glomerular Filtration Rate less than 5 mL per minute)

When the GFR declines below 5 mL per min, uremic symptoms can develop despite dietary protein restriction. Such patients must be repeatedly evaluated to ensure that they are taking the required amounts of protein and calories. If they cannot achieve these goals, then dialysis therapy or transplantation is required. One particular problem, anorexia, deserves special emphasis. Fortunately, relying solely on a patient's perception of hunger is not necessary. If anorexia is suspected, the amount of protein actually consumed should be calculated as described in Table 6-1.

Role of Phytoestrogens and Vegetable-based Proteins

Evidence suggests that phytoestrogens and plant proteins may retard the progression of CKD. Evidence from animal experiments and small groups of patients indicates that consumption of soy protein, rich in isoflavones, and of flaxseed, rich in lignans, can prevent progressive CKD. A randomized cross-over trial by Soroka et al. compared vegetable proteins with animal proteins in an LPD regimen. Patients with stage IV CKD had significantly lower values of SUN and 24-hour creatinine and phosphate excretion rates with the vegetarian diet than with the nonvegetarian diet. However, the number of patients was small, and no additional benefits on renal function were seen.

Angiotensin-Converting Enzyme Inhibitors and Low Protein Diets

The beneficial effects of agents that inhibit the renin-angiotensin system on proteinuria and progression of CKD is widely accepted. Proteinuria is closely linked to the severity of CKD, yielding another indication for dietary protein restriction. Combining an ACEI with an LPD produced a significant additive effect in reducing proteinuria and slowing the progression of kidney disease.

Exercise in Chronic Renal Impairment

Resistance training can have multiple important benefits for healthy individuals and for patients with CKD. These benefits include increased nitrogen retention and the expression of insulin-like growth factor 1 in skeletal muscle. The result is suppressed muscle loss in patients with CKD. A randomized controlled trial of resistance training in patients with CKD showed improved nitrogen retention, with increased serum prealbumin levels, hypertrophy of types 1 and 2 muscle fibers, and improved use of dietary protein. Similar results occur in patients treated with dialysis.

A potential mechanism is that resistance training can reduce levels of inflammatory markers like C-reactive protein and IL-6. For these reasons, resistance training for 45 minutes at least 3 times per week should be used as a nonpharmacologic intervention to offset the catabolic effects of chronic uremia.

Treating Hyperlipidemia in Chronic Renal Insufficiency

By extrapolation from results of primary and secondary intervention trials in otherwise healthy subjects, lipid-lowering therapy seems to be a rational approach to reducing the risk for coronary artery and peripheral vascular disease in patients with CKD. Unfortunately, some drugs used for this problem can cause adverse reactions in patients with CKD. Despite the absence of conclusive evidence that demonstrates a benefit of lipid-lowering drug therapy in patients with CKD, guidelines are available for managing dyslipidemias in patients with CKD (Table 6-3). As with otherwise healthy adults, dietary modification is an initial step in managing hyperlipidemia: the National Cholesterol Education Program (NCEP) guidelines seem appropriate for hyperlipidemic patients with CKD. Patients with a total cholesterol level more than 200 mg per dL on two occasions should be instructed in a diet similar to that shown in Table 6-3. The diet provides less than 30% of total calories from fat: saturated fat should be below 10% of calories, and cholesterol intake should be below 300 mg per day. All subjects should eliminate other cardiovascular disease risk factors, such as smoking, obesity, and hypertension. Improving glycemic control in diabetic patients and avoiding excessive alcohol intake are also prudent.

HMG CoA reductase inhibitors should be considered as initial therapy for hypercholesterinemia, because the drugs can be given daily, are potent, and have few side effects. This class of drugs raises hepatic LDL-receptor activity and decreases hepatic production of LDL cholesterol. Removal of LDL, IDL, and VLDL is increased by receptor-induced uptake of LDL, the precursor of IDL and VLDL. The decrease in VLDL explains the modest decrease in triglycerides that occurs with these agents. A retrospective analysis of one large clinical trial indicated that pravastatin may slow the loss of kidney function in patients with proteinuria who have moderate CKD. Regarding adverse effects, early reports suggested that HMG CoA reductase inhibitors could cause hepatotoxicity, myopathy, and occasionally myoglobinuria in patients with CKD. More extensive experience indicates, however, that these agents are generally well tolerated. Another consideration relates to transplant rejection, because after cardiac transplantation, these drugs are associated with a decrease in serum cholesterol level and in acute rejection and coronary vasculopathy; a similar benefit was seen on lipid levels and in the incidence of acute rejection episodes in renal transplant recipients.

If a patient with CKD still has high cholesterol levels, combination therapy with an HMG CoA reductase inhibitor and either a bile acid sequestrant or nicotinic acid should be considered. However, when an HMG CoA reductase inhibitor is combined with nicotinic acid, gemfibriozil, or cyclosporine, creatine phosphokinase (CPK) levels must be monitored because of an increased risk for rhabdomyolysis. Unfortunately, cyclosporine absorption is impaired by bile acid sequestrants, and these agents should not be prescribed for patients who have undergone renal transplant and are receiving cyclosporine. Other problems with bile acid sequestrants include constipation and abdominal gas. Probucol can reduce total and LDL cholesterol levels in patients with nephrotic syndrome, but HDL cholesterol also may decrease; however, probucol can have a beneficial effect on atherosclerosis by acting as an antioxidant. In patients with the nephrotic syndrome, 10 mg per day atorvastatin can improve the plasma lipids. Fibric acids, clofibrate and gemfibrozil, mainly act to reduce serum triglycerides, but use of these agents can cause an increase in LDL-cholesterol with an increased risk for myopathy in patients with nephrotic syndrome. Consequently, using these agents in patients with CKD andhyperlipidemia is not advised.

CONCLUSION

In summary, manipulation of the diet remains integral to the management of patients with CKD, because a properly designed diet is both safe and effective. The dietary prescription should be based on each patient's protein and energy requirements. Dietary adherence and nutritional adequacy must be monitored regularly to ensure that the patient's diet is adequate. Successful therapy by this regimen, like any therapeutic strategy, requires motivation, but many patients welcome the opportunity to have "control" over their illness. Tangible rewards of nutritional therapy include reduced uremic symptoms and metabolic complications, plus the potential for slowing the progression of CKD.

ACKNOWLEDGMENT

This work was supported in part by National Institute of Health grant DK37175.

SELECTED READINGS

Aparicio M, Chauveau P, de Precigout V, et al. Nutrition and outcome on renal replacement therapy of patients with chronic renal failure treated by a supplemented very low-protein diet. *J Am Soc Nephrol* 2000;11:719–727.

Avesani CM, Draibe SA, Kamimura MA, et al. Resting energy expenditure of chronic kidney disease patients: influence of renal function and subclinical inflammation. *Am J Kidney Dis* 2004;44:1008–1016.

Gansevoort RT, De Zeeuw D, De Jong PE. Additive antiproteinuric effect of ACE inhibition and a low-protein diet in human renal disease. *Nephrol Dial Transplant* 1995;10:497–504.

Kaysen GA, Dubin JA, Muller HG, et al. Inflamation and reduced albumin synthesis associated with stable decline in serum albumin in hemodialysis patients. *Kidney Int* 2004;65:1408–1415.

Maroni BJ, Staffeld C, Young VR, et al. Mechanisms permitting nephritic patients to achieve nitrogen equilibrium with a protein-restricted diet. *J Clin Invest* 1997;99:2479–2487.

Masud T, Manatunga A, Cotsonis G, et al. The precision of estimating protein intake of patients with chronic renal failure. *Kidney Int* 2002;62:1750–1756.

Mitch WE. Malnutrition: a frequent misdiagnosis for hemodialysis patients. *J Clin Invest* 2002;110:437–439.

Mitch WE, Remuzzi G. Diets for patients with chronic kidney disease, still worth prescribing. *J Am Soc Nephrol* 2004;15:234–237.

Soroka N, Silverberg DS, Greemland M, et al. Comparison of vegetable-based (SOYA) and an animal-based low-protein diet in predialysis chronic renal failure patients. *Nephron* 1998;79:173–180.

Walser M, Mitch WE, Maroni BJ, et al. Should protein be restricted in predialysis patients? *Kidney Int* 1999;55:771–777.

Nutritional Requirements of Diabetics with Nephropathy

Ralf Dikow and Eberhard Ritz

With an excess of fat diabetes begins and from an excess of fat diabetics die, formerly of coma, recently of atherosclerosis.
Joslin, EP. Atherosclerosis and diabetes. *Annals of Clinical Medicine* 1927;5:1061–1079.

WHAT IS DIABETES?

Diabetes is a heterogeneous disease. Currently, one distinguishes two major types of diabetes. Type 1 diabetes (insulinopenic), which is usually secondary to the autoimmune destruction of the insulin secreting β cells in the pancreas (insulitis), usually begins at a young age. These patients require insulin treatment within the first year after the onset of diabetes. Type 2 diabetes is usually seen in elderly individuals. Increasingly, however, it is also seen in the obese young. Type 2 diabetes is characterized by insulin resistance, which is, to a large extent, genetically determined. After years or decades, the secretory capacity of the pancreatic islets is exhausted. The patients respond initially to weight reduction, oral hypoglycemic agents, or both. As the disease progresses, these patients usually require insulin.

Matters are much more complex than this simple scheme suggests; up to 10% of elderly patients with diabetes have an autoimmune illness [Late Autoimmune Diabetes in Adults (LADA)]. On the other hand, 10% to 15% of patients with type 2 diabetes develop diabetes at a relatively young age as a result of genetic abnormalities of insulin secretion [Maturity Onset Diabetes of the Young (MODY)]. The major health problem in Western populations is currently type 2 diabetes. It affects approximately 6% to 10% of the general population. In some populations, the prevalence is much higher. For instance, in Saudi women aged 50 years, the prevalence is no less than 50%. The prevalence increases with advancing age. Currently, the prevalence of type 2 diabetes is increasing throughout the Western world.

Both type 1 and type 2 diabetes cause similar long-term complications, namely, *macrovascular disease* [coronary heart disease (CHD), cerebrovascular disease, and peripheral arterial disease] and *microvascular disease* (retinopathy and nephropathy).

THE EPIDEMIOLOGY OF NEPHROPATHY AND END-STAGE RENAL DISEASE IN DIABETES

Diabetic nephropathy, usually in patients with type 2 diabetes, recently has become the single most common cause of end-stage renal disease. Currently, more than 50% of patients admitted to start renal replacement therapy at the University of Heidelberg have type 2 diabetes. Comparable figures have been reported from the United States, where the incidence of diabetic nephropathy is 334 per million population per year, according to the The United States Renal Data System (USRDS) report 2003 (www.USRDS.org). These high rates of diabetic nephropathy not only impose a burden on the health budget but are also associated with immense human suffering as a result of amputation, blindness, heart disease, and so on.

WHY IS THE PREVALENCE OF TYPE 2 DIABETES RISING?

Undoubtedly, a strong genetic predisposition plays an important role, as illustrated by family studies and, more specifically, by twin studies, although the genes that are responsible have not been identified. Despite the strong genetic determination, the risk for developing type 2 diabetes is considerably influenced by lifestyle factors. That lifestyle, particularly the diet, plays an important role is illustrated by observations that indicate that the prevalence of type 2 diabetes is very low in periods of nutritional deprivation, for example, during and after World War II in Europe. Conversely, type 2 diabetes becomes extremely prevalent when indigenous populations adopt a Western lifestyle, for example, Pima Indians, inhabitants of the Pacific island of Nauru, or Australian aboriginals.

The current epidemic of obesity throughout the Western world, particularly in the United States, is certainly a major predisposing factor for type 2 diabetes. Why did the predisposition for such an adverse condition as diabetes not disappear during evolution by natural selection? One very persuasive explanation is assigned to the so-called "thrifty gene hypothesis," which proposes that when periods of nutritional deprivation (with a low insulin level) or insulin resistance are followed by high insulin levels after refeeding, storing energy in adipose tissue, rather than simply using it, provides a survival advantage. Consequently, when individuals whose ancestors had been genetically programmed for survival in a lean environment are exposed to an environment with excessive calorie supply and physical inactivity, this metabolic program causes insulin resistance, central obesity, dyslipidemia, and hypertension. This constellation has been called *metabolic syndrome* or *syndrome X* and is thought to be the forerunner of type 2 diabetes.

Several observations suggest that lifestyle modification has a major benefit once type 2 diabetes has developed. Australian investigators sent diabetic Australian aborigines back into the desert to adopt the lifestyle of their ancestors as hunters and gatherers. Within several weeks, glycemia and dyslipidemia were reversed. The salutary effects of dietary restriction and physical exercise have been known for several millenia. Wise ancient Indians advised individuals whose glycosuric urine attracted flies to visit on foot at least 100 villages—a therapy that involved physical exercise and weight reduction.

THE ROLE OF NUTRITION THERAPY IN THE MANAGEMENT OF DIABETES MELLITUS

Nutrition therapy is not only one of the most challenging aspects of diabetes care but is also an essential component of successful diabetes management. Current thinking about nutrition and diabetes is reviewed in the recent statements of Franz et al. and Sheard in the nutrition recommendations of the American Diabetes Association (ADA). The interested reader is referred to these excellent in-depth reviews.

The goals of nutrition therapy are summarized in Table 7-1. One major goal is to achieve and maintain near-normal glucose concentrations.

A second goal is to manage dyslipidemia, particularly in view of the excessive cardiovascular risk of the patient with diabetes, a risk comparable to that of the survivor of a myocardial infarction. Recognition of this risk has prompted a marked downward revision of acceptable low-density lipoproteins (LDL) cholesterol concentrations in the Third Report of the National Cholesterol Education Program.

Table 7-2 summarizes the recommended lipid concentrations for a patient with diabetes.

Another goal is to control or even reverse obesity in type 2 diabetics through lifestyle modifications that include caloric restriction and physical exercise. Clinical data strongly support the potential for moderate weight loss to reduce the risk for developing diabetes. The benefit from loss of weight is improved control of glycemia, of dyslipidemia, and of blood pressure; these interventions often become less effective, however, as the disease progresses.

The dietary recommendations about the relative proportions of carbohydrates, protein, and fat have changed with greater insights into the pathologic mechanisms. Table 7-3 shows that the recommended relative contribution of calories from carbohydrates has progressively increased, whereas the recommended proportion of fat has progressively decreased. The currently accepted recommendations can be summarized as follows.

CARBOHYDRATE. In contrast to previous opinion, the total amount of carbohydrate in a diet rather than the type of carbohydrate is what is important in controlling postprandial glucose levels. Individuals with diabetes should reduce their intake of low molecular weight sugars (mono- and disaccharides) to the same extent as, but no more than, individuals without diabetes. The general philosophy is that patients with diabetes should eat the same prudent diet that is recommended for the general

Table 7-1. Optimal glycemic control for individuals with diabetes according to the recommendations of the American Diabetes Association (ADA)

	Goal	Action Suggested
Preprandial glucose (mg/dL)[a]	80–120	<80 or >140
Bedtime glucose (mg/dL)[a]	100–140	<100 or >160
HbA1c (%)	<7	>8

[a] whole blood values.

From Sheard NF, Nathaniel GC. The role of nutrition therapy in the management of diabetes mellitus. *Nutr Clin Care* 2000;6:334–348, with permission.

Table 7-2.   Goals for treating plasma lipid disorders
in diabetic patients according to the third report of
the National Cholesterol Education Program (NCEP)

- Diabetes is a CHD risk equivalent
- Patients with CHD or CHD risk equivalents have an LDL cholesterol goal of <100 mg/dL
- In diabetic patients with high triglycerides (≥200 mg/dL) the sum of LDL + VLDL (equivalent to total cholesterol–HDL cholesterol) is a secondary target. The goal value is <130 mg/dL
- A low HDL (<40 mg/dL) should receive clinical attention; currently, insufficient evidence exists to specify a goal of therapy

CHD, coronary heart disease; LDL, low-density lipoproteins; VLDL, very–low-density lipoproteins; HDL, high-density lipoproteins.
From Executive Summary of the Third Report of the National Cholesterol Education Program (NCEP). Expert panel on detection, evaluation, and treatment of high blood cholesterol in adults (Adult Treatment Panel III). *JAMA* 2001;285:2486–2497, with permission.

population. The problem is to adjust the insulin dose, or oral hypoglycemic agents, to dietary carbohydrates, taking into account the effectiveness of insulin (the insulin sensitivity). Although carbohydrates do have differing glycemic responses, evidence of a long-term benefit is insufficient to recommend the use of low–glycemic-index diets as a primary strategy in dietary advice.

FAT.   Hyperlipemia and, to a major extent, hypertriglyceridemia in patients with type 1 diabetes can be reversed by tight glycemic control. In contrast, type 2 diabetic dyslipidemia is demonstrable before the onset of diabetes and, although somewhat improved by adequate glycemic control, usually persists despite such measures. Difficulties with lipid control are aggravated with the onset of renal disease and proteinuria, particularly at nephrotic levels of proteinuria. Specifically in individuals with diabetes and elevated LDL cholesterol, decreasing saturated fat intake to less than 7% of total calories is recommended. In individuals with pronounced hyperglycemia, weight reduction and decreasing intake

Table 7-3.   History of dietary
recommendations for diabetes mellitus

Year	Carbohydrate (%kcal)	Protein (%kcal)	Fat (%kcal)
1921	20	10	70
1950	40	20	40
1971	45	20	35
1986	Up to 60	12–20	<30
1994	Variable[a]	10–20	Variable[b]

[a] Based on nutritional assessment and treatment goals.
[b] Less than 10% from saturated fats.
From Sheard NF, Nathaniel GC. The role of nutrition therapy in the management of diabetes mellitus. *Nutr Clin Care* 2000;6:334–348, with permission.

of sucrose, total carbohydrates, and alcohol are recommended; carbohydrates should be exchanged for more mono-unsaturated fat (olive oil or canola oil) in the diet.

PROTEIN. The recommended dietary allowance (RDA) for protein in the general population is 0.8 g per kg b.w., or approximately 10% of total calories. The usual protein intake in Europe and in the United States is far greater than RDA. The nutritional requirement for protein in the patient with well-controlled diabetes is not different from that recommended for the general population. However, in hyperglycemic individuals, protein synthesis is decreased and protein breakdown is increased, thus leading to a negative nitrogen balance. During periods of hyperglycemia or weight loss, somewhat higher protein intakes may improve nitrogen balance, but this theory is not proved.

SODIUM CHLORIDE. Blood pressure in diabetic individuals tends to be sodium-sensitive. It is wise to follow the recommendation of the Joint National Committee on Prevention, Detection, Evaluation and Treatment of High Blood Pressure for individuals with hypertension and lower the sodium chloride intake to 6 g per day; the importance of reducing dietary sodium intake has been illustrated by recent studies, which show that reduced sodium intake lowers blood pressure and that sodium intake even predicts cardiovascular mortality.

The salient features of the nutritional recommendations by the ADA for individuals with diabetes mellitus are summarized in Table 7-4.

WHAT ARE THE NUTRITIONAL REQUIREMENTS OF PATIENTS WITH DIABETES AND NEPHROPATHY?

To answer this question one has to address several different issues:

• Do dietary factors contribute to the development or progression of diabetic nephropathy?
• Does the presence of advanced diabetic nephropathy necessitate changes in the management of patients with diabetes?
• Does renal replacement therapy have an effect on the management of patients with diabetes?

In this context, it is helpful to first describe the natural history of diabetic nephropathy, because the interventions depend on the stage of nephropathy. At the time of diagnosis, when the patient is markedly hyperglycemic, renal function is increased (renal hyperfunction), as shown in Table 7-5. This abnormality is ameliorated, but not normalized, during the so-called phase of clinical latency. The first indication of renal damage is the appearance of albumin ("microalbuminuria") in the urine at concentrations that are not detected by routine measurements of urine protein but can be detected using sensitive techniques [Elisa, Radioimmunoassay (RIA), specific dipsticks]. With the increase of urinary albumin excretion, blood pressure also increases. This stage is a window of opportunity, because renal function is still normal, but the high-risk patient can be identified and given specific therapy, primarily administration of ACE inhibitors or angiotensin receptor blockers (pharmacologic blockade of the renal angiotensin system). After several years,

**Table 7-4. Nutritional recommendations
of the American Diabetes Association (ADA)**

General recommendations
- Moderate caloric restriction (250–500 calories less than average daily intake) for individuals with type 2 diabetes
- Increase in physical activity

Protein
- 10%–20% of daily caloric intake (both animal and vegetable sources)
- 0.8 g/kg b.w./d in patients with overt nephropathy
- Once GFR decreases, further restriction to 0.6 g/kg b.w./d)

Total fat
- <10% of calories from saturated fats (<7% in individuals with high LDL cholesterol)
- <10% of calories from polyunsaturated fats
- 10%–15% of calories from monounsaturated fats
- Limitation of dietary cholesterol to <300 mg daily (<200 mg daily in individuals with high LDL cholesterol)
- Two to three servings of fish/w provide dietary n-3 polyunsaturated fat and can be recommended

Carbohydrates and sweeteners
- Carbohydrates from whole grains, fruits, vegetables, and low-fat milk should be included
- Regarding the glycemic effects of carbohydrates, the total amount is more important than the source or type
- Avoid excessive simple sugars
- Sucrose, if used, must be substituted for, not simply added to, other carbohydrates
- Moderate consumption of fructose-sweetened food is allowed
- Calories from all nutritive sweeteners must be accounted for in the meal plan

Fiber
- Daily consumption of 20–35 g dietary fiber from both soluble and insoluble fibers is recommended

Sodium chloride
- 6–7.5 g/d (approx. 100–130 mmol/d) in individuals without hypertension
- <6 g/d (<100 mmol/d) in individuals with mild to moderate hypertension
- <5 g/d (<85 mmol/d) in individuals with hypertension and nephropathy

Alcohol
- No more than two drinks/d for men and one drink/d for women
- To reduce the risk of hypoglycemia, alcohol should be consumed with food

Vitamins and minerals
- Generally no need for additional vitamin and mineral supplementation for the majority of individuals with diabetes

LDL, low-density lipoproteins.
From American Diabetes Association. Nutrition principles and recommendations in diabetes. *Diabetes Care* 2004;27:S36–S46, with permission.

Table 7-5. The stages of diabetic nephropathy

Stage	Glomerular Filtration	Albuminuria	Blood Pressure	Time Course (years after diagnosis)
Renal hyperfunction	Elevated High/normal	Absent	Normal	At diagnosis
Clinical latency	Within the normal range	Absent		
Microalbuminuria (incipient nephropathy)		20–200 µg/min (30–300 mg/d)	Rising within or above the normal range	5–15
Macroalbuminuria or persisting proteinuria (overt nephropathy)	Decreasing	200 µg/min (300 mg/d)	Increased	10–15
Renal failure	Diminished	Massive	Increased	15–30

frank proteinuria supervenes. From this time it will take an average of only 7 years before patients are in end-stage renal disease requiring renal replacement therapy.

Do Dietary Factors Contribute to the Development and Progression of Diabetic Nephropathy?

Development of Diabetic Nephropathy

As shown in Table 7-6, apart from genetic predisposition and nonmodifiable factors such as gender (higher risk in men than in premenopausal women) and ethnicity (higher risk in Blacks, Hispanics, and Asians than in other ethnic groups), several modifiable factors increase the risk that individuals with type 1 and type 2 diabetes will develop diabetic nephropathy.

THE ROLE OF HYPERGLYCEMIA. Diabetic nephropathy cannot develop in the absence of hyperglycemia. An important risk factor is the quality of glycemic control, as documented in type 1 diabetes by the DCCT (Diabetes Control and Complications Trial) and in type 2 diabetes by the Kumamoto study in Japan and the UK-PDS study in the United Kingdom. Notably, no safe cut-off value exists for blood glucose concentration (see Table 7-7). Glycemic control is reflected by the level of hemoglobin A1c, that is, the proportion of hemoglobin molecules that have undergone postribosomal modification by glycation. The normal value is about 6.1% (depending on the method used). The risk of diabetic nephropathy (and retinopathy) rises with increasing levels of hemoglobin A1c. The hemoglobin A1c value is superior to spot measurements of blood glucose, because it reflects the level of glycemia in the past 4 to 6 weeks, that is, it is the integral of glucose concentrations (preprandial and postprandial) over time.

THE ROLE OF HYPERTENSION. Another important risk factor is blood pressure. At least in type 2 diabetes, the presence of hypertension before the onset of diabetes clearly determines the ultimate risk for developing diabetic nephropathy. Recent evidence indicates that lowering blood pressure reduces the risk for developing diabetic nephropathy in type 2 diabetes. Furthermore, the evidence is overwhelming that lowering blood pressure is effective in attenuating the rate of progression in established diabetic nephropathy. Hypertension is strongly modified by body weight and salt intake, two aspects that have obvious implications for the dietary management of patients.

Blood pressure is influenced by salt intake, as shown in the recent DASH study (Dietary Approach to Stop Hypertension). Reducing sodium intake from 144 ± 58 mmol per day to 67 ± 46

Table 7-6. Factors that increase the risk to develop diabetic nephropathy

- Hyperglycemia
- Smoking
- Hypertension
- High protein intake?
- Dyslipidemia?

Table 7-7. Effect of intensified insulin treatment on development (primary prevention) and progression (secondary prevention) of nephropathy in Japanese type 2 diabetic patients

	Conventional Insulin Treatment (n = 55)	Intensified Insulin Treatment (n = 55)	
	(Percent of patients after 6 years)		p
Primary prevention (development)	28%	7.7%	0.03
Secondary prevention (progression)	32%	11.5%	0.04

From Ohkubo Y, Kishikawa H, Araki E. Intensive insulin therapy prevents the progression of diabetic microvascular complications in Japanese patients with non-insulin-dependent diabetes mellitus: a randomized prospective 6-year study. *Diabetes Res* 1995;28:103–117, with permission.

mmol per day by eating a diet rich in vegetables, fruits, and low-fat dairy products reduced systolic blood pressure by 7.1 mm Hg in normotensive individuals and no less than 11.5 mm Hg in hypertensive individuals. The salt dependency of blood pressure is particularly pronounced in individuals with diabetes. We had shown that blood pressure was "salt sensitive," that is, increased by more than 3 mm Hg when salt intake was increased from 20 to 200 mmol per day, in no less than 43% of patients with type 1 diabetes, regardless of the presence or absence of microalbuminuria. There are several potential reasons for this finding. One reason is that insulin is an antinatriuretic hormone and acutely lowers sodium excretion. Second, in the presence of hyperglycemia, increased amounts of glucose and sodium are reabsorbed in the proximal tubule via the glucose–sodium cotransporter. As a result, exchangeable sodium and extracellular fluid volume tend to be higher in patients with diabetes than in healthy individuals. Salt-sensitivity of blood pressure and volume expansion is even more pronounced once patients develop renal disease and renal failure. Conversely, dietary sodium restriction, administration of diuretics, or both are particularly effective in reducing the blood pressure of patients with diabetes.

In a recent prospective study, high sodium intake also predicted mortality and risk for CHD, independent of other cardiovascular factors, including blood pressure. The cardiovascular risk is extremely high in the patient with diabetes. These considerations provide a further rationale to recommend reducing dietary salt intake in patients with diabetes.

Patients with type 2 diabetes tend to be obese. In obese individuals without diabetes, blood pressure is sodium sensitive as well; in several small clinical trials, even moderate weight loss diminished salt sensitivity. This observation is less surprising in view of recent molecular evidence, which indicates that adipose tissue is not only a storehouse of energy but is also an active endocrine organ, with a complete local renin-angiotensin system and the capacity to synthesize endocrine factors, including estrogens, leptin, adiponectin, and others. When motivating patients to lose weight, it is important to emphasize that complete normalization of body weight is not necessary to achieve at least some benefits against hypertension. Even a reduction of several kg can be associated with a marked decrease in blood pressure.

The Joint National Committee on Prevention, Detection, Evaluation, and Treatment of High Blood Pressure and the ADA and its European counterparts recommend an average of 6 g sodium chloride per day, that is, approximately 100 mmol per day. Patients should be instructed that this goal can be achieved by reducing the consumption of cured meat, canned food, salted varieties of bread, hard cheese, and seafood. Obviously, meals should be prepared without adding salt, and soups are a notorious source of salt. Monitoring compliance, by occasionally measuring sodium excretion in 24-hour urine collections, would be prudent.

THE ROLE OF DIETARY INTAKE OF PROTEIN. That high protein intake increases the renal risk in different animal models of renal damage is well known. Conversely, restricting protein intake reduces hyperfiltration and intraglomular pressure. As a result, the increase of proteinuria, glomerulosclerosis, and hypertension is lessened, and progression is slowed.

𝑣 In patients with diabetes who do not have nephropathy, only fragmentary evidence exists that high protein intake increases the renal risk for developing microalbuminuria. In one important cross-sectional study (EURODIAB study) Toeller et al. examined 2,696 patients with type 1 diabetes in 16 European countries. The authors noted that in individuals whose protein consumption was more than 20% of total energy intake, the albumin excretion rates were higher, particularly in individuals with hypertension and poor metabolic control. This association was found specifically for animal protein; no association was found for vegetable protein. In animal experiments, manipulation of dietary protein intake was particularly effective early in the course of progressive renal disease. Therefore, recommending a reduction of protein consumption to less than 20% of total energy intake (as proposed by the EURODIAB investigators) would seem prudent. This advice is also in line with the recommendations of the ADA. Whether a more drastic reduction of dietary protein is effective when renal function is already markedly impaired will be discussed. Long-term adherence to dietary restriction of protein is notoriously poor. This is one more argument against waiting until incipient proteinuria indicates that the patient is at high renal risk, and for educating the patient from the very beginning of diabetes to stick to a prudent diet; that is, reducing protein intake to the RDA of 0.8 g/kg b.w./d and emphasizing substitution of vegetable protein for protein from animal sources. An added benefit of this policy is that the consumption of total fat and saturated fat will also be reduced.

✦ THE HYPOTHETICAL ROLE OF DYSLIPIDEMIA. A potential renal risk factor is dyslipidemia. This risk has been well documented in cross-sectional and longitudinal association studies, in which dyslipidemia was found to be a potent predictor of progressive loss of renal function. Furthermore, a large body of experimental evidence in different models of renal damage suggests that a high intake of fat (in particular, oxidized fat) aggravates progression of renal disease, whereas dietary restriction of fat (or lowering of fat by antilipidemic agents) attenuates progression. Controlled evidence for such a relationship is missing, however.

The renal benefit of lipid lowering by dietary measures (and by administering lipid lowering medication) has not been definitely proven, but a strong rationale for it exists because of the excessive coronary risk among patients with diabetes. Recent recommendations of the National Cholesterol Education Program (see Table 7-2), including the stringent goals for LDL cholesterol, can usually be achieved safely and economically only with a combination of dietary measures and lipid-lowering agents, particularly statins. Whether the so-called pleiotropic effects of these agents also plays a role, apart from their lipid-lowering effects, is currently unclear.

The fact that in the WOSCOPS study (West of Scotland Coronary Prevention Study) the risk of new onset type 2 diabetes was reduced by 30% when subjects at high cardiovascular risk were treated with pravastatin is of interest. This reduction may indicate that lipids play a role even in the genesis of type 2 diabetes, perhaps by affecting the free fatty acid concentrations that reduce insulin sensitivity. This finding has not been confirmed in other studies, such as the Heart Protection Study.

What practical dietary recommendations should be given to the patient with diabetes and incipient nephropathy?

Patients with diabetes should follow a prudent diet and, in principle, follow the recommendations outlined in Table 7-4.

Progression of Diabetic Nephropathy

The factors involved in the progression of established diabetic nephropathy differ from the factors operative in the development of diabetic nephropathy, not in principle, but with respect to their relative importance, as summarized in Table 7-6. The factors that are important for progression of diabetic nephropathy are listed in Table 7-8. See results in Chapter 9.

THE ROLE OF HYPERTENSION. An overwhelming body of evidence documents that the single most important factor that determines progression of established diabetic nephropathy is hypertension. Blood pressure rises when the patient develops microalbuminuria. In particular, the usual decrease of blood pressure during nighttime is attenuated or even reversed. In recent years, the fact that conventional levels of "normotension" are not good

Table 7-8. Factors that increase the risk of progression of diabetic nephropathy to end-stage renal disease

- Hypertension
- Proteinuria
- Smoking
- Poor glycemic control
- Dyslipidemia?
- High dietary intake of protein?

enough for the patient with diabetes and renal disease has become apparent. Several national committees propose a target blood pressure less than or equal to 125/75 mm Hg in patients with diabetes who have proteinuria. However, in the highly comorbid population of the Irbesartan Diabetic Nephropathy Trial (IDNT), mortality was substantially higher than in the general population, if the systolic blood pressure achieved was below 120 mm Hg. Although it is uncertain whether the relationship is causal, caution against excessive blood pressure lowering is sensible. The 125/75 mm Hg blood pressure target can usually be reached only if one administers more than one class of antihypertensive agents; ACE inhibitors or angiotensin receptor blockers are the medication of first choice. Nevertheless, dietary salt restriction remains a very important component of antihypertensive management in patients with diabetic nephropathy. Although diuretics must usually be administered in addition to restricting salt intake, the side effects of diuretic treatment, particularly hypokalemia and hypomagnesemia, are reduced if the patient is on a low salt intake. Blood pressure control with antihypertensive agents is markedly facilitated by a low-salt diet, so that less antihypertensive medication is required. With the exception of calcium channel blockers, the blood pressure-lowering effect of all antihypertensive agents is increased by low-salt intake and reversal of hypervolemia. Notably, diuretics, particularly in patients with hyperkalemia, may cause or aggravate insulin resistance and dyslipidemia.

THE ROLE OF PROTEINURIA. In the past, optimal renal protection was assumed to have been achieved when blood pressure was lowered to the target level, that is less than or equal to 125/75 mm Hg (see preceding text). More recently, in addition to lowering blood pressure, reducing proteinuria has become another important therapeutic goal. Proteinuria can be considered a "nephrotoxin." Several studies in patients with diabetic and nondiabetic renal disease have shown that long-term protection of renal function was greatest in those patients in whom the most pronounced reduction of proteinuria could be achieved. For this reason, when administering ACE inhibitors or angiotensin receptor blockers, urinary protein excretion should be monitored. When the reduction of proteinuria is not satisfactory, a further increase in the dosage of ACE inhibitor or angiotensin receptor blocker (ARB) is recommended, even when target blood pressure has been reached. Notably, several studies have shown that reduction of proteinuria by ACE inhibitors was amplified by a low protein intake. One novel approach, based on preliminary data, is the use of ACE inhibitors plus angiotensin receptor blockers and the administration of aldosterone receptor blockers in patients with "aldosterone escape" (i.e., those patients with a secondary increase in the level of serum or urinary aldosterone occurring after the initial decrease in aldosterone production that follows administration of ACE inhibitors or ARBs). However, in patients with diabetic nephropathy, a well-controlled study of the efficacy of these maneuvres has not been conducted yet

THE ROLE OF DIETARY PROTEIN INTAKE. The Modification of Diet in Renal Disease (MDRD) study, which enrolled mostly patients without diabetes, showed a slight delay in dialysis dependency when patients with advanced renal failure were given a very low-protein diet (0.58 g/kg b.w./d), but the benefit was not impressive and certainly was much smaller than the benefit derived from aggressive lowering of blood pressure. The results of this controlled trial are in striking contrast to those of a few uncontrolled studies that had shown marked benefit from protein restriction. The meta-analysis of Kasiske showed that the effect of protein restriction was greater in 11 nonrandomized studies comprising 2,248 patients than in 13 randomized studies comprising 1,919 patients. Ruggenenti et al. concluded that "the benefit of a low-protein diet on slowing the progression of renal failure is negligible and that the delay of dialysis for a few months, i.e., short-lasting freedom from dialysis, is not cost-effective, particularly since it may lead to poor nutritional status."

Specific information is available on the effect of protein restriction in patients with diabetes. In a prospective parallel group study, Zeller et al. studied patients with type 1 and manifest nephropathy. Of these patients, 20 were given a low-protein (0.6 g/kg b.w./d) diet with 500 to 1,000 mg phosphorus and 2,000 mg of sodium. The control group of 15 patients received 1 g protein/kg b.w./d and the same amount of phosphorus and sodium. The glomerular filtration rate (GFR) was measured using the iothalamate clearance. Iothalamate clearance decreased by 3.1 mL/min/mo with the low-protein diet and by 12.1 mL/min/mo in the control diet group. Although the difference between groups was statistically significant ($p = 0.02$), large interindividual differences were observed.

In a cross-over study, Walker et al. switched patients with type 1 diabetes and overt nephropathy from a normal protein diet (NPD) (1.13 g/kg b.w./d) to a low-protein diet (0.67 g/kg b.w./d). As shown in Figure 7-1 the rate of loss of GFR, measured by the radiochelate method, was markedly attenuated when patients were on the low-protein diet, and this change was associated with a decrease in albuminuria. The study is confounded, however, by lower blood pressure with low-protein diet, the possibility of carry-over effects, and nonstandardized concurrent treatment.

Almost all studies showed that albuminuria (a surrogate marker of glomerular damage) decreases with a low-protein diet, but the effect on GFR is not entirely consistent. To this result must be added the fact that Brodsky et al. found a decrease in muscle strength, an increase in fat mass, and reduced whole body leucine oxidation when patients with type 1 diabetes and early nephropathy were given 0.6 g protein/kg b.w./d. This finding illustrates the potential danger of malnutrition and is of particular concern because malnutrition is a potent predictor of cardiovascular death in patients with uremia. The issue is complex, however, because indices of malnutrition may also be attributable to a state of microinflammation with increased expression of inflammatory cytokines, as illustrated in Table 7-9.

THE ROLE OF GLYCEMIC CONTROL. Although blood pressure control is of overwhelming importance, the rate of progression is also determined to a minor degree by the quality of glycemic control. Hemoglobin A1c concentrations have been shown to correlate with the rate of loss of GFR at any given level of blood pressure. Good glycemic control is also important for other reasons. Because cells shrink in a hyperosmolar milieu, hyperglycemia

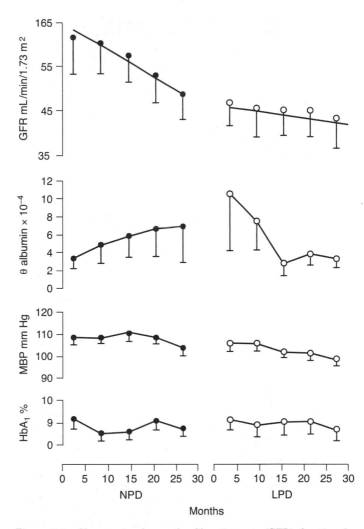

Figure 7-1. Changes in glomerular filtration rate (GFR), fractional clearance of albumin [calculated as clearance (UV/P) of albumin divided by the GFR)], mean blood pressure (MBP), and glycosylated haemoglobin (HbA1) in 19 proteinuric insulin-dependent diabetic patients on normal protein diets (NPD) (closed circles) and [low-protein diets (LPD)] (open circles). (From Walker JD, Dodds RA, Murrells TJ, et al. Restriction of dietary protein and progression of renal failure in diabetic nephropathy. *Lancet* 1989;2:1411–1415, with permission.)

Table 7-9.   Two different types of
malnutrition in chronic renal failure

	Type 1 "Uremia-induced"	Type 2 "Cytokine-driven"
Comorbidity (for example, chronic heart failure)	Low association	High association
Serum albumin	Normal/low	Low
Presence of inflammatory markers (high levels of CRP and cytokines)	No	Yes
Food intake	Low	Low/normal
Resting energy expenditure	Normal	Elevated
Oxidative stress	Increased	Markedly increased
Protein catabolism	Decreased	Increased
Optimal treatment strategy	Dialysis/nutritional support	First priority elimination of the sources of chronic inflammation

From Stenvinkel P, Heimburger O, Lindholm B, et al. Are there two types of malnutrition in chronic renal failure? Evidence for relationships between malnutrition, inflammation and atherosclerosis (MIA syndrome). *Nephrol Dial Transplant* 2000;15:953–960, with permission.

causes translocation of potassium from the intracellular to the extracellular compartment as part of a homeostatic effort to hold intracellular solute content constant. Therefore, hyperglycemia predisposes the patient to hyperkalemia. In patients with impaired renal function, the amount of glucose lost in the urine (glucosuria) is limited, so glycemic decompensation may also cause excessive hyperglycemia and predispose patients to hyperosmolar coma. Finally, catabolism and impaired infection control are common in patients with poor glycemic control.

As shown in Figure 7-2, Chinese authors documented that patients with type 2 diabetes who were treated with dialysis had substantially poorer survival when glycemic control was poor in the 6 months preceding the start of dialysis. In patients with diabetes who were undergoing dialysis, several other trials showed higher mortality in patients with higher HbA1c levels than in patients with good blood glucose control.

Does Presence of Advanced Diabetic Nephropathy Necessitate Changes in a Patient's Dietary Management?

In the patient with advanced diabetic nephropathy, the most important components of medical management are

- maintaining glycemic control
- maintaining blood pressure control

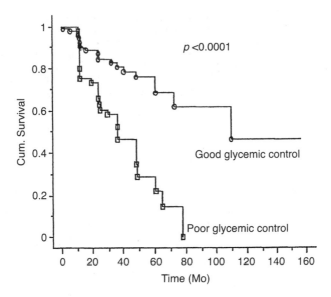

Figure 7-2. **Cumulative survival with hemodialysis therapy in Taiwanese patients with type 2 diabetes having good glycemic control (HbA1c 5% to 10%) and poor glycemic control (HbA1c >10%) in the 6 months preceding dialysis.** (From Wu MS, Yu CC, Yang CW, et al. Poor predialysis glycemic control is a predictor of mortality in type II diabetic patients on maintenance hemodialysis. *Nephrol Dial Transplant* 1997;12:2105–2110, with permission.)

- monitoring progression
- controlling dyslipidemia
- avoiding malnutrition

Maintaining Glycemic Control

When the GFR is reduced, the half-life of insulin is prolonged, because the renal and the extrarenal clearances of insulin are diminished. This relation holds for both endogenous insulin (e.g., released by sulfonylureas) and exogenous insulin (i.e., insulin injection). As a result, when the dosage of insulin is not adjusted, the patient with renal disease is at risk for developing hypoglycemia.

The propensity to develop hypoglycemia is modulated by additional factors. Patients with impaired renal function tend to be anorectic. A diminished diet predisposes patients to hypoglycemia. Anorexogenic factors are excreted in normal urine and, presumably, these factors accumulate in renal failure. Furthermore, the plasma concentration of leptin, an adipocyte hormone that reduces appetite, is increased in renal failure.

Most sulfonylurea compounds (or their active metabolites) accumulate in renal failure, with the exception of gliquidone and glimepiride. This accumulation is particularly pronounced for glibenclamid, which may cause prolonged episodes of hypoglycemia and necessitate prolonged infusion of large quantities of glucose. Some of the newer oral antihyperglycemic agents, for example, glinides and thiazolidiones, do not accumulate in renal failure, so no dosage adaptation is required.

On the other hand, the action of insulin is impaired in renal failure. Because of aggravated insulin resistance, the patient with diabetes and renal failure is prone to develop hyperglycemia. Insulin resistance is caused by low-molecular-weight, water-soluble substances that are removed by dialysis (subsequent text). In the individual patient, the net effect of the opposing tendencies to develop hypoglycemia or hyperglycemia cannot be safely predicted. Consequently, strict monitoring of glycemia is necessary in the patient with diabetes and renal failure.

Because of the risks associated with oral hypoglycemic agents, and to avoid catabolism, it is wise to be more liberal about the decision to begin insulin therapy. The use of insulin is indispensable in the patient with intercurrent disease, particularly infection or surgical intervention. One important factor that may render glycemic control particularly difficult is gastroparesis, the disturbance in gastric emptying as a result of autonomic polyneuropathy. Delayed transfer of food from the stomach to the intestine may make dietary management difficult. After the patient with diabetic gastroparesis has eaten, up to several hours may be required for the glucose derived from food items to enter the circulation.

When managing glycemia in patients with diabetes and advanced nephropathy, be aware that HbA1c levels may be artefactually increased and reflect not only glycation but also carbamylation of hemoglobin. If the patient is receiving erythropoietin, younger erythrocytes are in the circulation, and HbA1c concentrations will decrease, even though glycemic control is unchanged. This artefact results from the fact that such young erythrocytes are exposed to a hyperglycemic milieu for shorter periods of time.

Maintaining Blood Pressure Control

As stated in the preceding text, dietary salt restriction, use of diuretics, or both are the cornerstone of blood pressure control. However, being aware that antihypertensive agents can influence the control of glycemia and lipidemia is important (see Table 7-10).

A physician who recommends salt restriction and administers diuretics must also be aware that hypovolemia is undesirable. This complication can be recognized from the constellation of hypokalemia, metabolic alkalosis (elevated serum bicarbonate concentration), increased uric acid concentration, and a tendency for an acute rise of serum urea and creatinine concentrations. The patient also tends to have orthostatic hypotension.

Hypovolemia is particularly undesirable in patients with diabetes and left ventricular hypertrophy (because a stiff left ventricle requires a higher filling pressure) or the patient with diabetes and autonomic polyneuropathy, who has impaired vasoconstriction when blood pressure decreases.

Monitoring Progression

Accurately measuring the rate of GFR loss requires the use of marker substances that are not available in clinical practice.

Table 7-10. Adverse effects of common antihypertensive drugs in the diabetic patient

Betablocker (nonspecific > β_1-selective)	Decreased glucose tolerance "masking" of the symptoms of hypoglycemia delayed recovery from hypoglycemia dyslipidemia
Diuretics (thiazides > furosemide)	Dyslipidemia hyperglycemia via insulin resistance and diminished glucosuria
ACE inhibitors/Ang II receptor blockers	Hypoglycemia (greater insulin sensitivity)? Hyperkalemia increase in serum creatinine (in patients with hypovolemia, renal artery stenosis)
α receptor blocker	Orthostatic hypotension congestive heart failure

Usually physicians rely on serum creatinine or endogenous creatinine clearance. In individuals with low muscle mass, particularly elderly, wasted, diabetic women, the serum creatinine concentration may grossly underestimate GFR. The explanation is that creatinine is chiefly derived from conversion of creatine to creatinine in muscle, and a wasted individual with a low muscle mass will produce less creatinine.

After ingestion of cooked meat, serum creatinine level increases transiently, because prolonged cooking can increase the production of creatinine from creatine in muscle. Serum creatinine (SCR) levels tend to decrease when patients are given meat-free diets.

A good index of GFR is the endogenous creatinine clearance (CCR), which requires a 24-hour urine collection. Because 24-hour urine collections for measurement of CCR are tedious and error-prone, algorithms have been proposed to assess GFR; for example, the Cockroft–Gault formula

$$CCR = (140 - age) (wt \text{ in kg})/72 \times SCR \text{ (mg/100 mL)}$$

or the MDRD formula for GFR based on serum creatinine and patient characteristics.

The rate of urinary protein excretion is an important surrogate marker to monitor the progression of diabetic nephropathy. Monitoring proteinuria enables assessing the effect of therapeutic interventions to retard progression; for example, blood pressure lowering and glycemic control.

Controlling Dyslipidemia

Patients with advanced diabetic nephropathy tend to have more dyslipidemia. This condition is the combined result of renal failure yielding hypertriglyceridemia and accumulation of incompletely catabolized lipoprotein particles [e.g., intermediate-density lipoproteins (IDL)] and chylomicrons. Severe proteinuria aggravates dyslipidemia through mechanisms analogous to the ones operative in the nephrotic syndrome.

In principle, hypertriglyceridemia would respond well to fibrates. Most fibrates, with the exception of gemfibrozil, accumulate in patients with renal failure, exposing them to the risk of muscle necrosis (rhabodomyolysis). Statins do not accumulate because of renal failure, which makes them safer.

An important clinical observation is that medications that reduce proteinuria (e.g., ACE inhibitors), also tend to improve dyslipidemia, so that blood pressure control by ACE inhibitors (or ARBs) can have clinically important benefits for the lipid status.

Avoiding Malnutrition

The main issue in the patient with advanced diabetic nephropathy is avoiding malnutrition and wasting. For any given degree of renal failure, patients with diabetes tend to be more wasted than patients without diabetes. One important reason for this observation is that insulin is an anabolic hormone, so the absence of, or the resistance to, its effects diminishes synthesis of muscle protein and predisposes individuals to loss of muscle. Important confounding factors are anorexia (common in renal failure), gastroparesis, and catabolism during intercurrent illness or surgery and, particularly, during long periods of fasting (often during ill-advised efforts to reduce weight). Experimental studies showed that breakdown of muscle protein in the fasting state is considerably greater in uremic animals than in nonuremic animals, so the combination of uremia and diabetes is particularly disadvantageous.

The risk of a negative protein balance is aggravated if the patient with diabetes has high levels of proteinuria.

Against this background, one has to discuss the use of low-protein diets to retard progression. Such diets are not safe unless calorie intake is strictly maintained (patients tend to eat less rather than to eat less protein when they are not properly instructed and monitored). The occurrence of catabolism can be recognized by monitoring serum urea concentrations and urinary urea excretion rates, but the simple clinical examination of inspecting the patient and assessing his muscle mass is usually sufficient. Anthropometric measurements are rarely required for this purpose.

Biochemical markers such as serum albumin concentration and concentrations of complement factors may be misleading in renal failure. Notably, many patients with uremia have signs of "microinflammation," including increased concentrations of CRP (C-reactive protein) and SAA (serum amyloid A protein). As shown in Table 7-9 Stenvinkel proposed to differentiate between malnutrition caused by uremia per se and malnutrition resulting from microinflammation (see Chapters 8 and 11).

According to consensus, renal replacement therapy, that is, continuous ambulatory peritoneal dialysis (CAPD) or hemodialysis, should be started earlier in the patient with diabetes and uremia than in the patient with uremia who does not have diabetes. Timely start of dialysis is often necessary not because of symptoms of uremia but because of fluid overload, vomiting because of gastroparesis, recurrent episodes of left ventricular dysfunction with pulmonary edema, or wasting. In this stage of renal failure, the most important task is to avoid malnutrition.

Does Renal Replacement Therapy Affect a Patient's Dietary Management?

☞ Hemodialysis has the beneficial effect of removing substances that interfere with the action of insulin, so that sensitivity to endogenous or exogenous insulin increases. As a consequence, patients tend to be less hyperglycemic. On the other hand, hemodialysis removes hypothetical anorexigenic substances, so that appetite increases and patients gain weight, with an increase in lean body mass. This increase may cause glycemic control to deteriorate. The net effect is difficult to predict, and monitoring of glycemia and of HbA1c concentrations is necessary.

Dialysates most often contain glucose in concentrations ranging from 100 to 200 mg per dL. The dialyzed and very often anuric patient is at particular risk if glucose concentrations increase to very high levels, because this event can cause hypervolemia, thirst, and hyperkalemia, as discussed. Another consequence of hemodialysis is loss of amino acids, so the protein requirement is higher than in patients without uremia. A dietary intake of 1.2 g/kg b.w./day is commonly recommended (see Chapter 11).

For patients treated with CAPD, the dialysate contains glucose in concentrations ranging from 1,500 mg per dL to 4,000 mg per dL. This high concentration is used to remove excess fluids from the patient (see Chapter 12). However, the net uptake of glucose ranges from 100 g and more per day. Because these are excess calories, obesity is common among patients treated with CAPD. CAPD may offer a unique advantage to offset this problem, because insulin can be administered intraperitoneally to imitate the natural secretion of insulin into the portal circulation. This mode of administration of insulin is not consistently used, however, and most patients are on subcutaneous insulin.

For the patient with diabetes who has successfully received a combined pancreas and kidney transplant, reversing diabetes and restoring normal insulin secretion does not pose specific dietetic problems, with the exception of the advice that patients should avoid major weight gain. The patient with diabetes who has received a kidney graft has several hazards like higher infection rates and a higher cardiovascular morbidity and mortality in the long run. The patient without diabetes who is treated with steroids and calcineurin inhibitors (e.g., cyclosporin A or tacrolimus) has a long-term risk of developing type 2 diabetes that is as much as 30%. Major culprits are presumably genetic predisposition, weight gain, and, specifically in the case of tacrolimus, disturbance of insulin secretion. The latter effect is dose dependent.

SELECTED READINGS

American Diabetes Association. Nutrition principles and recommendations in diabetes. *Diabetes Care* 2004;27:S36–S46.

Brodsky I, Robbins DC, Hiser E, et al. Effects of low-protein diets on protein metabolism in insulin-dependent diabetes mellitus patients with early nephropathy. *J Clin Endocrinol Metab* 1992;75: 351–357.

DCCT Research Group. The effect of intensive treatment of diabetes on the development and progression of long-term complications in insulin-dependent diabetes mellitus. *N Engl J Med* 1993;329: 977–986.

Diabetes Prevention Program Research Group. Reduction in the incidence of type 2 diabetes with lifestyle intervention or metformin. *N Engl J Med* 2003;346:393–403.

Dullaart RPF, Beusekamp BJ, Meijer S, et al. Long-term effects of protein restricted diet on albuminuria and renal function in IDDM patients without clinical nephropathy and hypertension. *Diabetes Care* 1993;16:483–492.

Executive Summary of the Third Report of the National Cholesterol Education Program (NCEP). Expert panel on detection, evaluation, and treatment of high blood cholesterol in adults (Adult Treatment Panel III). *JAMA* 2001;285:2486–2497.

Franz MJ, Bantle JP, Beebe CA, et al. Evidence-based nutrition principles and recommendations for the treatment and prevention of diabetes and related complications (technical review). *Diabetes Care* 2002;25:148–198.

Freeman DJ, Norrie J, Sattar N, et al. Pravastatin and the development of diabetes mellitus. *Circulation* 2001;103:357–362.

Kasiske BL, Lakatua JD, Ma JZ, et al. A meta-analysis of the effects of dietary protein restriction on the rate of decline in renal function. *Am J Kidney Dis* 1998;31:954–961.

Klahr S, Levey AS, Beck GJ, et al. Modification of Diet in Renal Disease Study Group. The effects of dietary protein restriction and blood-pressure control on the progression of chronic renal disease. *N Engl J Med* 1994;330:877–884.

Nakao N, Yoshimura A, Morita H, et al. Combination treatment of angiotensin-II receptor blocker and angiotensin-converting-enzyme inhibitor in non-diabetic renal disease (COOPERATE): a randomized controlled trial. *Lancet* 2003;361:117–124.

Ohkubo Y, Kishikawa H, Araki E. Intensive insulin therapy prevents the progression of diabetic microvascular complications in Japanese patients with non-insulin-dependent diabetes mellitus: a randomized prospective 6-year study. *Diabetes Res* 1995;28: 103–117.

Ritz E, Orth SR. Nephropathy in patients with type 2 diabetes mellitus. *N Engl J Med* 1999;341:1127–1133.

Ritz E, Rychlik I, Locatelli F, et al. End-stage renal failure in type 2 diabetes: a medical catastrophe of worldwide dimensions. *Am J Kidney Dis* 1999;34:795–808.

Ruggenenti P, Schieppati A, Remuzzi G. Progression, remission, regression of chronic renal diseases. *Lancet* 2001;357:1601–1608.

Sacks FM, Svetkey LP, Vollmer WM, et al. Effects on blood pressure of reduced dietary sodium and the Dietary Approaches to Stop Hypertension (DASH) diet. *N Engl J Med* 2001;344:3–10.

Sato A, Hayashi K, Naruse M, et al. Effectiveness of aldosterone blockade in patients with diabetic nephropathy. *Hypertension* 2003;41:64–68.

Sheard NF, Nathaniel GC. The role of nutrition therapy in the management of diabetes mellitus. *Nutr Clin Care* 2000;6:334–348.

Stenvinkel P, Heimburger O, Lindholm B, et al. Are there two types of malnutrition in chronic renal failure? Evidence for relationships between malnutrition, inflammation and atherosclerosis (MIA syndrome). *Nephrol Dial Transplant* 2000;15:953–960.

Steppan CM, Bailey ST, Bhat S, et al. The hormone resistin links obesity to diabetes. *Nature* 2001;409:307–312.

Toeller M, Buyken A, Heitkamp G, et al, EURODIAB IDDM Complications Study Group. Protein intake and urinary albumin excretion rates in the EURODIAB IDDM complications study. *Diabetologia* 1997;40:1219–1226.

Tuomilehto J, Jousilahti P, Rastenyte D, et al. Urinary sodium excretion and cardiovascular mortality in Finland: a prospective study. *Lancet* 2001;357:848–851.

UK Prospective Diabetes Study (UKPDS) Group. Intensive blood-glucose control with sulphonylureas or insulin compared with conventional treatment and risk of complications in patients with type 2 diabetes (UKPDS 33). *Lancet* 1998;352:837–853.

Vedovato M, Coracina A, Mazzon C, et al. Impact of salt intake on 24hr-blood pressure and albuminuria in type 2 diabetes. Abstract on the 14th Annual Meeting of the European Diabetic Nephropathy Study Group. Redworth Hall, UK, 2001.

Walker JD, Dodds RA, Murrells TJ, et al. Restriction of dietary protein and progression of renal failure in diabetic nephropathy. *Lancet* 1989;2:1411–1415.

Wu MS, Yu CC, Yang CW, et al. Poor pre-dialysis glycemic control is a predictor of mortality in type II diabetic patients on maintenance hemodialysis. *Nephrol Dial Transplant* 1997;12:2105–2110.

Zeller K, Whittaker E, Sullivan L, et al. Effect of restricting dietary protein on the progression of renal failure with insulin-dependent diabetes mellitus. *N Engl J Med* 1991;324:78–84.

8

Nephrotic Syndrome: Nutritional Consequences and Dietary Management

Jane Y. Yeun and George A. Kaysen

Nephrotic syndrome results from urinary loss of albumin and other plasma proteins of similar size and is characterized by hypoalbuminemia, hyperlipidemia, and edema formation. Quantifying the loss of tissue protein in the urine is more difficult than quantifying the urinary loss of albumin and other plasma proteins. However, marked muscle wasting (sometimes obscured by edema) has been described in patients with continuous and massive proteinuria. Micronutrients such as vitamin D, iron, and zinc are bound to plasma proteins and are lost into the urine in nephrotic syndrome, making it possible for depletion syndromes to occur when proteinuria is massive and continuous. Not only does altered lipid metabolism in nephrotic syndrome result in hyperlipidemia, but it also may lead to progressive renal failure from interstitial fibrosis and to accelerated atherosclerosis.

The major rationales for changing a patient's diet, then, are to blunt manifestations of the syndrome (such as edema and hyperlipidemia), to replace nutrients lost in the urine, and to reduce risks for progressive renal disease and atherosclerosis. Rarely, specific allergens in food may cause renal disease in some patients, and dietary modification might be curative.

DIETARY PROTEIN

Metabolic abnormalities in nephrotic syndrome include depletion of plasma and tissue protein pools. Superficially, nephrotic syndrome resembles protein–calorie malnutrition (i.e., kwashiorkor). In both cases, the plasma albumin concentration is reduced, plasma volume is expanded, and albumin pools shift from the extravascular to the vascular compartment. In protein–calorie malnutrition, providing the needed protein and calories will correct all of the manifestations of malnutrition, whereas this is not the case in nephrotic syndrome.

In patients with nephrotic syndrome, the main causes of hypoalbuminemia are albumin loss in the urine, an inappropriate increase in the fractional catabolic rate of albumin, and an insufficient increase in the synthesis rate of albumin to replace the loss. Although average values for urinary protein losses are approximately 6 to 8 g per day (the amount contained in a hen's egg), simply increasing dietary protein is of little demonstrable benefit. Dietary protein supplementation causes an increase in the defect in the filtration barrier of the glomerular capillary when compared to low-protein diets and results in increased urinary protein losses (see Fig. 8-1). Dietary protein restriction, in contrast, reduces urinary protein excretion, decreases protein degradation

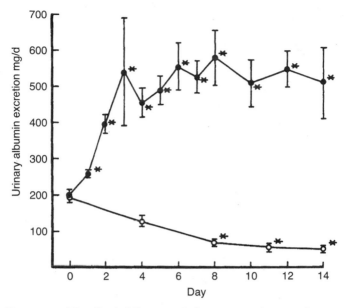

Figure 8-1. The effect of dietary protein augmentation on urinary albumin excretion (UAE) in rats with nephrotic syndrome. Nephrotic syndrome was induced by injection of anti-FX 1A antibody to produce passive Heymann nephritis. Twenty-eight rats were initially fed a diet containing 8.5% protein as sodium caseinate. On day 0, 15 animals had dietary protein increased to 40% casein (solid circles), and 13 animals remained on the 8.5% casein diet (open circles). Urinary albumin excretion increased significantly in the animals fed a high-protein diet by the second day and remained significantly greater thereafter, whereas urinary albumin excretion decreased in the low-protein diet by day 8. *p <0.05 versus time 0.

and amino acid oxidation, maintains nitrogen balance, and may have a salutary effect on the rate of progression of renal disease.

Reducing urinary protein excretion is desirable for several reasons. In addition to its effect on protein metabolism, reducing urinary protein excretion also reduces the blood lipid level, because the degree of hyperlipidemia varies directly with urinary protein losses. Proteinuria itself is thought to damage the renal interstitium directly through a variety of putative mechanisms. Filtered proteins are reabsorbed by the tubule and carry iron, complement components, and biologically active lipids into the interstitial space. Once lipids reach the interstitial space, they may act as chemoattractants for monocytes and cause renal injury. Reabsorbed iron from proteinuria is biologically active and may act as an oxidant to injure the kidney. Diets that are high in protein also are high in acid content, leading to acidosis and resulting in increased ammoniagenesis in the kidney. The accelerated rates of renal ammonia production also may lead to renal injury. The reduction in urinary protein excretion that follows the initiation of a low-protein diet can have a potentially salutary effect on progressive renal injury through any or all of these mechanisms (see Table 8-1).

Table 8-1.   Benefits of reducing proteinuria

Increases serum albumin levels
Decreases serum lipid levels
Retards progression of renal failure and interstitial fibrosis
    Decreases tubular exposure to complement factors
    Decreases tubular exposure to iron
    Decreases tubular exposure to oxidized lipids
    Decreases exposure to growth factors that cause maladaptive renal
        hypertrophy
Improves edema
    Improves renal response to atrial natriuretic factor
Preserves growth in children

Several studies have suggested that the composition of proteins in the diet may be as important as its absolute nitrogen content. In experimental studies in rats, dietary augmentation with some amino acids caused a prompt increase in urinary albumin excretion (UAE), whereas branched-chain amino acid supplementation did not affect proteinuria. Studies in animal models of nephrotic syndrome and in humans with renal disease also suggested that specific types of dietary proteins may be of particular importance. When patients with nephrotic syndrome were fed a vegetarian soy diet, urinary protein excretion decreased, as did blood lipid levels. In rats with puromycin-induced nephrotic syndrome, not only did a 20% soy protein diet lower proteinuria and blood lipid levels, but it also improved the creatinine clearance and decreased glomerular sclerosis and reduced the level of proinflammatory cytokines in the kidney. Because the soy protein diet was low in fat (28% of calories) and protein (0.71 g per kg ideal body weight), distinguishing whether the beneficial effects of a soy-based diet in patients with nephrotic syndrome are from the amino acid composition alone, or from the lower fat and protein content, is difficult. Studies of nephrotic rats suggested, however, that much of the benefit of a soy-based diet derived from a direct effect of soy proteins on the kidney (possibly through reducing the degree of nitrotyrosine formation), rather than through changes in hepatic lipid metabolism. Curiously, little difference was observed in effects on urinary protein excretion between diets containing 1.1 and those containing 0.7 g soy protein/kg/d.

More recent animal studies suggest that a flaxseed-based protein diet may offer even more benefit than soy protein. Velasquez et al. studied the effects of 20% casein, 20% soy protein, or 20% flaxseed meal on a rat model of diabetic nephropathy, using the obese spontaneously hypertensive rat developed by the National Institute of Health (NIH). Flaxseed meal reduced proteinuria and glomerular and tubulointerstitial injury more than a casein- or soy protein–based diet, although creatinine clearance and plasma creatinine levels did not differ. The common pathway for the beneficial effects of plant-protein diets may be the phytoestrogens, present in soybeans as isoflavones and in flaxseed as lignans. These compounds are estrogen-like and may exert their effects through binding to the estrogen receptor; however, much work remains to be done in this area.

In human studies, concomitant use of an angiotensin-converting enzyme (ACE) inhibitor with a high-protein diet (1.3 to 1.6 g protein/kg/d) prevented the diet-induced increase in urinary protein excretion. Serum protein and albumin levels increased significantly in eight patients after they crossed over to the high-protein diet with ACE inhibitor, compared with a mildly protein-restricted diet (0.8 g per day). The use of ACE inhibitor or angiotensin receptor blocker (ARB) in patients with normal to moderately restricted protein intake (0.8 g per day) also lowered levels of proteinuria, triglycerides, total cholesterol, and low-density lipoprotein (LDL) cholesterol.

Nephrotic syndrome is characterized by high levels of protein in the urine (proteinuria), but a much larger number of patients have low levels of urinary albumin loss (microalbuminuria) Microalbuminuria is found in hypertensive and diabetic subjects and predicts progression of renal disease and cardiovascular risk in both populations. The amount of dietary protein, measured as a fraction of total calorie intake, is related to the level of risk for UAE in hypertensive diabetic subjects. Restriction of total protein intake reduces UAE in both noninsulin-dependent and insulin-dependent diabetic subjects. The type of protein consumed also has an effect on UAE in diabetic subjects, suggesting that either the amino acid composition or the lipid composition of the food ingested contributes to the effect of a protein-rich meal.

Recommendations

Because urinary protein excretion varies from day to day in individual patients, we collect three separate 24-hour urine specimens, with simultaneous measurements of serum albumin and protein, to establish baseline values. Patients are then placed on a 35-kcal per kg diet that contains 0.8 to 1.0 g protein per kg and is restricted to 2 g of sodium. We then monitor 24-hour urinary urea excretion every 2 to 3 months to ensure that patients are not eating more (or less) protein than recommended. The goal is to decrease proteinuria without reducing serum albumin and protein concentration. This goal is usually attainable when dietary protein intake is restricted to these levels (see Table 8-2).

Dietary protein intake can be estimated because, in steady state, it is equal to protein catabolic rate (PCR). If total body urea pools do not change during the 24-hour period [blood urea nitrogen (BUN) and weight are stable], estimating the amount of protein ingested is possible by the formula.

PCR = [10.7 + 24-hour urine urea nitrogen excretion/0.14] g/d
      + 24-hour urine protein excretion

For example, if urinary urea nitrogen excretion is 6 g nitrogen per day and the patient is in steady state, then protein intake is equal to PCR, or 53.6 g per day plus urinary protein excretion. If the prescribed diet varies, an accurate nutritional history should be obtained and the diet adjusted accordingly.

Although "high-quality" protein (meat and dairy products) is usually recommended, vegetarian diets based on soy protein are more effective in reducing urinary protein loss, increasing serum protein levels, correcting hyperlipidemia, and reducing renal inflammation and fibrosis. Consequently, we recommend soy-based

Table 8-2. Dietary recommendations in nephrotic syndrome

Calorie	35 kcal/kg/d
Protein	0.8–1.0 g/kg/d
	Soy protein may be more beneficial than "high-quality protein"
Fat	<30% of total calories
	Cholesterol <200 mg/d
	Higher proportion of polyunsaturated fatty acids (10% of energy)
	Fish oil may be beneficial for IgA nephropathy (12 g/d)
Minerals	<2 g Na
	Iron only when clearly iron deficient
	Calcium, if vitamin D deficient (2 g/d)
Vitamins	1,25-$(OH)_2$-vitamin D, if vitamin D deficient

IgA, immunoglobulin A.

protein in the diet. A plant-based diet may be even more useful in preventing diabetes and the development of diabetic renal disease, in ameliorating the progression of diabetic nephropathy, and in preventing obesity-related kidney diseases.

An ACE inhibitor or ARB should be used concomitantly to prevent excessive dietary protein restriction.

LIPIDS

Several lipid and biochemical abnormalities occur in nephrotic syndrome (see Table 8-3). In the patient without renal disease, the same abnormalities are associated with accelerated atherosclerosis. Although patients with nephrotic syndrome have not been shown definitively to be at increased risk for developing accelerated atherosclerosis, this is most likely the case.

One hallmark of nephrotic syndrome is hyperlipidemia, characterized by high serum levels of total cholesterol and triglycerides, mostly in the LDL, very–low-density lipoprotein (VLDL), and intermediate-density lipoprotein (IDL) fractions. Clearances of triglycerides, VLDL, and IDL are decreased because of (a) reduced lipoprotein lipase (the enzyme responsible for the metabolism of lipoproteins) on the vascular endothelium in the setting

Table 8-3. Proatherogenic factors in nephrotic syndrome

High cholesterol	Increased low-density lipoprotein
	Increased very–low-density lipoprotein
	Increased intermediate-density lipoprotein
	Normal to low high-density lipoprotein
Altered high-density lipoprotein structure	
High lipoprotein(a)	
High triglycerides	
Increased fibrinogen	

of hypoalbuminemia, and (b) a proteinuria-induced alteration in the structure of the lipoproteins. Thus, reducing proteinuria would be expected to reduce the levels of these lipoproteins, independent of the effect on albumin concentration. LDL synthesis is increased but does not correlate with serum albumin levels, suggesting that LDL synthesis is not driven by a general increase in protein synthesis in the liver. The high-density lipoprotein (HDL) cholesterol levels are either unaffected or are reduced, leading to an increased ratio of LDL/HDL cholesterol. In addition, maturation of HDL is impaired, resulting in smaller HDL moieties that are more atherogenic.

Plasma lipoprotein(a) [Lp(a)] levels also are increased in patients with nephrotic syndrome. The concentration of plasma Lp(a) is genetically determined in patients without kidney disease and largely depends on the specific isoform of the apolipoprotein(a) moiety synthesized by the liver. In patients with nephrotic syndrome, plasma Lp(a) levels are increased, regardless of the isoform, as are plasma fibrinogen levels. The increased levels of both are associated with atherosclerosis and are high because of increased hepatic synthesis. As with lipids, the plasma Lp(a) and fibrinogen levels decrease when proteinuria abates.

In experimental animals with renal disease, elevated lipid levels alone can induce severe and progressive renal injury, and reducing plasma lipid levels favorably alters the course of the renal damage. Even though the influence of hyperlipidemia on the progression of renal disease in humans is less certain, evidence exists that lipids play a role in human renal disease.

First, hereditary lecithin cholesterol acyl transferase (LCAT) deficiency may be linked to progressive mesangial and glomerular sclerosis. Patients with lipoprotein glomerulopathy, presumably from an inherited abnormality in apolipoprotein E, develop nephrotic syndrome, progressive renal failure, and glomerular lipoprotein thrombi. Second, exposing human proximal tubular cells to albumin-bound fatty acids results in apoptosis. Third, hypercholesterolemia is an independent risk factor for progression of renal disease in insulin-dependent diabetic patients and predicts the onset of microalbuminuria. Fourth, several small observational clinical studies showed that treating patients with nephrotic syndrome with a cholesterol-lowering agent [a 3-hydroxy-3-methyl-glutaryl-coenzyme A (HMG CoA) reductase inhibitor or statin] lowered urinary protein excretion and increased serum albumin levels compared with baseline values but had no effect on serum creatinine levels. The largest of these studies randomly allocated 43 patients with nephrotic syndrome to usual therapy or to usual therapy plus fluvastatin. After 1 year of follow-up, total cholesterol, LDL, and triglyceride levels had decreased significantly in the fluvastatin group. Urinary protein excretion decreased, serum albumin levels increased, and creatinine clearance was greater in the statin group. Results of biopsy showed less interstitial fibrosis and significantly less renal fat deposits in the fluvastatin group, although the degree of glomerular sclerosis was not different. Fifth, several case reports and small case series reported that selective removal of LDL with apheresis reduced LDL and Lp(a) levels, increased serum albumin level, and ameliorated the proteinuria or caused remission of proteinuria in patients with nephrotic syndrome. Although these studies were prospective, none was randomized or blinded. In addition, these studies were too brief to allow a meaningful assessment of the effects of treating hyperlipidemia on ultimate renal outcome (death or dialysis), although a reduction in urinary protein excretion is a reasonable surrogate for an improved outcome. Finally, a recent study found elevated levels of lipid peroxidation products in the glomeruli of patients with congenital nephrotic syndrome of the Finnish type, associated with down-regulation of antioxidant systems in the kidney.

Therefore, reversing the changes in plasma lipid levels and biochemical composition is desirable in patients with nephrotic syndrome, (a) to reduce the risk for cardiovascular disease and (b) to retard the progression of renal injury. Consequently, efforts should be made to reduce high plasma lipid levels, both by nutritional and by pharmacologic means, in patients anticipated to have a prolonged nephrotic syndrome. If the underlying disease can be easily treated (e.g., minimal change disease), the primary goal should be to reduce plasma lipid levels. Although no basis exists for providing lipid-lowering drugs to patients with nephrotic syndrome who have a normal lipid profile, those with nephrotic syndrome who have elevated LDL cholesterol and reduced HDL cholesterol levels should be treated.

As with protein intake, the types of lipids ingested may be important. Lipids include compounds such as prostaglandins (PGs) and leukotrienes, important regulators of vascular resistance. These compounds are products of the metabolism of polyunsaturated fatty acids (PUFAs), which are not synthesized by mammals and are available only through the diet. Thus, dietary supplementation with specific PUFAs could affect the levels of these important vasoactive compounds. Lipids derived from marine sources are rich in ω-3 PUFAs (e.g., eicosapentaenoic acid), whereas those derived from vegetable oils are rich in ω-6 PUFAs (e.g., arachidonic acid). Eicosapentaenoic acid competes with arachidonic acid as a substrate for cyclooxygenase and lipoxygenase.

Cyclooxygenase converts arachidonic acid and eicosapentaenoic acid to the diene [e.g., prostaglandin I2 (PGI2), thromboxane (TX)A$_2$] and triene metabolites (e.g., PGI$_3$ and TXA$_3$), respectively. TXA$_2$ is a potent vasoconstrictor, whereas TXA$_3$ is biologically inert. In contrast, the vasodilators PGI$_2$ and PGI$_3$ are equipotent. Alterations in the generation of both vasodilatory prostaglandins (PGE$_2$, PGI$_2$) and vasoconstricting cyclooxygenase metabolites (TXA$_2$) can occur during renal injury or during a physiologic stress, such as plasma volume contraction.

Lipoxygenase converts arachidonic acid and eicosapentaenoic acid to the four and five series of leukotrienes, which also can cause vasoconstriction or vasodilatation. Although changes in eicosanoid metabolism may support the glomerular filtration rate during adaptation to renal injury or plasma volume contraction, these changes also may play a pathogenic role. Because of the differences in the biologic activity of their vasoconstrictive and vasodilative metabolites, substituting eicosapentaenoic acid for arachidonic acid in the diet may alter the expression of renal injury.

The use of specific PUFAs has been shown to alter the course of renal injury and to reduce blood lipid levels in experimental animals. In human studies, the results are equivocal. Low doses of fish oil (5 g per day) added to a vegetarian soy diet, given to patients with nephrotic syndrome, had no added beneficial effect on either proteinuria or blood lipid levels compared with the soy diet alone. Higher doses of fish oil (15 g per day) for subjects given an unrestricted diet caused a decrease in levels of plasma total triglycerides and LDL triglycerides and an increase in LDL cholesterol levels. Donadio et al. treated 55 patients with immunoglobulin A (IgA) nephropathy with 12 g of fish oil per day in a prospective, randomized, placebo-controlled study and found a significant reduction in the rate of progression of renal disease. At the end of the treatment period, the fish oil–treated group had a lower prevalence of hypertension, a slower increase in serum creatinine levels, and fewer cases of nephrotic-range proteinuria.

Recommendations

Dietary fat restriction has been shown to be partially effective in reducing blood lipid levels in patients with nephrotic syndrome. Diets low in fat (less than 30% of total calories) and cholesterol (less than 200 mg per day) and rich in polyunsaturated fatty acids and in linoleic acid (10% of energy) can reduce blood lipid levels (Table 8-2).

If the serum total cholesterol level remains elevated (more than 200 mg per dL) after dietary lipid restriction and attempts to minimize urinary protein excretion, then pharmacologic therapy should be instituted. Giving fish oil supplements can be beneficial for patients with IgA nephropathy (Table 8-2).

ANTIOXIDANTS

Oxidized lipoproteins are known to cause progressive atherosclerosis and are postulated to cause progressive renal failure through glomerular and interstitial damage. In animal studies, clear evidence exists that reducing the lipid levels or administering dietary antioxidants such as selenium and vitamin E reduces the proteinuria and hypoalbuminemia, retards progression of renal failure, and variably ameliorates the renal pathology. However, in humans, no definitive benefit has been shown.

Recommendations

Given the paucity of data in humans, selenium and vitamin E supplementation is not recommended.

SALT AND WATER

Edema formation is one of the most bothersome symptoms of nephrotic syndrome and frequently brings the patient to the attention of the nephrologist. Edema results from pathologic retention of salt and water.

The classic model of edema formation in nephrotic syndrome proposes that the lower plasma albumin concentration decreases the difference between the interstitial and plasma oncotic pressure ($\Delta\pi$) and favors fluid shifts from plasma to the interstitium. Ultimately, plasma volume contracts. Edema occurs when the amount of fluid entering the interstitium exceeds maximal lymph flow, further decreasing circulatory volume. The plasma volume contraction then activates the renin–angiotensin–aldosterone axis and causes secondary renal sodium retention. Because plasma volume contraction also increases vasopressin release, water is retained, leading to hyponatremia (as seen in other edema-forming states such as congestive heart failure and liver disease). Recent data suggest that low oncotic pressure is a less common mechanism for edema formation in nephrotic syndrome and occurs only when serum albumin levels are less than 1.5 to 2.0 g per dL. When "underfilling" is present, dietary sodium restriction and amelioration of the hypoalbuminemia may play an important role in managing edema in patients with nephrotic syndrome.

A second and more important mechanism proposed for edema formation is the reduced ability of the patients with nephrotic syndrome to excrete a sodium load in response to either plasma volume expansion or atrial natriuretic peptide (ANP). Experimentally, this problem appears to be intrinsic to the nephrotic kidney and unrelated to changes in circulating blood volume. For example, the normal increase in urinary cyclic guanosine monophosphate during saline infusion is blunted in nephrotic rats because of increased phosphodiesterase activity in the inner medullary collecting duct cells. The increase in phosphodiesterase activity accelerates the hydrolysis of cyclic guanosine monophosphate, the effector of ANP, thereby reducing the response of the kidney to ANP. The reduced ability of the proteinuric kidney to excrete sodium leads to salt retention and edema. Consequently, hydrostatic pressure increases in the systemic capillary bed, even though defense mechanisms to counteract edema formation (such as increased lymphatic flow and decreased interstitial protein concentration) have already been activated. Thus, the effective plasma volume may not be reduced, unlike that in liver disease. Diuretics and restriction of dietary sodium chloride are effective in treating edema. Recent data in humans suggest that renal production of natriuretic peptide is increased in nephrotic syndrome and that a low-protein diet ameliorates its rise. However, whether these findings translate into a direct effect on avid renal sodium and water retention is not clear.

Recommendations

A low-sodium (2 g per day) diet is recommended. Patients with hyponatremia should be restricted to less than 1 L of fluid per day. Concomitant diuretic use is usually necessary.

VITAMIN D

Hypocalcemia, including a reduced serum ionized calcium level and a total calcium level, is common in patients with nephrotic syndrome. Hypocalcemia does not result entirely from a reduced fraction of calcium bound to albumin. Plasma levels of vitamin D are reduced, and the degree of this abnormality correlates inversely with UAE and directly with plasma albumin. Hypovitaminosis D is not the result of a loss of functioning renal mass, because plasma vitamin D levels also are low in patients with nephrotic syndrome who have normal renal function. Synthesis of vitamin D by the proximal nephron can be impaired in some experimental models of nephrotic syndrome in the rat. How or whether this applies to patients with nephrotic syndrome is unknown. Vitamin D–binding protein is a 52 kDa protein and a member of the albumin supergene family. The protein is lost into the urine of patients with nephrotic syndrome, and vitamin D levels normalize when proteinuria resolves. Whether the synthesis of vitamin D–binding protein increases in response to its urinary loss or is modulated by changes in dietary protein is unknown. Labeled vitamin D administered to subjects with nephrotic syndrome appears rapidly in their urine, suggesting that vitamin D loss, presumably by loss of its binding protein, is the cause of hypovitaminosis D.

The clinical significance of hypovitaminosis D is controversial. Some investigators find that although total 1,25-dihydroxyvitamin D is reduced, free vitamin D is not. However, serum parathyroid levels are often increased in relation to the level of ionized calcium and vitamin D, suggesting functional hypovitaminosis D. Patients with nephrotic syndrome malabsorb calcium, a defect that can be corrected by exogenously administered vitamin D. Hypovitaminosis D in patients with nephrotic syndrome can cause rickets, especially in children. Unlike many of the other manifestations of nephrotic syndrome, hypovitaminosis D can be treated with replacement therapy.

Recommendations

Measure the plasma parathyroid hormone level. If the level is high, treat with 1,25-dihydroxyvitamin D and calcium supplements. Alternatively, plasma free 1,25-dihydroxyvitamin D level can be measured (see Chapter 3).

IRON

Although urinary iron losses in transferrin increase, the anemia is more likely to be caused by decreased levels of erythropoietin than by decreased levels of iron. Unless unequivocal evidence of iron deficiency exists, do not administer iron, because filtered transferrin releases iron in the renal tubule, especially when urine pH is lower than 6. The renal tubular cells may reabsorb the released iron, causing or contributing to renal injury and interstitial fibrosis.

Recommendations

Anemia associated with nephrotic syndrome should not be assumed to be a consequence of iron deficiency. Iron should not be administered unless iron deficiency is documented.

ZINC AND COPPER

The most important zinc-binding protein is albumin, and urinary zinc losses can be substantial in nephrotic syndrome. Documented zinc deficiency, however, is probably a consequence of both reduced absorption and urinary loss of zinc. The effect of proteinuria on zinc metabolism has been largely ignored. The extent to which zinc depletion plays a role in the clinical manifestations of nephrotic syndrome is not known.

Copper, like iron, is also bound to ceruloplasmin, a circulating plasma protein. Although the urinary loss of this 151-kDa protein may cause a decrease in blood copper levels, no clinically recognized manifestations result.

Recommendations

If zinc deficiency is documented, oral replacement is indicated.

CONCLUSION AND SAMPLE DIETS

In summary, the loss of protein in patients with nephrotic syndrome could result directly or indirectly in a compromised nutritional status, accelerated atherosclerosis, progressive renal injury, and excessive losses of several ions, trace elements, and vitamins. Because the urinary protein loss is responsible for many of the manifestations and complications of nephrotic syndrome, maneuvers to decrease urinary protein losses are very important. Mildly restricting protein to 0.8 to 1.0 g/kg/d, eating a soy vegetarian diet, restricting fat intake to less than 30% of calories, and increasing the proportion of polyunsaturated fatty acids, in conjunction with using ACE inhibitors, ARBs, or both, are the mainstays of therapy. Sodium restriction and diuretic use are crucial in treating edema. Although trace elements and vitamins also may be lost in the urine, the importance of these losses to the clinical manifestations of nephrotic syndrome is not established. Given the potential harmful effects of replacement, especially iron, routine supplementation is not recommended. If a specific deficit is documented, replacement therapy is appropriate. The principal effects of dietary manipulation in nephrotic syndrome are summarized in Table 8-4. These concepts are particularly important in the pediatric population, because growth in children with steroid-resistant nephrotic syndrome seems to depend on the preservation of renal function, the cumulative dose of steroids, and the severity of hypoalbuminemia.

The following suggested diets are a 2-day diet using a high-quality protein source and a 2-day diet using a vegetarian soy

Table 8-4. Beneficial effects of dietary restrictions on the expression of nephrotic syndrome

Type of Restriction	Effects
Protein	Reduces proteinuria
	Increases serum albumin levels
	Decreases hyperfiltration
	Decreases tubular exposure to complement, iron, other toxins
	Retards the rate of progression of renal disease
Lipid	Decreases tubular exposure to oxidized lipids
	Decreases risk for atherosclerosis
	Retards the rate of progression of renal disease
Sodium	Reduces edema
	Optimizes diuretic effect
Water	Corrects hyponatremia

protein source for a 65-kg man who participates in moderate physical activity. We have made no adjustment for urinary protein losses and generally have not advised adjustment for urinary protein losses. The amounts of food may be adjusted for patients of different weights.

Nonvegetarian High-quality Protein

DAY 1

Breakfast

> 2 waffles, plain (4 tbsp fat-free Cool Whip, 1/2 cup frozen strawberries)
> 1/2 cup low-fat yogurt, plain
> 6 oz apple juice

Lunch

> 1 chicken-salad sandwich (2 oz chicken salad, 1 tbsp mayonnaise, 2 slices whole wheat bread)
> 1 cup romaine lettuce, shredded (2 tbsp oil-and-vinegar dressing)
> 1 blueberry muffin
> 1 cup 1% milk

Dinner

> 3 oz. lean roast beef (cooked with 1/8 tsp salt)
> 1/2 cup mashed potatoes (1 tsp margarine)
> 1/2 cup broccoli, seasoned
> 2 dinner rolls (2 tsp margarine)
> 1 orange
> 1 cup tea/coffee (2 tsp sugar)

DAY 2

Breakfast

> 1/4 cup Egg Beaters (1 tsp vegetable oil)
> 1 cup oatmeal (2 tsp sugar)
> 1 slice whole wheat toast (1 tsp jelly)
> 1 cup 1% milk

Lunch

> 1 tuna sandwich (2 oz tuna, 1 tsp mayonnaise, 2 slices whole wheat bread)
> 4 carrot sticks
> 1 apple
> 4 graham crackers
> 1 cup tea/coffee (2 tsp sugar)

Dinner

> 3 oz baked chicken, seasoned (cooked with 1/8 tsp salt)
> 1/2 cup rice
> 1/2 cup boiled cabbage
> 1/2 cup corn
> 1/12 angel-food cake
> 6 oz grape juice

Strict Vegetarian Soy Diet

DAY 1

Breakfast

2 oz tofu scramble
1 cup oatmeal (2 tsp sugar)
1/2 English muffin (2 tsp jelly)
1 medium orange
1 cup soy milk

Lunch

1 tempeh burger (soy product, 1/4 cup tempeh, 1 hamburger bun, 1 tbsp mayonnaise)
1/2 cup baked beans, homemade (1/2 tsp salt)
1/2 cup applesauce
1 cup grape juice

Dinner

8 oz soy spaghetti
2 oz soy cheese
4 oz fruit salad
1 medium baked potato (1 tbsp margarine)
Tea/coffee (nondairy creamer, 2 tsp sugar)

DAY 2

Breakfast

1/2 cup soy sausage
2 pancakes (4 tbsp syrup)
1/2 cup applesauce
6 oz orange juice

Lunch

3 oz soy bologna (2 slices whole wheat bread, 1 tbsp mayonnaise)
1/2 cup corn
1/2 cup carrot/raisin salad (2 tsp mayonnaise, 1 tsp sour cream substitute)

Dinner

6 oz tofu stir-fry
1 cup mixed vegetables (1/2 cup broccoli, 1/2 cup cauliflower, 1 tsp oil, 1/8 tsp salt)
1/2 cup stewed potatoes (1/8 tsp salt)
1 cup soy milk
2 oatmeal raisin cookies

Soy Products

BREAKFAST

Soy milk (8 oz)
Protein = 7 g
Fat = 5 g

Na = 40 mg
Carbohydrate = 5 g
Tempeh (soy bacon)
Soy sausage (per serving)
Protein = 9 g
Fat = 0 g
Na = 240 mg
Carbohydrate = 8 g
Soy pancake mix
Tofu scramble

LUNCH

Soy bologna (per serving)
Protein = 14 g
Fat = 0 g
Na = 335 mg
Carbohydrate = 8 g

DINNER

Tofu stir fry (3 oz.)
Protein = 5 g
Fat = 1 g
Na = 70 mg
Carbohydrate = 19 g

SELECTED READINGS

Alfrey AC. Role of iron and oxygen radicals in the progression of chronic renal failure. *Am J Kidney Dis* 1994;23:183–187.

Arici M, Chana R, Lewington A, et al. Stimulation of proximal tubular cell apoptosis by albumin-bound fatty acids mediated by peroxisome proliferators activated receptor-gamma. *J Am Soc Nephrol* 2003;14(1):17–27.

Azadbakht L, Shakerhosseini R, Atabak S, et al. Beneficiary effect of dietary soy protein on lowering plasma levels of lipid and improving kidney function in type II diabetes with nephropathy. *Eur J Clin Nutr* 2003;57(10):1292–1294.

Cataliotti A, Giordano M, De Pascale E, et al. CNP production in the kidney and effects of protein intake restriction in nephrotic syndrome. *Am J Physiol Renal Physiol* 2002;283(3):F464–F472.

D'Amico G, Gentile MG, Manna G, et al. Effect of vegetarian soy diet on hyperlipidemia in nephrotic syndrome. *Lancet* 1992;-339:1131–1134.

Don BR, Kaysen GA, Hutchison FN, et al. The effect of angiotensin-converting enzyme inhibition and dietary protein restriction in the treatment of proteinuria. *Am J Kidney Dis* 1991;17:10–17.

Donadio JV Jr, Bergstralh EJ, Offord KP, et al. A controlled trial of fish oil in IgA nephropathy. *N Engl J Med* 1994;331:1194–1199.

Garini G, Mazzi A, Allegri L, et al. Effectiveness of dietary protein augmentation associated with angiotensin-converting enzyme inhibition in the management of the nephrotic syndrome. *Miner Electrol Metab* 1996;22:123–127.

Gentile MG, Fellin G, Cofano F, et al. Treatment of proteinuric patients with a vegetarian soy diet and fish oil. *Clin Nephrol* 1993;40:315–320.

Gross JL, Zelmanovitz T, Moulin CC, et al. Effect of a chicken-based diet on renal function and lipid profile in patients with type 2 diabetes. *Diabetes Care* 2002;25:645–651.

Hansen HP, Christensen PK, Tauber-Lassen E, et al. Low-protein diet and kidney function in insulin-dependent diabetic patients with diabetic nephropathy. *Kidney Int* 1999;55(2):621–628.

Harris RC, Ismail N. Extrarenal complications of the nephrotic syndrome. *Am J Kidney Dis* 1994;23:477–497.

Jenkins DJ, Kendall CW, Marchie A, et al. Type 2 diabetes and the vegetarian diet. *Am J Clin Nutr* 2003;78(Suppl. 3):610S–616S.

Kaysen GA. Albumin turnover in renal disease. *Miner Electrol Metab* 1998;24:55–63.

Kaysen GA, de Sain-van der Velden MG. New insights into lipid metabolism in the nephrotic syndrome. *Kidney Int Suppl* 1999;71:S18–S21.

Keane WF. Proteinuria: its clinical importance and role in progressive renal disease. *Am J Kidney Dis* 2000;35(Suppl. 1):S97–S105.

Levey AS, Greene T, Beck GJ, et al. Dietary protein restriction and the progression of chronic renal disease: what have all of the results of the MDRD study shown? Modification of diet in renal disease study group. *J Am Soc Nephrol* 1999;10(11):2426–2439.

Lim VS, Wolfson M, Yarasheski KE, et al. Leucine turnover in patients with nephrotic syndrome: evidence suggesting body protein conservation. *J Am Soc Nephrol* 1998;9:1067–1073.

Maddox DA, Alavi FK, Silbernick EM, et al. Protective effects of a soy diet in preventing obesity-linked renal disease. *Kidney Int* 2002;61(1):96–104.

Mittal SK, Dash SC, Tiwari SC, et al. Bone histology in patients with nephrotic syndrome and normal renal function. *Kidney Int* 1999;55(5):1912–1919.

Mollsten AV, Dahlquist GG, Stattin EL, et al. Higher intakes of fish protein are related to a lower risk of microalbuminuria in young Swedish type 1 diabetic patients. *Diabetes Care* 2001;24:805–810.

Neverov NI, Kaysen GA, Tareyeva IE. Effect of lipid-lowering therapy on the progression of renal disease in nondiabetic nephrotic patients. *Contrib Nephrol* 1997;120:68–78.

Pedraza-Chaverri J, Barrera D, Hernandez-Pando R, et al. Soy protein diet ameliorates renal nitrotyrosine formation and chronic nephropathy induced by puromycin aminonucleoside. *Life Sci* 2004;74(8):987–999.

Pijls LTJ, de Vries H, Donker AJM, et al. The effect of protein restriction on albuminuria in patients with type 2 diabetes mellitus: a randomized trial. *Nephrol Dial Transplant* 1999;14:1445–1453.

Rodrigo R, Bravo I, Pino M. Proteinuria and albumin homeostasis in the nephrotic syndrome: effect of dietary protein intake. *Nutr Rev* 1996;54:337–347.

Ruggenenti P, Mise N, Pisoni R, et al. Diverse effects of increasing lisinorpil doses on lipid abnormalities in chronic nephropathies. *Circulation* 2003;107(4):586–592.

Samuels R, Mani UV, Iyer UM, et al. Hypocholesterolemic effect of spirulina in patients with hyperlipidemic nephrotic syndrome. *J Med Food* 2002;5(2):91–96.

Scharer K, Essigmann HC, Schaefer F. Body growth of children with steroid-resistant nephrotic syndrome. *Pediatr Nephrol* 1999; 13:928–934.

Solin ML, Ahola H, Haltia A, et al. Lipid peroxidation in human proteinuric disease. *Kidney Int* 2001;59(2):481–487.

Stec J, Podracka L, Pavkovcekova O, et al. Zinc and copper metabolism in nephrotic syndrome. *Nephron* 1990;56:186–187.

Sulowicz W, Stompor T. LDL-apheresis and immunoadsorption: novel methods in the treatment of renal diseases refractory to conventional therapy. *Nephrol Dial Transplant* 2003;13(Suppl. 5): 59–62.

Taal MW, Brenner BM. Combination ACEI and ARB therapy: additional benefit in renoprotection? *Curr Opin Nephrol Hypertens* 2002;11(4):377–381.

Thompson GR. LDL apheresis. *Atherosclerosis* 2003;167(1):1–13.

Tovar AR, Murguia F, Cruz C, et al. A soy protein diet alters hepatic lipid metabolism gene expression and reduces serum lipids and renal fibrogenic cytokines in rats with chronic nephrotic syndrome. *J Nutr* 2002;132:2562–2569.

Vaziri ND. Molecular mechanisms of lipid disorders in nephrotic syndrome. *Kidney Int* 2003;63(5):1964–1976.

Velasquez MT, Bhathena SJ. Dietary phytoestrogens: a possible role in renal disease protection. *Am J Kidney Dis* 2001;37(5): 1056–1068.

Velasquez MT, Bhathena SJ, Ranich T, et al. Dietary flaxseed meal reduces proteinuria and ameliorates nephropathy in an animal model of type II diabetes mellitus. *Kidney Int* 2003;64(6): 2100–2107.

Walls J. Relationship between proteinuria and progressive renal disease. *Am J Kidney Dis* 2001;37(Suppl):S13–S16.

Wilmer WA, Rovin BH, Hebert CJ, et al. Management of glomerular proteinuria: a commentary. *J Am Soc Nephrol* 2003;14(12): 3217–3232.

Wrone EM, Camethon MR, Palaniappan L, et al. Association of dietary protein intake and microalbuminuria in healthy adults: third National Health and Nutrition Examination Survey. *Am J Kidney Dis* 2003;41(3):580–587.

9

Nutritional Strategies in Progressive Renal Insufficiency

Denis Fouque

The kidney accounts for excretion of most metabolites derived from food and beverage intake. Because lipids and carbohydrates are completely processed or stored in the body, protein and its nitrogen derivatives are the most important nutritional compounds handled by the kidney. Indeed, nitrogen compounds are not stored in the adult body in a steady metabolic state. Thus, at equilibrium, every gram of nitrogen absorbed is rapidly eliminated into the urine after adequate metabolic process.

In healthy adults, increasing protein intake is associated with a concomitant increase in nitrogen output, whereas a diet extremely poor in protein is associated with a markedly reduced urinary urea nitrogen output. However, this adaptation presents some limitation, in that the body has obligatory daily nitrogen losses that are not entirely influenced by protein intake, for example, losses from fecal matter, perspiration, hair, and nails. In patients with renal disease, this loss has been estimated to be approximately 0.031 mg nitrogen per kg of body weight. Further, protein needs estimated by gold standard methods, such as nitrogen balance or labeled *amino acid turnover*, have precisely characterized the body nitrogen metabolism and the subsequent optimal level of protein intake in healthy adults and in patients with chronic kidney disease (CKD). From these data, safe and acceptable diets can be proposed for patients with varying levels of renal insufficiency.

In addition, recent research data have confirmed that protein intake can regulate proteinuria, as seen in Figure 9-1. Because proteinuria has been identified as one of the most important and independent risk factors for CKD progression, every attempt to lower proteinuria to a minimal level seems worthwhile. In this chapter, we address the potential role of protein intake on renal function, the optimal protein diet in patients with CKD who have various levels of renal function, the ways to monitor such diets, the potential side effects, and the results of large clinical trials and meta-analyses of low-protein interventions in chronic renal insufficiency.

PROTEIN METABOLISM AND KIDNEY DISEASE

Overnutrition is associated with altered renal hemodynamics, particularly if the excess consists of high protein intake, high amino acid intake, or both. Whether lipids or carbohydrates directly affect renal function or disease is unclear; however, ample evidence exists that a high protein load acutely increases glomerular filtration rate (GFR), microalbuminuria, and over

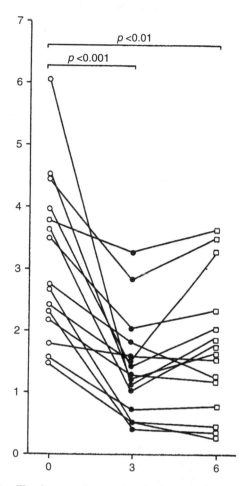

Figure 9-1.   The decrease in proteinuria (left panel) and the concomitant increase in serum albumin (right panel) during 3 and 6 months' treatment with a very–low-protein diet (0.3 g/kg b.w./d) in 15 patients with stage 4 chronic renal disease [From Aparicio M, Bouchet JL, Gin H, et al. Effect of a low-protein diet on urinary albumin excretion in uremic patients. *Nephron* 1988;50(4):288–291, with permission.]

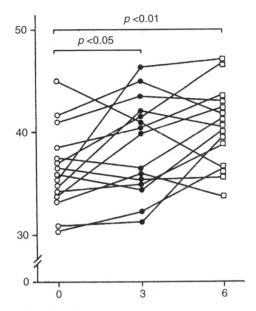

Figure 9-1. *Continued.*

the long-term, glomerulosclerosis in animals and in humans. By contrast, reducing the protein load may stop, or even induce remission in, the progression of experimental renal scarring. A number of mechanisms or compounds have been nominated to explain these alterations, for example, glucagon, insulin, insulin-like growth factor-1, angiotension II, prostaglandins, and kinins. Sodium retention may be associated with protein-induced hyperfiltration in response to stimulation of the proximal sodium–amino acid cotransporter. Notably, the hemodynamic changes observed during chronic renal insufficiency closely match those of protein-induced hyperfiltration. In this context, protein restriction almost ablates all hemodynamic changes observed after 5/6 nephrectomy by reducing glomerular pressure and flow. In long-term experimental studies in animals, low protein intake retarded the onset of proteinuria and renal fibrosis, extended survival, and seemed quite independent of the severity of existing renal damage. In almost all studies, however, the animals were hypertensive, and proteinuria was not considered as important a prognostic factor as it is today.

Glomerular protein trafficking induces hypermetabolism and oxidant stress, and a low-protein diet (LPD) is associated with reduced oxygen consumption and malondialdehyde production. The nature of protein absorbed may also influence the renal response. For decades, the GFR in vegetarians has been reported to be lower than in omnivores. When rats with chronic renal failure (CRF) were fed casein or soy proteins, proteinuria and histologic renal damage were always more severe in the group of rats that was fed protein of animal origin (e.g., casein).

Levels of growth factors and profibrotic agents, such as transforming growth factor (TGF)-β, fibronectin, and plasminogen activator inhibitor-1 PAI-1 can be experimentally modulated by an LPD, resulting in less renal injury and reduced proteinuria. Finally, albuminuria *per se* seems to possess a persistent pathogenic effect that results in tubulointerstitial lesions and apoptosis. Besides the well-known effects of angiotensin-converting-enzyme (ACE) inhibitors and angiotensin II receptor antagonists ARA-II, an LPD that is known to independently decrease glomerular capillary pressure and albuminuria may therefore add to the protective antifibrotic and antiapoptotic effects obtained by lowering proteinuria.

Clinically, whether reducing protein intake will efficiently protect the kidney from progressive injury is less clear, for several reasons. First, experimental studies are designed to assess the effects of diets with extreme differences in protein intake with a magnitude of one to five. Obviously, this is not the case in clinical practice. Second, protein in food is rarely pure and is associated with other factors, such as phosphorus, sodium, energy, and water, that could affect kidney function. Thus, modulating protein intake also affects other nutrients. Third, in experimental conditions, one single intervention can be studied; however, in clinical settings, patients should follow a dietary protocol and receive a cocktail of nephroprotective interventions that mask, to some extent, the true effect of any single intervention.

OPTIMAL LEVEL OF DIETARY PROTEIN AND ENERGY INTAKE

In adults, a Western diet contains approximately 1.3 g protein/kg b.w./d. Women have a protein intake 35% to 50% lower than men of the same age. This intake is spontaneously reduced by about 15% by the age of 70. However, the mean optimal protein intake, as defined (on the basis of nitrogen balance) by the Food and Agriculture Organization (FAO) in 1985, is 0.50 g protein/kg b.w./d. To ensure that 97.5% of individuals maintain nitrogen balance, researchers have added to this value two standard deviations of the mean, which raises the optimal daily intake to 0.75 g protein/kg b.w./d. Eventually to correct for the vegetal nature of protein, which may be less absorbed by a factor of 10%, the protein intake can be subsequently raised to 0.8 g protein/kg b.w./d. Other more recent research data using different techniques have confirmed these values. However, the Gaussian distribution of daily protein requirements might explain why some patients do well with protein intakes that are less than the average recommended values. Finally, these protein requirements were estimated in healthy adults or in patients with renal disease who were receiving a controlled energy intake of at least 35 kcal/kg b.w./d. These results would not be applicable in healthy adults or in individuals with CRF whose energy intake is inadequate.

Increasing or decreasing energy requirements is not necessary for patients with CKD before end-stage renal disease (ESRD) develops. Indeed, research data show that basal rate metabolism and energy requirements in these patients do not differ from those in healthy adults, and nitrogen balance is obtained with a protein intake of 0.6 g/kg b.w./d. Recently, the Kidney Disease Outcomes Quality Initiatives (K/DOQI) have developed a set of guidelines, and they recommend that protein and energy intake should be 0.6 g protein/kg b.w./d (Guideline 24) and that energy intake should be 35 kcal/kg b.w./d for patients with CRF younger than 60 years and 30 to 35 kcal/kg b.w./d for those older than 60 (Guideline 25), who do not require maintenance dialysis treatment.

However, the average spontaneous intakes of patients with kidney disease are somewhat different. Indeed, spontaneous reductions in energy and protein intake have been reported when renal function is impaired, and intake values as low as 21 kcal and 0.85 g protein/kg b.w./d have been observed in patients with stage 3 CKD; that is, a GFR less than 30 mL per minute. A recent report showed that for an equal amount of protein, a diet that derives 70% of protein from vegetable sources enables a greater amount of calories to be consumed than a diet that derives 70% of its protein from animal sources. These observations are of particular importance, as these patients cannot adapt their protein metabolism because of a deficient energy intake. Obviously, such individuals will do worse than if they received an optimal, moderately low protein intake and adequate energy intake.

METABOLIC CONSEQUENCES OF REDUCED PROTEIN INTAKE IN RENAL DISEASE

Nature of Protein Restricted Diets

During the past 50 years, various levels of protein restriction have been studied. Indeed, the protein metabolism of a healthy adult enables individual adaptation to a protein intake that is as low as 0.3 g protein/kg b.w./d, if energy and essential amino acid (EAA) supplies are present; these levels of protein intake have also been studied in patients with CKD. In specific trials, to avoid nutritional deficits, supplements have been distributed as EAA pills or keto acids (KA) of amino acids; amino acids can recapture nitrogen from waste endogenous uremic products and synthesize the corresponding EAAs. Research data suggest that up to 0.6 g protein/kg b.w./d can be safely prescribed if at least 50% of the protein is of high biologic value (i.e., from an animal source), and energy intake meets the recommended goal (i.e., 35 kcal/kg b.w./d for patients younger than 65 and 30 to 35 kcal/kg b.w./d for those older than 65). If lower levels of protein intake are to be prescribed, supplements (EAA or KA) should be added to avoid EAA deficit. Currently, estimating the number of patients who receive low protein intake counseling, and the level of intake that they are prescribed, is difficult. Finally, by dramatically reducing blood urea nitrogen, a low protein intake could alleviate uremic symptoms and postpone the start of dialysis or prolong survival in countries with limited dialysis resources.

Adaptation to Protein Metabolism

An adaptive response (i.e., a decrease in whole body leucine flux and oxidation) has been observed in patients with stage 3 to 4 CRF who were prescribed a 40% reduction in protein intake (from 1.0 to 0.6 g/kg b.w./d or 1.1 to 0.7 g/kg/d) during 1 week or 3 months, with no sign of body composition alteration. With a more restricted protein intake (0.35 g/kg b.w./d supplemented with KA or EAAs) for an extended period of 16 months, this adaptive response was still observed, while neutral nitrogen balance and body composition was maintained. This adaptation is also observed in patients with the nephrotic syndrome: a reduction of protein intake from 1.85 to 1.0 g protein/kg b.w./d was well tolerated. Reducing protein intake was even more beneficial for seven patients with nephrotic syndrome, when their intake was reduced from 1.2 to 0.66 g protein/kg b.w./d, because not only was their leucine metabolism adapted, but a strong reduction in proteinuria was also achieved that consequently increased serum albumin levels. Thus, with adequate energy supply, the uremic body correctly regulates protein metabolism.

Glucose Metabolism

Insulin resistance has been commonly reported during the course of CRF and may impair glycemic control. After a 3-month LPD, patients have improved insulin sensibility, reduced fasting serum insulin or daily insulin needs, and reduced blood glucose and endogenous glucose production, possibly because of decreased interaction between uremic toxins and glucose metabolism.

Control of Osteodystrophy (Decrease in Serum Parathormone Levels)

Because proteins of animal origin are strongly associated with phosphorus (1 g protein approximately contains 13 mg of phosphorus), reducing protein intake obviously reduces phosphate load. In addition, in some very–low-protein diets, a keto analog supplement is added as a calcium salt. Both low phosphate intake and adjunction of calcium reduce serum parathormone (PTH) levels and improve renal osteodystrophy before ESRD. Particularly, renal osteomalacia and osteofibrosis were improved after 12 months of an LPD supplemented with keto analogs.

Improvement in Lipid Profile

Because a reduced protein intake generally entails eating less protein of animal origin (e.g., meat and dairy products), the accompanying saturated lipids are concomitantly decreased, resulting in an improved serum lipid profile. For instance, reducing protein intake from 1.1 to 0.7 g/kg b.w./d for 3 months induced an increase in serum lipoprotein AI levels and in the Apo-AI/Apo-B ratio. In another report, a 6-month LPD improved patients' oxidative status by decreasing red cell malondiadehyde and increasing polyunsaturated fatty acids, particularly C22:4 and C22:5.

Reduction in Proteinuria

As seen in Figure 9-1, a reduced protein intake induces a decrease in proteinuria. This decrease is important, because proteinuria is now well identified as an independent risk factor for progressive renal disease, and every attempt to reverse proteinuria seems worthwhile. The fact that the most efficient interventions are made by ACE inhibitors, ARA-II, or both is well established; however, adding an LPD confers additional protection to the kidney and may further postpone end-stage renal failure.

Hypocaloric Risk

Guidelines for patients to reduce the protein content of a diet without decreasing the whole daily intake are not entirely straightforward. Without adequate counseling, a risk for hypocaloric intake is present as well, which can supersede the spontaneous decline observed when GFR falls below 50 mL per minute. However, the general experience is that, with adequate supervision, energy intakes recorded are usually more than 30 kcal/kg b.w./d, and body composition is adequate, in patients receiving a long-term LPD. The K/DOQI guidelines have reinforced the need for a dietary care plan to be started as early as possible during CKD and obviously before starting dialysis.

Overall Safety

Although starting an LPD requires skilled dietitians, trained staff, and patient involvement, adherence can be obtained after a few weeks or months, provided that regular dietary interviews and urinary urea measurements are done. Patients will do better if their diet is monitored than if they are not followed at all. Although clinical trials reported fairly low energy intakes during low protein intervention, long-term nutritional status, as measured by dual-energy x-ray absorptiometry (DEXA) or anthropometry, does not reflect alteration in body composition. Furthermore, patients who received a low protein intake for years before ESRD had a survival rate during maintenance dialysis that was similar to those achieved by other therapies.

MONITORING NUTRITIONAL INTAKE

A selective reduction of protein, without decreasing total food, energy intake, or both, is rather technical. Indeed, studies reported that patients might reduce their global daily food intake, rather than selectively reducing protein intake. Furthermore, clinical experience shows that anorectic patients spontaneously reduce their intake of energy-containing food rather than reducing protein intake, because energy requires larger volumes to be absorbed. A randomized 6-month dietetic intervention showed that patients who received an educational course on protein food content increased their serum albumin level and improved their body composition compared with patients who did not receive this dietary intervention.

Protein intake can be estimated from two sources: (i) intake from dietary reports and (ii) output from urinary urea excretion in patients without ESRD, or protein nitrogen appearance (PNA), formerly called protein catabolic rate (PCR) in patients with ESRD. At present, two formulas are routinely used to assess nitrogen (N) and thus protein intake in CKD:

Eq 1:   N intake (g/d) = UNA (g/d) + $0.031 \times$ b.w. (kg)

Eq 2:   N intake (g/d) = $1.20 \times$ UNA (g/d) + 1.74

where b.w. is the actual patient's body weight.

Table 9-1. Example of patient's adherence assessment: Estimation of dietary protein intake (DPI) in a stable noncatabolic 80-kg adult patient undertaking a 0.6 g protein/kg b.w./d diet, based on a daily urinary nitrogen appearance (UNA)

Patient's UNA = 5.2 g/d

Eq 1:   UNA + 0.031 × 80 kg = 5.2 + 2.48 = 7.68 g N

DPI = 7.68 g × 6.25 = 48 g; thus, DPI/kg = 48 g/80 kg = 0.60 g/kg b.w./d

Or

Eq 2:   1.2 × UNA + 1.74 = 6.24 + 1.74 = 7.98 g N

DPI = 7.98 × 6.25 = 49.9 g; thus, DPI /kg = 49.9/80 = 0.62 g/kg b.w./d

Adherence to the diet, e.g., an actual protein intake not greater than 20% more than prescribed intake, is considered acceptable if this patient presents a UNA not greater than 6.3 g per day.
From Masud T, Manatunga A, Cotsonis G, et al. The precision of estimating protein intake of patients with chronic renal failure. *Kidney Int* 2002;62:1750–1756, with permission.

To convert into protein, multiply N intake by 6.25. See the example in Table 9-1.

Adherence to an LPD is defined by an actual intake equal to ± 20% of prescribed intake. In well-controlled studies, the actual intake tends to be greater by 10% to 20%. In most clinical trials, 40% to 70% of enrolled patients meet the required intakes, and on a day-to-day basis, not more than 70% of patients in experienced teams will meet this goal. Thus, a constant effort seems necessary and should be set up to support the nutritional care of patients with CKD.

Whereas energy expenditure can be reliably assessed through indirect calorimetry, Harris–Benedict formula, or physical activity questionnaires, energy intake is more difficult to monitor, because it can only be deduced from dietary interviews or records. The optimal energy intake to achieve is 35 kcal/kg b.w./d and 30 to 35 kcal/kg b.w./d in patients older than 60 years. Thus, regular interviews between patient and dietitian are mandatory, and we have estimated that at least four interviews are necessary to ensure good understanding of what a low-protein optimal energy intake is and how an adequate home food record should be performed. The K/DOQI guidelines have recommended that a dietary care plan should be designed and implemented early in the course of CKD. These guidelines recommend that at least one dietetic interview be performed every 3 to 4 months. A general patient follow-up is proposed in Table 9-2.

EVIDENCE FOR AN OPTIMAL PROTEIN INTAKE FOR PATIENTS WITH PROGRESSIVE CHRONIC KIDNEY DISEASE

As demonstrated in the preceding text, protein intake plays an important role in renal structure and function, and numerous

Table 9-2.   Nutritional follow-up and dietary counseling in chronic renal failure (CRF) patients before end-stage renal disease (ESRD)

Time Span	To Do	Result
Every mo for 4 mo; then every 3–4 mo	Dietary interview	Develop a care plan; tailor diet to patient taste and economic situation
	Home 3-d food record	Record energy intake; verify adequate understanding of diet and adherence from urinary urea
	24-h urinary urea	Estimate protein intake
Every 3 mo	Body weight Anthropometry (optional) SGA (optional)	
	Serum albumin; serum prealbumin; serum cholesterol C-reactive protein	

If GFR is below 15 mL per minute, survey can be more frequent, particularly if superimposed disease occurs; consider starting supplementary treatment if follow-up does not show alteration in nutritional status or laboratory markers.

trials have tried to assess the relationship between the level of protein intake and the potential deleterious or protective effects on the kidney. However, some concessions have to be made when interpreting the findings of these trials.

Estimating Renal Damage

One of the major caveats for quantifying renal damage in humans is that repeated histologic analyses are not available, for ethical reasons. Thus, during dietary interventions, researchers are left with outcomes such as serial measures of renal function over time. The next cornerstone is the unfortunate interaction between most commonly used renal function markers (e.g., serum creatinine, 1/serum creatinine, urinary creatinine clearance, or formula-derived creatinine clearance) and the protein intake itself. Indeed, protein intake, and the accompanying creatine and creatinine load, interferes with the muscle creatinine pool and creatinine generation. As a consequence, creatinine delivered to the plasma will not be constant, a condition required to measure renal function adequately. In addition, serum creatinine and creatinine clearance can be affected by a number of medications, such as cimetidine, that act on tubular excretion of creatinine and that generally were not controlled during clinical trials. Third, and more importantly, a change in protein load acutely changes GFR. Thus, reducing protein intake toward a new plateau will rapidly reduce GFR by 10% to 20% before a new equilibrium can be reached. As a consequence, even with the use of a perfect GFR marker, a delay of 3 to 4 months is mandatory when an effect of protein intake is expected to occur before any conclusion can be drawn about changes in GFR. This observation has been clearly illustrated in the first phase of the Modification of Diet in Renal Disease (MDRD) study.

Methodologic Caveats

Another important aspect of clinical research relies on the methodologic quality, design, and reports of trials. Indeed, a number of criteria now exist for rating trials, generating evidence, and producing clinical guidelines that should be used to clarify the effects of a given treatment. Evidence level A is obtained from the best-quality, large, randomized and controlled trials (RCT) and meta—analyses (grades 1 or 2); evidence level B from prospective controlled clinical trials (CCT) (grade 3); and evidence level C, the lowest rank, acquired from retrospective trials, case reports, or expert opinion (grades 4 and 5). After extensively searching the literature published since 1974, we excluded more than 50 low-quality studies (too small in size or uncontrolled) and identified only seven randomized controlled trials and four meta-analyses.

Results of Major RCTs and Meta-analyses

Randomized Clinical Trials

Rosman et al. studied protein restriction in 247 patients during a period of 2 and 4 years. Protein intake was 0.90 to 0.95 g/kg b.w./d in patients whose GFR was between 60 and 30 mL per minute, and protein intake was 0.70 to 0.80 g/kg b.w./d in patients whose GFR was between 30 and 10 mL per minute; protein intake in the control groups was not restricted. After 2 years, restricted diets had significantly slowed GFR only in men; however, patients with polycystic kidney disease did not improve with a restricted diet. After 4 years, a marked improvement in survival was observed in patients treated with the more restricted protein intake (survival off-dialysis, 60% protein restricted group versus 30% protein unrestricted group, p <0.025). Adherence to the LPDs was very good after a short period of training and sustained over time, and protein restriction did not cause malnutrition.

Ihle et al. studied 72 patients with advanced renal failure for 18 months, randomized to receive a protein-unrestricted control diet or 0.4 g protein/kg b.w./d. Actual protein intake, estimated from urinary urea, was 0.8 or 0.6 g/kg b.w./d. The GFR [^{51}Cr-ethylenediaminetetra-acetate (^{51}Cr-EDTA)] decreased only in the control group, whereas no decrease occurred in the LPD group. The number of patients who started dialysis during the trial was significantly greater in the control group (p <0.005). Body composition somewhat varied, with a loss of body weight in the LPD group, whereas no change was observed in other anthropometric measures or in serum albumin levels in either group. No food record was made, so an insufficient energy intake cannot be ruled out to explain weight loss under LPD. The authors concluded that this moderate reduction in protein intake had a beneficial effect.

Williams et al. studied the effects of three different interventions for 18 months in 95 patients with advanced renal failure. Patients randomly received a diet that supplied 0.6 g protein/kg b.w./d and 800 mg phosphate (LPD group); a diet that provided 1,000 mg phosphate per day plus phosphate binders, without specific protein restriction (low-phosphate group); or diet with no protein or phosphate restrictions. Dietary adherence, estimated both by urinary urea output and diet recalls, averaged 0.7, 1.02, and 1.14 g protein/kg b.w./d and 815, 1,000, and 1,400 mg phosphorus per day, respectively. Slight weight losses were observed in the protein- and phosphate-restricted groups (−1.3 and −1.65 kg b.w. for the LPD and low-phosphate group, respectively). No difference was observed among any of the three groups in the decrease in creatinine clearance over time. Death or the commencement of dialysis therapy did not differ among the three groups. Both the small size of the study and the GFR estimation by creatinine clearance greatly limit the value of this study.

By contrast, the Northern Italian Cooperative Study Group was a large randomized controlled study in 456 patients with GFRs lower than 60 mL per minute, followed for 2 years. Patients were prescribed 1 g/kg b.w./d (control group) or 0.6 g/kg b.w./d (LPD); both diets provided at least 30 kcal/kg b.w./d. Actual protein intakes were rather close, because the control group ate 0.90 g protein/kg b.w./d and the low-protein group ate 0.78 g/kg b.w./d, and a large overlap occurred between groups. The main outcome was "renal survival," defined as the start of dialysis or the doubling of serum creatinine levels. Only a borderline difference existed between control and LPD groups, with slightly fewer patients in the LPD group reaching a renal endpoint ($p = 0.059$).

Malvy et al. examined a more severe protein restriction (0.3 g protein/kg b.w./d) supplemented with keto analogues (Ketosteril, 0.17 g/kg b.w./d) versus 0.65 g protein/kg b.w./d in 50 patients with severe renal insufficiency (creatinine clearance ≤20 mL/min). Patients were followed until dialysis or until creatinine clearance was less than 5 mL/min/1.73 m². Renal survival did not differ between diets, but the size of the study prevented any valid conclusion being made. For the patients with the most advanced disease at inclusion (GFR of 15 mL/min/1.73 m²), the "half-life" for renal death was 9 months in the 0.65 g protein/kg b.w./d, compared with 21 months in the group with the most restricted diet (0.3 g protein/kg b.w./d), which may indicate that tight protein restriction might be worthwhile for patients with advanced disease. A loss of 2.7 kg b.w. occurred over 3 years in the group assigned to the very−low-protein diet, lost equally from fat and lean body mass. No weight loss or body composition change occurred in the group assigned to the 0.65 g protein per kg b.w. diet.

The MDRD study tested the effects of low protein intake and strict blood pressure control on the progression of renal disease in more than 800 patients separated in two groups: Study A, GFR: 25 to 55 mL/min/1.73 m² of body surface area, and Study B, GFR: 13 to 24 mL/min/1.73 m² of body surface area. In Study A, patients received 1 g protein/kg b.w./d or more and were to reach a mean blood pressure of 105 mm Hg, compared to the low-protein group, who received 0.6 protein/kg b.w./d and achieved a mean blood pressure of 92 mm Hg; in Study B, patients received 0.6 g protein/kg b.w./d or 0.3 g protein/kg b.w./d, plus a keto acid supplement, and had blood pressure goals comparable to those in Study A. GFR decrease was estimated by the slope of ^{125}I-iothalamate clearance, measured every 4 months over 2 years; mean follow-up was 2.2 years. Actual protein intakes were 1.11 g protein/kg b.w./d versus 0.73 g protein/kg b.w./d in Study A (n = 585), and 0.69 versus 0.46 g protein/kg b.w./d in Study B (n = 255). No difference was observed in GFR decline between groups in Study A, whereas a borderline greater decline in GFR was observed in the group receiving 0.69 g protein/ kg b.w./d diet as compared with the 0.46 g/kg b.w./d plus keto acid group in Study B (p = 0.07).

At first glance, these results were disappointing to the renal community, but some caveats should be pointed out. First, during the first 4 months in Study A, a sharp decrease in GFR was observed in the group with the more restricted protein intake (0.73 g/kg b.w./d) in response to the physiologic reduction in glomerular hemodynamics that follows protein restriction. This result was followed by a slower linear decrease than was observed in the group with higher protein intake (1.11 g/kg b.w./d). If a run-in period is considered, during follow-up (from 4 months after the start until 3 years), the slope of GFR decrease was significantly lower in the more restricted protein group, and renal survival improved (p = 0.009). Secondly, the actual progression of renal failure was lower than expected from the pilot study, and thus a 3-month follow-up should have been added to correct for this inadequacy. In the Diabetes Control and Complications Trial (DCCT) trial for strict blood glucose control, however, no renal effect was detected at 2 years, and the protective consequence of strict glucose control on microalbuminuria or proteinuria was observed only after 4 years.

Secondary MDRD analyses, although less robust, are of interest. When patients were analyzed according to protein intake, a strong relation was found between actual protein intake and GFR slope (p = 0.011) or renal death (p = 0.001). Indeed, for every reduction in 0.2 g protein/kg b.w./d of intake, a 1.15 mL/min/yr reduction was observed in GFR decline and a 49% reduction in renal death. Thus, these analyses support a moderate beneficial effect of reduced protein intakes in patients with CRF; these effects were attributed to a reduced protein intake rather than to a well-identified level of protein restriction that was necessary to slow progression.

Meta-analyses

To clarify these issues, a series of meta-analyses have been performed. The criterion analyzed was renal death, for example, the occurrence of death, the need to start dialysis, or a GFR decrease during the study. Literature since 1974 was searched, using exhaustive databases. To reduce biases, for quality purpose and robustness of conclusions, only randomized controlled trials were kept for final analysis. The renal death results are reported in Figure 9-2. Odds ratios (i.e., treatment effect estimate between treated and control group) and the overall pooled analysis are shown for each trial in Figure 9-3. Among more than 1,400 patients (753 in LPD groups and 741 in control or larger protein intake groups), a 39% reduction in renal death (p <0.006) was seen for patients consuming a low-protein diet. When addressing the effect of low protein intake on GFR,

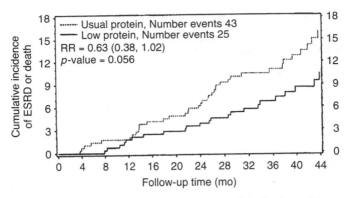

Figure 9-2. **Occurrence of renal failure or death in Study A of the Modification of Diet in Renal Disease Study including a 10-month additional follow-up after completion of the study ($p = 0.056$ between the two levels of protein intake). [From Levey AS, Greene T, Beck GJ, et al. Dietary protein restriction and the progression of chronic renal disease: what have all of the results of the MDRD study shown? Modification of Diet in Renal Disease Study Group.** *J Am Soc Nephrol* **1999;10(11):2426–2439, with permission.]**

Kasiske et al. showed, in more than 1,900 patients, a beneficial effect in patients with lower protein intakes who spared 0.53 mL/min/yr of GFR ($p < 0.05$). The number needed to treat (NNT) among patients with an LPD to prevent one renal death per year was calculated to be 18, a number that compares favorably with the well-accepted mortality reductions observed with statins in the 4S trial (NNT = 30) and the WOSCOPS study (NNT = 111).

The case for protein restriction in patients with diabetes is somewhat less clear. Indeed, most clinical trials are of shorter duration, during which renal death cannot be taken into account. Furthermore, they address surrogate criteria such as reductions in microalbuminuria, proteinuria, and creatinine clearance. In addition, in many older trials, ACE inhibitors were not equally distributed, and blood pressure control was not strictly comparable between groups. Zeller et al. compared 1 g protein/kg b.w./d versus 0.6 g protein/kg b.w./d in 36 patients with type 1 diabetes for at least 1 year (mean follow-up, 35 months). Actual protein intake was 1.08 g protein/kg b.w./d versus 0.72 g protein/kg b.w./d. The investigators observed a strong reduction in iothalamate-estimated GFR decline in the group with low protein intake ($p < 0.02$), but only in the subgroup of patients with a GFR greater than 45 mL per minute. Hansen et al. reported recently the longest randomized trial to date in patients with type 1 diabetes. Patients were given their usual protein intake or 0.6 g protein/kg b.w./d and followed for 4 years. Actual protein intake during the entire trial duration was 1.02 g/kg b.w./d versus 0.89 g/kg b.w./d, a slight but significant difference. No difference in proteinuria was observed,

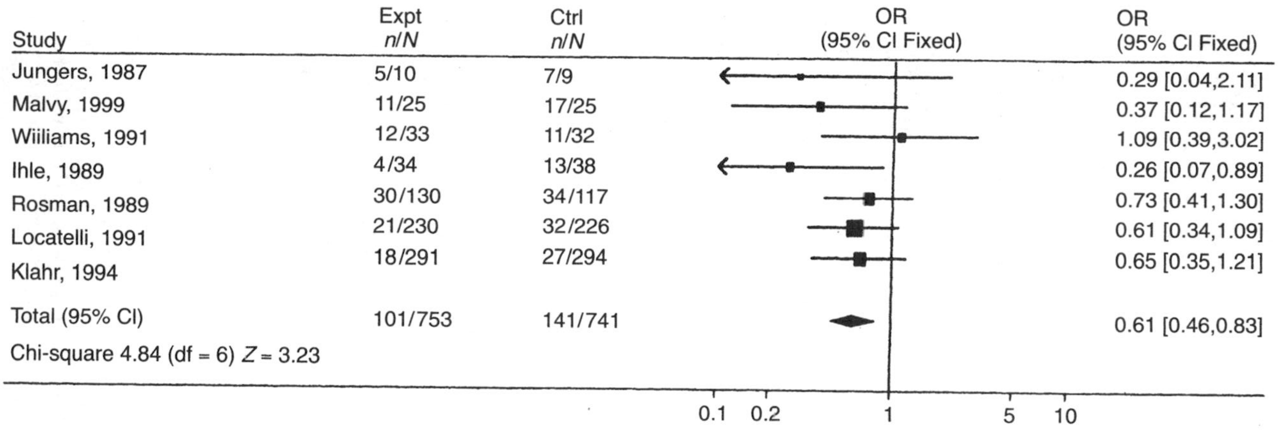

Study	Expt n/N	Ctrl n/N	OR (95% CI Fixed)	OR (95% CI Fixed)
Jungers, 1987	5/10	7/9		0.29 [0.04,2.11]
Malvy, 1999	11/25	17/25		0.37 [0.12,1.17]
Wiiliams, 1991	12/33	11/32		1.09 [0.39,3.02]
Ihle, 1989	4/34	13/38		0.26 [0.07,0.89]
Rosman, 1989	30/130	34/117		0.73 [0.41,1.30]
Locatelli, 1991	21/230	32/226		0.61 [0.34,1.09]
Klahr, 1994	18/291	27/294		0.65 [0.35,1.21]
Total (95% CI)	101/753	141/741		0.61 [0.46,0.83]
Chi-square 4.84 (df = 6) $Z = 3.23$				

Figure 9-3. Meta-analysis of the results of low-protein diets in chronic kidney disease patients. A square denotes the odds ratio (treatment/control) for each trial, and the diamond indicates the overall results of the seven trials combined. 95% confidence intervals are represented by horizontal lines. Overall "common" odds ratio = 0.61 (95% CI: 0.46, 0.83), $p = 0.006$. [From Fouque D, Wang P, Laville M, et al. Low-protein diets delay end-stage renal disease in nondiabetic adults with chronic renal failure. *Nephrol Dial Transplant* 2000;15(12):1986–1992, with permission.]

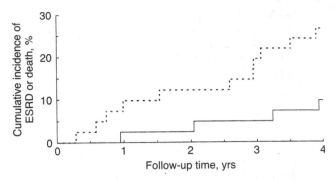

Figure 9-4. **Cumulative incidence of end-stage renal disease or death in patients with type 1 diabetes receiving usual protein diet (1.02 g/kg b.w./d, dashed line) or low protein diet (0.89 g/kg b.w./d, solid line) during 4 years; $p = 0.042$, log rank [From Hansen HP, Tauber–Lassen E, Jensen BR, et al. Effect of dietary protein restriction on prognosis in patients with diabetic nephropathy.** *Kidney Int* **2002;62(1):220–228, with permission.]**

but renal death was reduced by 36% in the moderately LPD, as seen in Figure 9-4. In addition, by Cox analysis after adjusting for cardiovascular disease, the difference was even more significant ($p = 0.01$). Finally, meta-analyzing a subgroup of patients with diabetes, Pedrini et al. showed that a combined criterion of microalbuminuria and renal function was improved by 44% ($p < 0.001$) by an LPD.

CONCLUSION

Patients with CKD will have to follow detailed dietary prescriptions during their entire lifetimes. A nutritional survey appears mandatory to verify that adequate energy will be provided, although recommendations for protein intake may evolve according to the stage of kidney disease. We have shown convincing evidence that during stage 3 and 4 CKD, for example, for a GFR between 60 and 15 mL per minute, protein intake should be reduced from Western unrestricted intake to 0.6 to 0.8 g/kg b.w./d, tailored to individual requirements, adherence, and body composition alteration through regular nutritional and dietary support.

SELECTED READINGS

Aparicio M, Bouchet JL, Gin H, et al. Effect of a low-protein diet on urinary albumin excretion in uremic patients. *Nephron* 1988; 50(4):288–291.

Aparicio M, Chauveau P, Combe C. Low protein diets and outcome of renal patients. *J Nephrol* 2001;14(6):433–439.

Aparicio M, Chauveau P, De Precigout V, et al. Nutrition and outcome on renal replacement therapy of patients with chronic renal failure treated by a supplemented very low protein diet. *J Am Soc Nephrol* 2000;11(4):708–716.

Aparicio M, Gin H, Merville P, et al. Parathormone activity and rate of progression of chronic renal failure in patients on low-protein diet. *Nephron* 1990;56(3):333–334.

Aparicio M, Lafage MH, Combe C, et al. Low-protein diet and renal osteodystrophy. *Nephron* 1991;58(2):250–252.

Bankir L, Kriz W. Adaptation of the kidney to protein intake and to urine concentrating activity: similar consequences in health and CRF. *Kidney Int* 1995;47(1):7–24.

Bergstrom J. Discovery and rediscovery of low protein diet. *Clin Nephrol* 1984;21(1):29–35.

Bernard S, Fouque D, Laville M, et al. Effects of low-protein diet supplemented with ketoacids on plasma lipids in adult chronic renal failure. *Miner Electrol Metab* 1996;22(1-3):143–146.

Bernhard J, Beaufrere B, Laville M, et al. Adaptive response to a low-protein diet in predialysis chronic renal failure patients. *J Am Soc Nephrol* 2001;12(6):1249–1254.

Brenner BM. Nephron adaptation to renal injury or ablation. *Am J Physiol* 1985;249(3 Pt 2):F324–F337.

Chauveau P, Barthe N, Rigalleau V, et al. Outcome of nutritional status and body composition of uremic patients on a very low protein diet. *Am J Kidney Dis* 1999;34(3):500–507.

Cirillo M, Anastasio P, Spitali L, et al. Effects of a meat meal on renal sodium handling and sodium balance. *Miner Electrol Metab* 1998;24(4):279–284.

Combé C, Deforges-Lasseur C, Caix J, et al. Compliance and effects of nutritional treatment on progression and metabolic disorders of chronic renal failure. *Nephrol Dial Transplant* 1993;8(5):412–418.

Coresh J, Walser M, Hill S. Survival on dialysis among chronic renal failure patients treated with a supplemented low-protein diet before dialysis. *J Am Soc Nephrol* 1995;6(5):1379–1385.

de Zeeuw D, Remuzzi G, Parving HH, et al. Proteinuria, a target for renoprotection in patients with type 2 diabetic nephropathy: lessons from RENAAL. *Kidney Int* 2004;65(6):2309–2320.

Diamond JR. Effects of dietary interventions on glomerular pathophysiology. *Am J Physiol* 1990;258(1 Pt 2):F1–F8.

Dixon R, Brunskill NJ. Activation of mitogenic pathways by albumin in kidney proximal tubule epithelial cells: implications for the pathophysiology of proteinuric states. *J Am Soc Nephrol* 1999; 10(7):1487–1497.

El-Nahas AM, Paraskevakou H, Zoob S, et al. Effect of dietary protein restriction on the development of renal failure after subtotal nephrectomy in rats. *Clin Sci (London)* 1983;65(4):399–406.

FAO/WHO (Food and Agriculture Organization/World Health Organization): Energy and Protein Requirements. Report of a Joint FAO/WHO Ad Hoc Expert Committee. Technical Report Services No. 552; FAO Nutrition Meetings Report Series 52. Rome, Italy: World Health Organization, 1973.

Fouque D, Laville M, Boissel JP, et al. Controlled low protein diets in chronic renal insufficiency: meta-analysis. *Br Med J* 1992; 304(6821):216–220.

Fouque D, Wang P, Laville M, et al. Low protein diets delay end-stage renal disease in non-diabetic adults with chronic renal failure. *Nephrol Dial Transplant* 2000;15(12):1986–1992.

Gansevoort RT, de Zeeuw D, de Jong PE. Additive antiproteinuric effect of ACE inhibition and a low-protein diet in human renal disease. *Nephrol Dial Transplant* 1995;10(4):497–504.

Garg AX, Blake PG, Clark WF, et al. Association between renal insufficiency and malnutrition in older adults: results from the NHANES III. *Kidney Int* 2001;60(5):1867–1874.

Giatras I, Lau J, Levey AS. Angiotensin-Converting-Enzyme Inhibition and Progressive Renal Disease Study Group. Effect of angiotensin-converting enzyme inhibitors on the progression of nondiabetic renal disease: a meta-analysis of randomized trials. *Ann Intern Med* 1997;127(5):337–345.

Gin H, Aparicio M, Potaux L, et al. Low-protein, low-phosphorus diet and tissue insulin sensitivity in insulin-dependent diabetic patients with chronic renal failure. *Nephron* 1991;57(4):411–415.

Gin H, Combe C, Rigalleau V, et al. Effects of a low-protein, low-phosphorus diet on metabolic insulin clearance in patients with chronic renal failure. *Am J Clin Nutr* 1994;59(3):663–666.

Giordano M, De Feo P, Lucidi P, et al. Effects of dietary protein restriction on fibrinogen and albumin metabolism in nephrotic patients. *Kidney Int* 2001;60(1):235–242.

Goodship TH, Mitch WE, Hoerr RA, et al. Adaptation to low-protein diets in renal failure: leucine turnover and nitrogen balance. *J Am Soc Nephrol* 1990;1(1):66–75.

Hadj-Aissa A, Bankir L, Fraysse M, et al. Influence of the level of hydration on the renal response to a protein meal. *Kidney Int* 1992;-42(5):1207–1216.

Hansen HP, Tauber-Lassen E, Jensen BR, et al. Effect of dietary protein restriction on prognosis in patients with diabetic nephropathy. *Kidney Int* 2002;62(1):220–228.

Harris DC, Tay C. Altered metabolism in the ex vivo remnant kidney. II. Effects of metabolic inhibitors and dietary protein. *Nephron* 1993;64(3):417–423.

Hostetter TH, Meyer TW, Rennke HG, et al. Chronic effects of dietary protein in the rat with intact and reduced renal mass. *Kidney Int* 1986;30(4):509–517.

Hostetter TH, Olson JL, Rennke HG, et al. Hyperfiltration in remnant nephrons: a potentially adverse response to renal ablation. *Am J Physiol* 1981;241(1):F85–F93.

Ihle BU, Becker GJ, Whitworth JA, et al. The effect of protein restriction on the progression of renal insufficiency. *N Engl J Med* 1989;321(26):1773–1777.

Ikizler TA, Greene JH, Wingard RL, et al. Spontaneous dietary protein intake during progression of chronic renal failure. *J Am Soc Nephrol* 1995;6(5):1386–1391.

Jafar TH, Stark PC, Schmid CH, et al. Proteinuria as a modifiable risk factor for the progression of non-diabetic renal disease. *Kidney Int* 2001;60(3):1131–1140.

Jarusiripipat C, Shapiro JI, Chan L, et al. Reduction of remnant nephron hypermetabolism by protein restriction. *Am J Kidney Dis* 1991;18(3):367–374.

Jungers P, Chauveau P, Ployard F, et al. Comparison of ketoacids and low protein diet on advanced chronic renal failure progression. *Kidney Int Suppl* 1987;22:S67–S71.

Kasiske BL, Lakatua JD, Ma JZ, et al. A meta-analysis of the effects of dietary protein restriction on the rate of decline in renal function. *Am J Kidney Dis* 1998;31:954–961.

Kenner CH, Evan AP, Blomgren P, et al. Effect of protein intake on renal function and structure in partially nephrectomized rats. *Kidney Int* 1985;27(5):739–750.

King AJ, Levey AS. Dietary protein and renal function. *J Am Soc Nephrol* 1993;3(11):1723–1737.

Klahr S, Levey AS, Beck GJ, et al. Modification of Diet in Renal Disease Study Group. The effects of dietary protein restriction and blood-pressure control on the progression of chronic renal disease. *N Engl J Med* 1994;330(13):877–884.

Kleinknecht C, Salusky I, Broyer M, et al. Effect of various protein diets on growth, renal function, and survival of uremic rats. *Kidney Int* 1979;15(5):534–541.

Kopple JD. Uses and limitations of the balance technique. *J Parenter Enteral Nutr* 1987;11(Suppl. 5):79S–85S.

Kopple JD. McCollum award lecture, 1996: protein-energy malnutrition in maintenance dialysis patients. *Am J Clin Nutr* 1997;65(5):1544–1557.

Kopple JD. The National Kidney Foundation K/DOQI clinical practice guidelines for dietary protein intake for chronic dialysis patients. *Am J Kidney Dis* 2001;38(4 Suppl. 1):S68–S73.

Kopple JD, Berg R, Houser H, et al. Modification of Diet in Renal Disease (MDRD) Study Group. Nutritional status of patients with different levels of chronic renal insufficiency. *Kidney Int* 1989;27:S184–S194.

Kopple JD, Greene T, Chumlea WC, et al. Relationship between nutritional status and the glomerular filtration rate: results from the MDRD study. *Kidney Int* 2000;57(4):1688–1703.

Kopple JD, Levey AS, Greene T, et al. Effect of dietary protein restriction on nutritional status in the Modification of Diet in Renal Disease Study. *Kidney Int* 1997;52(3):778–791.

Kopple JD, Monteon FJ, Shaib JK. Effect of energy intake on nitrogen metabolism in nondialyzed patients with chronic renal failure. *Kidney Int* 1986;29(3):734–742.

Laville M, Fouque D. Nutritional aspects in hemodialysis. *Kidney Int Suppl* 2000;76:S133–S139.

Leon JB, Majerle AD, Soinski JA, et al. Can a nutrition intervention improve albumin levels among hemodialysis patients? A pilot study. *J Ren Nutr* 2001;11(1):9–15.

Levey AS, Greene T, Beck GJ, et al. Dietary protein restriction and the progression of chronic renal disease: what have all of the results of the MDRD study shown? Modification of Diet in Renal Disease Study Group. *J Am Soc Nephrol* 1999;10(11):2426–2439.

Lindenau K, Abendroth K, Kokot F, et al. Therapeutic effect of keto acids on renal osteodystrophy. A prospective controlled study. *Nephron* 1990;55(2):133–135.

Locatelli F, Alberti D, Graziani G, et al. Northern Italian Cooperative Study Group. Prospective, randomised, multicentre trial of effect of protein restriction on progression of chronic renal insufficiency. *Lancet* 1991;337(8753):1299–1304.

Locatelli F, Del Vecchio L. How long can dialysis be postponed by low protein diet and ACE inhibitors? *Nephrol Dial Transplant* 1999;14(6):1360–1364.

Maiorca R, Brunori G, Viola BF, et al. Diet or dialysis in the elderly? The DODE study: a prospective randomized multicenter trial. *J Nephrol* 2000;13(4):267–270.

Malvy D, Maingourd C, Pengloan J, et al. Effects of severe protein restriction with in advanced renal failure. *J Am Coll Nutr* 1999; 18(5):481–486.

Maroni B, Steinman TI, Mitch W. A method for estimating nitrogen intake of patients with chronic renal failure. *Kidney int* 1985; 27:58–65.

Maroni BJ, Staffeld C, Young VR, et al. Mechanisms permitting nephrotic patients to achieve nitrogen equilibrium with a protein-restricted diet. *J Clin Invest* 1997;99(10):2479–2487.

Masud T, Manatunga A, Cotsonis G, et al. The precision of estimating protein intake of patients with chronic renal failure. *Kidney int* 2002;62:1750–1756.

Mauer SM, Steffes MW, Azar S, et al. Effects of dietary protein content in streptozotocin-diabetic rats. *Kidney Int* 1989;35(1):48–59.

Mitch WE, Remuzzi G. Diets for patients with chronic kidney disease, still worth prescribing. *J Am Soc Nephrol* 2004;15(1):234–237.

Mitch WE, Walser M, Steinman TI, et al. The effect of a keto acid-amino acid supplement on the progression of chronic renal failure. *N Engl J Med* 1984;311(10):623–629.

Munro HN, McGandy RB, Hartz SC, et al. Protein nutriture of a group of free-living elderly. *Am J Clin Nutr* 1987;46(4):586–592.

Nakayama M, Okuda S, Tamaki K, et al. Short-or long-term effects of a low-protein diet on fibronectin and transforming growth factor-beta synthesis in Adriamycin-induced nephropathy. *J Lab Clin Med* 1996;127(1):29–39.

Nath KA, Kren SM, Hostetter TH. Dietary protein restriction in established renal injury in the rat. Selective role of glomerular capillary pressure in progressive glomerular dysfunction. *J Clin Invest* 1986;78(5):1199–1205.

National Kidney Foundation. K/DOQI Clinical practice guidelines for nutrition in chronic renal failure. *Am J Kidney Dis* 2000;35(6 Suppl. 2):S1–140.

Passey C, Bunker V, Jackson A, et al. Energy balance in predialysis patients on a low-protein diet. *J Ren Nutr* 2003;13(2):120–125.

Pedrini MT, Levey AS, Lau J, et al. The effect of dietary protein restriction on the progression of diabetic and nondiabetic renal diseases: a meta-analysis. *Ann Intern Med* 1996;124(7):627–632.

Peters H, Border WA, Noble NA. Angiotensin II blockade and low-protein diet produce additive therapeutic effects in experimental glomerulonephritis. *Kidney Int* 2000;57(4):1493–1501.

Peuchant E, Delmas-Beauvieux MC, Dubourg L, et al. Antioxidant effects of a supplemented very low protein diet in chronic renal failure. *Free Radic Biol Med* 1997;22(1-2):313–320.

Pollock CA, Ibels LS, Zhu FY, et al. Protein intake in renal disease. *J Am Soc Nephrol* 1997;8(5):777–783.

Premen AJ. Potential mechanisms mediating postprandial renal hyperemia and hyperfiltration. *FASEB J* 1988;2(2):131–137.

Rand WM, Pellett PL, Young VR. Meta-analysis of nitrogen balance studies for estimating protein requirements in healthy adults. *Am J Clin Nutr* 2003;77(1):109–127.

Rigalleau V, Baillet L, Lasseur C, et al. Splanchnic tissues play a crucial role in uremic glucose intolerance. *J Ren Nutr* 2003; 13(3):212–218.

Rigalleau V, Blanchetier V, Combe C, et al. A low-protein diet improves insulin sensitivity of endogenous glucose production in predialytic uremic patients. *Am J Clin Nutr* 1997;65(5):1512–1516.

Rosman JB, Langer K, Brandl M, et al. Protein-restricted diets in chronic renal failure: a four year follow-up shows limited indications. *Kidney Int Suppl* 1989;27:S96–102.

Rosman JB, ter Wee PM, Meijer S, et al. Prospective randomised trial of early dietary protein restriction in chronic renal failure. *Lancet* 1984;2(8415):1291–1296.

Schneeweiss B, Graninger W, Stockenhuber F, et al. Energy metabolism in acute and chronic renal failure. *Am J Clin Nutr* 1990;-52(4):596–601.

The Diabetes Control and Complications Trial Research Group. The effect of intensive treatment of diabetes on the development and progression of long-term complications in insulin-dependent diabetes mellitus. *N Engl J Med* 1993;329(14):977–986.

Thomas ME, Brunskill NJ, Harris KP, et al. Proteinuria induces tubular cell turnover: a potential mechanism for tubular atrophy. *Kidney Int* 1999;55(3):890–898.

Toigo G, Aparicio M, Attman PO, et al. Expert Working Group report on nutrition in adult patients with renal insufficiency (part 1 of 2). *Clin Nutr* 2000a;19(3):197–207.

Toigo G, Aparicio M, Attman PO, et al. Expert working group report on nutrition in adult patients with renal insufficiency (part 2 of 2). *Clin Nutr* 2000b;19(4):281–291.

Tom K, Young VR, Chapman T, et al. Long-term adaptive responses to dietary protein restriction in chronic renal failure. *Am J Physiol* 1995;268(4 Pt 1):E668–E677.

Vendrely B, Chauveau P, Barthe N, et al. Nutrition in hemodialysis patients previously on a supplemented very low protein diet. *Kidney Int* 2003;63(4):1491–1498.

Walser M, Hill S. Can renal replacement be deferred by a supplemented very low protein diet? *J Am Soc Nephrol* 1999;10(1):110–116.

Wang S, Denichilo M, Brubaker C, et al. Connective tissue growth factor in tubulointerstitial injury of diabetic nephropathy. *Kidney Int* 2001;60(1):96–105.

Williams AJ, Baker F, Walls J. Effect of varying quantity and quality of dietary protein intake in experimental renal disease in rats. *Nephron* 1987;46(1):83–90.

Williams PS, Stevens ME, Fass G, et al. Failure of dietary protein and phosphate restriction to retard the rate of progression of chronic renal failure: a prospective, randomized, controlled trial. *Q J Med* 1991;81(294):837–855.

Wiseman MJ, Hunt R, Goodwin A, et al. Dietary composition and renal function in healthy subjects. *Nephron* 1987;46(1):37–42.

Zeller K, Whittaker E, Sullivan L, et al. Effect of restricting dietary protein on the progression of renal failure in patients with insulin-dependent diabetes mellitus. *N Engl J Med* 1991;324(2):78–84.

Trace Elements and Vitamins in Renal Disease

Tahsin Masud

Trace elements and vitamins are micronutrients that are necessary for energy production, organ function, food metabolism, cell growth, and protection from harmful oxygen-free radicals. Unlike the macronutrients, trace elements and vitamins do not provide energy, but without sufficient quantities of micronutrients, the energy of the macronutrients cannot be released. Patients with chronic kidney disease (CKD) are at risk for developing a deficiency or excess of one or more of the micronutrients because of inadequate intake, interference with micronutrient absorption either by drugs or uremic toxins, altered metabolism, or loss or gain during dialysis. Because micronutrients function at the cellular level, the effect of deficiency or excess is generally subclinical and unrecognized until later stages of the deficiency state.

Blood and tissue levels of important trace elements and vitamins differ between healthy adults and patients with renal disease (see Table 10-1). Not all reports agree on the direction and magnitude of the changes seen in serum and tissue concentrations of these micronutrients among patients with CKD and those treated with hemodialysis (HD) or chronic peritoneal dialysis (CPD) compared with healthy adults. Further, acceptable micronutrient levels and the clinical consequences of altered concentrations of trace elements on the health of patients with renal disease are not established. The reasons for this relative lack of knowledge are that (a) most of the evidence for the body's requirements of many micronutrients is circumstantial and based on observations of deficiency symptoms (from either accidental or induced deficiencies) and the response of these symptoms to dietary supplementation with an element, rather than more direct evidence of a biochemical role played by the elements; (b) methodologic difficulties exist in precisely measuring these micronutrients; and (c) renal disease affects the excretion or accumulation of trace elements and vitamins. Much of the quantitative data available are inaccurate, and the absolute requirements for trace elements and vitamins in renal disease have not been studied; the guidelines for micronutrient intake and the need for supplements for patients with CKD were extrapolated from the recommendations for healthy adults. The Food and Nutrition Board of the Institute of Medicine recently developed Dietary Reference Intakes (DRIs) of most of the micronutrients for healthy US and Canadian adults. The term DRIs, relatively new to the field of nutrition, refers to a set of four nutrient-based reference values that can be used to assess and plan diets. These values include *estimated average requirement* (EAR), *recommended dietary allowance* (RDA), *adequate intake* (AI), and *tolerable upper level of intake* (UL) to provide insight into the risks for inadequacy

Table 10-1. Commonly recognized abnormalities in micronutrients found in patients with renal failure

Micronutrient	Effect of Renal Failure
Zinc	Serum ↓-↑, RBC ↑, leukocyte ↓, no change in patients undergoing CPD
Selenium	Serum and tissue ↓ in CRF, HD, and CPD
Iron	Tissue stores ↓
Aluminum	Serum N-↑ in CRF, serum and tissue ↑ in HD and CPD
Copper	Serum ↓-N in CRF, HD, and CPD, RBC N-↓
Thiamine	Serum ↓ in CRF, HD, and CPD
Riboflavin	Serum ↓-N in CRF, HD, and CPD, RBC ↓ in nephrotic syndrome
Pyridoxine	Serum ↓-N in CRF, HD, and CPD, RBC ↓ with high-flux HD and EPO therapy
Cobalamine	Serum ↑ in CRF, serum N in HD and CPD
Folic acid	Serum and RBC N-↑ in CRF, HD, and CPD
Ascorbic acid	Serum ↓-N in CRF, HD, and CPD
Vitamin A	Serum ↑ in CRF, HD, and CPD
Vitamin E	Serum ↓-N-↑ in CRF, HD, and CPD, RBC ↓ in HD and CPD

N, no change from; ↓, decreased; ↑, increased; RBC, erythrocytes; CRF, chronic renal failure; HD, hemodialysis; CPD, chronic peritoneal dialysis; EPO, erythropoietin.

or adverse events (see Fig. 10-1). The RDA and UL of most of the micronutrients for patients with kidney diseases are not established. This chapter examines the trace elements and vitamins whose metabolism, function, requirements, and toxicity are affected by renal disease or its treatment: HD, CPD, or renal transplantation.

TRACE ELEMENTS

Trace elements, as the name implies, are those substances that are required in only tiny amounts, to maintain levels conducive to good health. The requirements are typically in the range of micrograms or milligrams per day. These elements are present in the body at concentrations less than 50 mg per kg. Trace elements play an important role in biologic systems because they are components of proteins, enzymes, and antioxidants.

The blood and tissue concentrations of trace elements in patients with kidney disease are affected by several factors. Loss of glomerular filtration can limit excretion, or impaired tubular function can cause excessive excretion. Protein-bound trace elements can be lost by patients with significant proteinuria. Poor nutritional status or altered gastrointestinal absorption in advanced uremia can limit absorption and hence use of trace elements present in the diet. In end-stage renal disease (ESRD), contamination of the dialysate by large amounts of trace elements can result from ineffective water purification or incorrect preparation

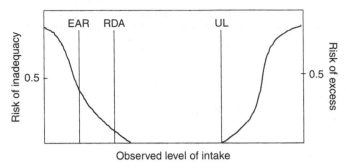

Figure 10-1. Dietary reference intakes and risks of inadequacy or excess. This figure shows that the Estimated Average Requirement (EAR) is the intake at which the risk of inadequacy is 0.5 (50%). The Recommended Dietary Allowance (RDA) is the intake at which the risk of inadequacy is very small, at 0.02 to 0.03 (only 2% to 3%). An Adequate Intake (AI) does not bear a consistent relation to the EAR or the RDA, but at an intake between RDA and the Tolerable Upper Intake Level (UL), the risks of inadequacy and of excess are both close to zero. At intakes greater than the UL, the risk of an adverse effect increases.

of the dialysate. Finally, the gain or loss of trace elements during dialysis depends on the gradient between the ultrafilterable fraction of an element in plasma, its concentration in the dialysate, and the type and permeability of the dialysis membrane.

Iron

Iron is the most widely studied and best understood essential element in humans. Iron is an essential cofactor of enzymes in the mitochondrial respiratory chain, in the citric acid cycle, and for enzymes needed for DNA synthesis; it is also central to the binding and transport of oxygen by hemoglobin and myoglobin. Conversely, cellular accumulation of metabolically active iron plays a key role in forming harmful oxygen radicals; these radicals cause peroxidative damage to vital cell structures.

Iron is absorbed almost exclusively in the duodenum and proximal jejunum. Besides the amount in the diet, intraluminal factors, erythropoietic activity, the functional capacity of intestinal mucosal cells, and the tissue–iron storage level regulate iron absorption. The total iron content of an adult ranges from 3 to 4 g; about one third of this amount is stored in the reticuloendothelial cells of the liver, spleen, and bone marrow or is bound to ferritin and hemosiderin. The remainder of the iron content is in a functional pool, composed of many essential proteins that use iron as a cofactor. Quantitatively, hemoglobin is by far the most important of these proteins, accounting for 65% of total body iron. Only 0.1% of iron is in the circulation bound to transferrin, a plasma glycoprotein that is normally about one-third saturated with iron. Since the introduction of recombinant human erythropoietin (rhEPO) to treat anemia, iron deficiency has become the most important secondary cause of anemia in patients who receive

Table 10-2. Factors leading to iron deficiency in patients undergoing dialysis

1. Increased demand of iron during erythropoiesis stimulated by rhEPO
2. Decreased iron uptake by intestinal mucosal cells
3. Occult gastrointestinal tract blood loss
4. External blood loss
   Blood retention in dialyzer and blood lines
   Frequent blood tests
   Accidental blood loss from vascular access

rhEPO, recombinant human erythropoietin.

dialysis treatment. Table 10-2 lists the important reasons patients undergoing dialysis develop iron deficiency.

Diagnosis of Iron Deficiency in End-Stage Renal Disease

No perfect indicators exist of iron deficiency or overload in humans, but serum ferritin and the percentage of transferrin saturation (TSAT) are the best available measures of body iron status. A serum ferritin level less than 30 ng per mL is highly predictive of iron deficiency in healthy subjects, but in patients with ESRD, especially those with inflammation, serum ferritin level is increased independently of total iron stores. Also, in patients with ESRD, iron tends to be sequestered in the storage pool and is not readily available for erythropoiesis. In such cases, the TSAT may be normal (see subsequent text), and the serum ferritin concentration actually underestimates the iron needs. The lower limit of normal for the serum ferritin in patients with ESRD is generally agreed to be 100 ng per mL, but no consensus exists on what upper limits of serum ferritin exclude a diagnosis of iron deficiency. The TSAT (the serum iron concentration multiplied by 100 and divided by the total iron-binding capacity) reflects iron that is readily available for erythropoiesis. Traditionally, a TSAT of less than 20% in patients undergoing HD is considered to indicate iron deficiency. Unfortunately, a TSAT of 20% or greater does not rule out the need for an iron supplement; many patients with TSAT of 20% or greater are still functionally iron deficient and will respond to iron administration with either an increase in hematocrit, despite a stable rhEPO dose, or maintain a stable hematocrit, with a lower rhEPO dose. Other tests of iron status, such as zinc protoporphyrin or erythrocyte ferritin, do not offer an improved diagnostic sensitivity or specificity over serum ferritin and TSAT. A value of hypochromic red cells of more than 10%, measured by automated red-cell analyzers, probably represents the best means of detecting functional iron deficiency at present, but this test is not always available.

Correction of Iron Deficiency

Oral iron is the safest, cheapest, and easiest means of iron supplementation, but parenteral doses are often necessary for patients undergoing dialysis, particularly those treated with

HD. Most oral iron supplements contain iron in the form of ferrous salts or iron polysaccharide (see Table 10-3); No clear evidence exists to support the superiority of any specific agent. Recommended dosages are at least 200 mg of elemental iron for adults, or 2 to 3 mg per kg b.w. for pediatric patients, administered at least 2 hours apart from meals or phosphate binders. A non–enteric-coated formulation is preferable, because enteric-coated forms may release iron beyond the duodenum and proximal jejunum, where it is maximally absorbed. Patients with ESRD who receive rhEPO therapy might not be able to maintain an adequate iron status with oral iron and might require parenteral preparations, such as iron dextran (Infed, DexFerum), iron gluconate (Ferrlecit), or iron sucrose (Venofer). The risk of a life-threatening anaphylactic reaction to iron dextran is reported to be approximately 0.6% to 0.7%; from 1976 to 1996, 31 deaths associated with iron dextran therapy were reported in the United States. In contrast, the risk for serious anaphylactic reaction with the use of iron gluconate and sucrose preparations is negligible; hypotension and flushing are the only important reported side effects. Intravenous iron gluconate or iron sucrose can be initiated safely, without a test dose, but a potential risk of transferrin oversaturation exists with rapid intravenous administration of either compound, even at the recommended dosages. Catalytically active, non–transferrin-bound iron has been detected in blood for 3.5 hours after a single bolus dose of 100 mg iron sucrose given intravenously. The potential harmful effects attributed to catalytically active iron are hydroxyl radical–mediated tissue injury and bacterial infection, but the magnitude of this risk is unknown. The National Kidney Foundation Kidney Disease Outcome Quality Initiative (K/DOQI) clinical practice guidelines for anemia in CKD suggest that the hemoglobin/hematocrit values should be maintained at 11 to 12 g per dL, or 33% to 36%; that iron should be administered to maintain a TSAT of 20% or greater; and that serum ferritin level should be maintained at 100 ng per mL or greater. Patients are unlikely to respond to iron administration (with a further increase in hemoglobin/hematocrit, a reduction in the rhEPO dose that is required to maintain the given hemoglobin/hematocrit, or both) if the TSAT increases to more than 50%, the serum ferritin level increases to more than 800 ng per mL, or both.

Table 10-3. Commercially available oral iron supplements

Oral Iron Supplements	Elemental Iron (mg/Tablet)	Tablets Per Day to Deliver ≥200 mg Elemental Iron
Ferrous sulfate	65	3
Ferrous gluconate	38	5
Niferex-150	150	2
Slow Fe	50	4
Feosol	65	3
Nu-Iron	150	2

Iron Overload in Patients Treated with Dialysis Therapy

Since the introduction of rhEPO, iron overload has become rare, and no consensus exists on the criteria for diagnosing iron overload in patients undergoing dialysis who receive intravenous iron therapy and rhEPO. A serum ferritin level consistently greater than 500 ng per mL is associated with severe hepatic iron overload by biomagnetic susceptometry, a noninvasive method of measuring tissue iron stores. Nevertheless, in one study of rhEPO-treated patients undergoing dialysis in whom bone marrow iron stores were measured, iron overload was not present with serum ferritin levels as high as 1,047 ± 445 ng per mL. Before the routine use of rhEPO in patients undergoing dialysis, bacterial infections associated with high serum ferritin levels were a matter of concern. This putative association did not take into account the role of other factors contributing to bacterial infections, such as anemia, transfusion-associated hepatitis, diabetes, and the immunosuppressive effect of blood transfusions. More worrisome are recent reports that serum ferritin is a marker of morbidity and mortality in patients undergoing HD and that administering large amounts of intravenous iron increases the risks for hospitalization and death. Iron overload has also been suggested to increase the risk of cardiovascular disease by increasing oxidation of low-density lipoprotein and promoting endothelial dysfunction. In summary, current K/DOQI recommendations on the upper limit of acceptable serum ferritin have to be reevaluated with regard to the long-term effect of iron administration on morbidity and mortality in patients with ESRD.

Aluminum

Human exposure to aluminum, a ubiquitous yet highly insoluble element, is through food, drinking water, and pharmaceuticals. No evidence exists that aluminum has any essential function in animals or humans; the main concern about aluminum is its potential toxicity. Patients with CKD are at risk for developing aluminum toxicity because urinary excretion is limited, and gastrointestinal absorption is unimpaired. An association exists between a high dialysate aluminum content and the dialysis encephalopathy syndrome, characterized by dysarthria–apraxia of speech, asterixis, myoclonus, dementia, focal seizures, and an abnormal electroencephalogram (EEG) that shows generalized slowing, with multifocal bursts of delta activity. In such patients, the aluminum content of gray matter was found to be threefold greater than that in patients undergoing dialysis who did not have dementia. Excess aluminum also affects the skeleton by markedly reducing bone formation, resulting in osteomalacia. Finally, aluminum toxicity causes microcytic anemia that is independent of iron deficiency. Such problems have practically disappeared as a result of the widespread use of aluminum-free deionized water for dialysis and eliminating the routine use of aluminum-based antacids for phosphate binding.

Diagnosis of Aluminum Toxicity

Patients with ESRD who are at risk for developing aluminum-related bone disease (ABD) include those who have undergone parathyroidectomy, a failed renal transplant, previous bilateral nephrectomy, and patients with diabetes mellitus. A bone biopsy remains the gold standard for diagnosing ABD, although serum aluminum levels below 40 μg per L are useful to exclude bone aluminum overload. Serum aluminum levels and the desferriox-amine (DFO) test, however, are not specific in diagnosing aluminum overload or ABD; but a DFO test producing an increment in serum aluminum level greater than 100 mg per L, combined with a serum parathyroid hormone (PTH) level less than 200 pg per mL, suggests the diagnosis of ABD. Bone biopsy is still required to confirm the diagnosis before initiating potentially risky deferrioxamine therapy. Aluminum-related encephalopathy is diagnosed by neurologic testing along with typical EEG findings; some correlation exists between high serum aluminum levels and signs of encephalopathy.

Therapy of Aluminum-Related Encephalopathy and Aluminum-Related Bone Disease

To prevent aluminum-related diseases, aluminum-based medications, such as the use of aluminum hydroxide as a phosphate binder or aluminum sucralfate for peptic ulcer, should be avoided in patients undergoing dialysis. When absolutely necessary, these medications should be used only for short periods and never in conjunction with any form of citrate (the citrate in fruit juices and effervescent analgesics sharply increases aluminum absorption). The quality of water in dialysis solutions should be monitored to keep the aluminum concentration virtually negligible. Vitamin D analogues should be withheld if the plasma aluminum is high, because vitamin D stimulates aluminum absorption by the gut and suppresses PTH secretion. Finally, a high serum PTH level protects the bone from aluminum deposition and may help mobilize aluminum from the body. Consequently, hyperparathyroidism should be ignored until the body and bone aluminum burden is reduced, and DFO therapy should be reserved for confirmed aluminum-related encephalopathy or bone disease.

Zinc

Zinc (Zn) is an essential element that is a component of enzymes necessary for essential biologic reactions. The prevalence of zinc deficiency in the general population or in patients with kidney disease has not been established, but this condition is extremely uncommon in North America. The important functions of Zinc include regulation of DNA and RNA synthesis; Zinc is involved in the function of the inflammatory cells, sex hormones, and the enzymes regulating carbohydrate tolerance; and Zinc acts as a stabilizer of biologic membranes, macromolecules, and organelles by protecting these molecules from oxidative damage. Zinc is also involved in hemoglobin synthesis, because Zinc deficiency may lead to anemia. Finally, Zinc deficiency is considered to play a role in the pathogenesis of some uremic symptoms (e.g., impaired smell and taste, anorexia, growth retardation, hypogonadism, and immunologic impairment).

Diagnosis of Zinc Deficiency

The physical examination should include an examination of fingernails for the presence of transverse grooves, called Beau lines, discoloration of nail plates, and paronychia, along with signs of generalized malnutrition. Blood zinc is found in two forms: tightly bound to α_2-macroglobulin and loosely bound to other proteins, primarily albumin. Variations in blood zinc levels usually reflect changes in the latter form. An assessment of the Zinc status is best made by measuring serum and neutrophil Zinc content, zinc-binding capacity, and serum or plasma alkaline phosphatase activity before and after zinc supplementation.

Alterations of Zinc Metabolism in Kidney Failure

In patients with CKD, serum or plasma Zinc levels are often decreased because of impaired intestinal absorption and a reduced affinity of albumin for Zinc. A decrease in animal protein in the diet or increased consumption of cereal and legumes (legumes are high in phytic acid, a potent inhibitor of zinc absorption) compromises availability of dietary Zinc. The serum Zinc level in patients undergoing HD is low or normal, because some loss of Zinc occurs through the dialyzer, but this loss can be balanced by release of Zinc from coil dialyzers. In patients treated with CPD therapy, the serum Zinc levels are more often normal, and the distribution of Zinc between erythrocytes and plasma is not altered. In patients treated with dialysis therapy, the erythrocyte Zinc concentration measured as Zinc protoporphyrin has been reported to be low, normal, or more often, high. This variability is attributed to the status of iron stores. Erythrocyte Zinc protoporphyrin is increased in iron deficiency, and its ratio to serum ferritin has been suggested as a useful diagnostic test for predicting erythropoietic response to iron supplementation. Likewise, significant correlations among plasma Zinc and serum iron and TSAT, Zinc erythrocyte, and parameters of iron deficiency are reported to be present in predialysis patients with CKD. These results suggest that low erythrocyte Zinc values reflect iron deficiency.

Zinc Supplementation

In patients with ESRD who have Zinc deficiency, a supplement has been shown to improve hypogeusia, nerve-conduction abnormalities, serum cholesterol levels, sperm count and libido, and the helper/suppressor (CD4/CD8) T-cell ratio. However, these studies were not carefully controlled, and conclusions about efficacy are suspect. Given the difficulties with diagnosing Zinc deficiency and the scanty evidence that Zinc supplements are effective, routine supplementation for patients with CKD, and for those undergoing dialysis or transplant, is not recommended. For patients who have findings that yield a high degree of clinical suspicion that Zinc deficiency is present and whose deficiency is confirmed by laboratory evidence, a trial of a Zinc supplement is warranted. Commercially available supplements are only in multivitamin–mineral preparations, with zinc content ranging from 15 to 25 mg per dose; if the clinical symptoms and laboratory test results do not improve, the supplement should be discontinued to avoid accumulation of Zinc or other components in the multivitamin.

Selenium

Selenium is an essential element for selenium-containing proteins called *selenoproteins*, such as selenomethionine and selenocysteine. The selenium-dependent glutathione peroxidases play important roles as antioxidants, and they seem to preserve elasticity by delaying the oxidation of polyunsaturated fatty acids. Other biologic functions include regulation of thyroid hormones and maintenance of the redox status of vitamin C and presumably other molecules.

Alterations of Selenium Metabolism in Kidney Failure

In patients with CKD and those undergoing HD and CPD, the serum or plasma levels of selenium are usually low. Reports about the erythrocyte concentration of selenium in patients with ESRD conflict. Evaluations indicate decreased selenium binding to albumin, with reduced transfer into erythrocytes. Impaired gastrointestinal absorption and selenium removal during dialysis also has been implicated as a possible reason for low plasma selenium levels. The clinical importance of low plasma glutathione peroxidase activity in patients undergoing dialysis is not known: Keshan disease, a cardiomyopathy that occurs almost exclusively in children, is the only human disease that has been firmly linked to selenium deficiency. However, the cardiovascular complications of patients undergoing dialysis are associated with reduced plasma and platelet selenium concentrations and low glutathione peroxidase activity, compared with that in patients undergoing dialysis who have no cardiovascular disease. A decreased half-life of erythrocytes and platelets plus thyroid abnormalities are associated with low serum selenium levels in patients undergoing dialysis. No case of selenium toxicity (selenosis) has been reported in patients undergoing dialysis.

Selenium Supplementation

Because the prevalence and clinical importance of selenium deficiency in causing uremic syndrome is not established, no routine supplementation of selenium is recommended.

Copper

Copper is widely distributed in biologic tissues, largely as a component of metalloenzymes. Early reports of high plasma copper levels in patients undergoing HD probably reflected copper release from ethylene oxide–sterilized, cuprophan dialysis membranes. Modern studies report normal levels and include normal plasma ceruloplasmin values in patients undergoing dialysis, unless inflammation is present (ceruloplasmin is an acute reactant protein). Although uncomplicated nutritional copper deficiency has not been unequivocally demonstrated in humans, hypochromic anemia, neutropenia, hypopigmentation of hair and skin, abnormal bone formation with skeletal fragility, and osteoporosis are associated with copper deficiency, so copper deficiency could play a role in the pathogenesis of anemia and growth retardation in patients treated with dialysis therapy. Patients undergoing dialysis therapy who are at risk for developing copper deficiency are those with enteropathies and those receiving prolonged parenteral nutrition with inadequate supplements. Apart from these situations, copper supplements are not necessary for patients with uremia.

Other Trace Elements

Alterations observed in serum or tissue concentration of other known trace elements in patients with CKD and those undergoing HD and CPD therapy, and the potential clinical consequences of these changes, are summarized in Table 10-4. The clinical importance of such changes is uncertain, and not enough information is available to formulate guidelines for routine monitoring of patients undergoing dialysis in terms of trace element abnormalities. The Association for the Advancement of Medical Instrumentation (AAMI) has developed the standards for maximum allowable trace element levels in the water and recommendations as to how frequently all important elements should be monitored during preparation of dialysates.

VITAMINS

Vitamins are organic compounds essential for normal metabolism, growth, and development; they regulate cell functions in conjunction with enzymes, cofactors, and other substances. With few exceptions, the body cannot manufacture or synthesize vitamins; hence, vitamins must be supplied in the diet or taken as dietary supplements. Vitamins are broadly categorized as water soluble or fat soluble; the water-soluble B and C vitamins are stored in the body only temporarily and then are eliminated, so frequent replenishment is necessary. The fat-soluble A, D, E, and K vitamins are stored in the body and need supplementation less frequently; accumulation of these vitamins causes toxicity. Regarding specific vitamins, vitamin D is discussed in Chapter 3. Vitamins C, E, and A (including β-carotene), along with mineral selenium, are considered antioxidant nutrients. These nutrients neutralize free radicals, the highly unstable molecules that cause oxidative damage in the body.

Water-Soluble Vitamins

Vitamin B₁ (Thiamine)

Thiamine exists mainly in various interconvertible forms, chiefly thiamine pyrophosphate. This coenzymatic form is involved in two main types of metabolic reactions: decarboxylation of α-keto acids (e.g., pyruvate, α-ketoglutarate, and branched-chain keto acids) and transketolation (e.g., among hexose and pentose phosphates). Thiamine deficiency results in anaerobic metabolism yielding lactic acidosis. Thiamine is present in vegetables, meats, legumes, and whole grains, but substantial loss of vitamin occurs during cooking above 100°C. After absorption (mainly in the jejunum), thiamine is transported in both erythrocytes and plasma; thiamine and its metabolites are readily excreted in urine.

ALTERATIONS OF THIAMINE METABOLISM IN RENAL FAILURE. Accelerated loss of thiamine may occur with diuretic therapy, HD, peritoneal dialysis, or diarrhea, but in one study, the thiamine status of patients with CKD or those undergoing HD (as assessed by plasma thiamine levels and erythrocyte transketolase activity coefficients) did not differ between thiamine-supplemented or nonsupplemented patients, and no change was seen after 14 days of no supplements. Another report indicated that impaired erythrocyte transketolase activity occurred in more than 50% of

Table 10-4. Summary of other trace element abnormalities in renal failure and their potential clinical consequences

	CRF	HD	CPD	Dialysis Induced	Clinical Consequences
Bromide	N	↓	↓	Yes	Disturbed sleep
Cadmium	Kidney↓liver↑ Serum N-↑	Kidney↓liver↑ Serum N-↑	N Serum N-↑		Growth retardation, hypertension, PTH↓
Chromium	N	↑	↑	Yes	Carcinogenic
Cobalt	N	↑	↑	?	?
Lead	↑	↑	↑	No	Hypertension, gastrointestinal, and neurologic diseases
Manganese	↓	↓-N	↓-N	No	Anemia, impaired glucose tolerance
Molybdenum	N-↑	↑	?	?	Arthropathy
Nickel	↑	↑-N-↓		Yes	Degeneration of heart muscle
Rubidium	N	↑-N-↓	?	Yes	Depression, central nervous system disturbance
Silicon	↑	↑	↑	Yes	Hypersilicemia protects against aluminum toxicity
Strontium	↑-↓	↑	?-↓	?	Osteomalacia
Tin	↓	↓↓	?	?	
Vanadium	N	↑	?	No	Bone disease, hypoglycemia

N, no change from normal; ↓, decreased; ↑, increased; ?, unknown; CRF, chronic renal failure; HD, hemodialysis; CPD, chronic ambulatory peritoneal dialysis; PTH, parathyroid hormone.

patients undergoing HD, but this problem may have been caused by inhibited enzyme activity rather than by a true vitamin deficiency. Patients with CKD who eat a diet restricted in protein or potassium are at risk for developing thiamine deficiency, and if it occurs, it could produce abnormalities as severe as Wernicke encephalopathy. This disorder can be subtle and might be confused with uremic symptoms or even dementia: in one study, 7 of 11 patients with this abnormality were diagnosed only at postmortem examination. A low serum thiamine concentration (less than or equal to 50 nmol per L) and low basal erythrocyte transketolase activity, which responds incrementally after adding thiamine, indicate thiamine deficiency. These tests are not routinely available, and clinical thiamine deficiency should be suspected in patients undergoing dialysis who have at least one of the clinical triad of Wernicke encephalopathy (ophthalmoplegia, ataxia, and disturbed consciousness). In one report, nine of ten patients who had unexplained encephalopathy while undergoing dialysis responded with significantly improved mental status when 100 mg per day of thiamine was given intravenously for several days. Another manifestation of thiamine deficiency, high-output heart failure (wet beriberi) has been reported in patients undergoing dialysis, but again, this manifestation is difficult to differentiate from other causes of heart failure. For these reasons, a daily thiamine supplement that contains the thiamine RDA for healthy subjects is indicated in patients with CKD or ESRD. The routine intravenous thiamine supplement should be considered for patients undergoing dialysis who have malnutrition and the slightest signs of altered mental status.

Vitamin B_2 (Riboflavin)

Riboflavin is an integral component of the coenzymes flavin mononucleotide and flavin adenine dinucleotide, functioning as a catalyst for redox reactions in numerous metabolic pathways and in energy use. Riboflavin is found mainly in meats; milk and dairy products; and green, leafy vegetables. Predominantly absorbed in proximal small intestine, riboflavin is largely bound to albumin, but a portion of riboflavin is associated with other proteins, mainly immunoglobulins; very little riboflavin is stored in body tissues. Any excess riboflavin or flavin-related products is excreted in urine. Riboflavin deficiency is characterized by sore throat, hyperemia, and edema of mucous membranes; cheilosis; angular stomatitis; glossitis; seborrheic dermatitis; and normocytic anemia. Riboflavin deficiency almost invariably occurs in combination with deficiencies of other water-soluble vitamins. ALTERATIONS OF RIBOFLAVIN METABOLISM IN KIDNEY FAILURE. As with thiamine, patients with CKD who eat a low-protein diet are at risk for developing riboflavin deficiency, and the riboflavin requirement is increased by dialysis. In patients with the nephrotic syndrome, erythrocyte riboflavin levels are reportedly reduced or normal. Riboflavin availability, as measured by erythrocyte glutathione–reductase activity, is proportional to fasting total homocysteine levels in patients undergoing dialysis. For these reasons, a daily riboflavin supplement at the RDA level for healthy subjects is recommended for patients with CKD or those being treated by dialysis. High doses of riboflavin are currently recommended for treating nucleoside reverse transcriptase–induced type B lactic acidosis, a condition reported in patients with the acquired immune deficiency syndrome.

Folic Acid

Folate is the generic term for this water-soluble vitamin. Fruits and vegetables constitute the primary dietary source of folate, but it can be destroyed by cooking. Folic acid, the oxidized and stable form of folate, is the form used in vitamin supplements and in fortified food products. Folate functions as a coenzyme in single-carbon transfer reactions that involve synthesis of nucleic acids or amino acid interconversions, including the catabolism of histidine to glutamic acid, interconversion of serine and glycine, and conversion of homocysteine to methionine. The erythrocyte folate concentration is considered to indicate tissue folate status, whereas the serum folate concentration reflects recent dietary intake and is best evaluated as fasting values measured repeatedly over time.

ALTERATIONS OF FOLATE METABOLISM IN RENAL FAILURE.   Nearly all patients with ESRD have homocysteine levels that are two- to threefold higher than those in age-matched controls with normal renal function. The cause of hyperhomocysteinemia is believed to be related to altered metabolism more than to reduced excretion. In patients with uremia, the conversion of homocysteine to methionine is substantially decreased. Homocysteine is formed from the metabolism of methionine as a result of methylation reaction involving the active form of methionine, S-adenosylmethionine (see Fig. 10-2). Homocysteine accumulates unless removed by two diverging pathways: in the transsulfuration pathway, homocysteine reacts with serine to form cystathionine and then cysteine, requiring vitamin B_6 as a cofactor. In the other, the transmethylation pathway, two reactions occur: one involving methionine synthetase, and a secondary reaction (not shown in the figure) in the liver, catalyzed by the enzyme betaine-homocysteine methyltransferase. In the methionine synthetase reaction, folate serves as a substrate in the form of 5-methyltetrahydrofolate, with methylcobalamin as a cofactor. Thus, folate is required in greater amounts; conversely, greater amounts of vitamin B_6 and B_{12} have no appreciable effect on reducing high homocysteine levels. Epidemiologic studies have unequivocally established an association between a high homocysteine level and cardiovascular and peripheral vascular morbidity and mortality in patients without kidney failure. In contrast, "reverse epidemiology" has been described for patients with ESRD, in whom higher total homocysteine levels are associated with lower cardiovascular risk. This finding is of particular interest, because reducing homocysteine levels by folic acid treatment in patients with ESRD is not associated with decreased cardiovascular event rates.

FOLIC ACID SUPPLEMENTATION.   In predialysis patients and in patients undergoing dialysis, 1 to 5 mg of folic acid daily reduces homocysteine levels by 25% to 30%, and this result should become evident within 4 to 6 weeks (intake of more than 10 mg per day of folic acid has not been shown to further reduce homocysteine levels in patients undergoing HD). Before folate is given for the long term, vitamin B_{12} status should be checked, and any deficiency

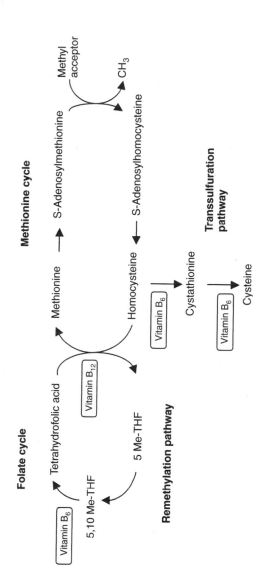

Figure 10-2. Metabolism of homocysteine through the transulfuration pathway to cysteine requires vitamin B_6 as a cofactor, whereas remethylation to methionine requires an adequate supply of folic acid with vitamins B_{12} and B_6 as cofactors. Me, methyl; THF, tetrahydrofolate.

corrected, because inappropriate treatment of vitamin B_{12} deficiency with folic acid can precipitate severe neurologic changes, including subacute combined degeneration of the spinal cord.

Vitamin B_6 (Pyridoxine)

Vitamin B_6 comprises a group of six related compounds: pyridoxine, pyridoxal, pyridoxamine, and their 5-phosphate esters. All these forms become active when converted to pyridoxal 5-phosphate (the active form of vitamin B_6), a cofactor for many enzymes involved in amino acid metabolism, including transaminases, synthetases, and hydroxylases. Vitamin B_6 plays an important part in the metabolism of tryptophan, glycine, glutamate, and the sulfur-containing amino acids, and pyridoxal 5-phosphate is a cofactor in reducing homocysteine levels by converting homocysteine to cysteine through the transulfuration pathway (Fig. 10-2).

Vitamin B_6 is available in meats, liver, vegetables, and the whole grain cereals. Gastrointestinal absorption involves phosphatase-mediated hydrolysis, followed by transport of the non-phosphorylated form into liver, where rephosphorylation occurs. Pyridoxal 5-phosphate is the major form of vitamin in plasma, and it is obtained entirely from the liver as an albumin complex. The major urinary excretory product is 4-pyridoxic acid, but with very high intake, much of the dose is excreted unchanged. Total urinary and fractional excretion of vitamin B_6 has been shown to increase significantly after 20 mg of furosemide in healthy controls and in patients with moderate CKD.

ALTERATIONS OF PYRIDOXINE METABOLISM IN RENAL FAILURE. Patients with CKD and those undergoing dialysis are at risk for developing vitamin B_6 deficiency. Symptoms of vitamin B_6 deficiency are peripheral neuropathies (including paresthesias), burning and painful dysesthesias, and other thermal sensations. To detect a deficiency, the erythrocyte vitamin B_6 content is determined by an indirect method, that is, by assessing the activity of erythrocyte aspartate aminotransferase before and after adding pyridoxal 5-phosphate. Results of this test are subnormal in patients treated with CPD therapy, even in the presence of normal plasma vitamin B_6 levels. No major differences in the peritoneal clearance of vitamin B_6 occur with either 1.5% or 2.5% dextrose-containing peritoneal dialysis solutions. The vitamin B_6 status of patients undergoing HD, as assessed by levels of serum pyridoxal 5-phosphate and erythrocyte vitamin B_6, shows low to normal values when patients are treated with conventional hemodialyzers, but subnormal values in patients treated with EPO dosing or dialysis with high-flux/high-efficiency dialyzers: vitamin B_6 is consumed during hemoglobin synthesis, so EPO causes a decrease in erythrocyte vitamin B_6 levels. A supplement of vitamin B_6 given for 4 weeks to patients undergoing HD increased pyridoxal 5-phosphate levels and symptomatically improved symptoms of peripheral neuropathy. Administering vitamin B_6 alone caused no appreciable decrease in homocysteine levels in patients undergoing dialysis.

SUPPLEMENTATION OF VITAMIN B_6. In summary, patients receiving prolonged diuretic therapy or dialysis patients, especially those receiving EPO, are at risk for developing vitamin B_6 deficiency. When peripheral neuropathy is suspected in elderly patients who receive dialysis therapy, especially CPD, vitamin B_6 deficiency should be considered. The recommended daily intake of vitamin B_6 in patients treated with dialysis is 100% of the RDA. Multivitamin preparations specifically marketed for patients with renal disease contain 10 mg of vitamin B_6, and the upper level of vitamin B_6 intake has been established as 100 mg daily; much higher doses can cause a sensory neuropathy.

Vitamin B_{12} (Cobalamin)

Cobalamin functions as a coenzyme for the critical transfer of methyl groups from methyl tetrahydrofolate to homocysteine, forming methionine and tetrahydrofolate. Impairment of this reaction results in deranged folate metabolism and is responsible for defects in DNA synthesis that lead to megaloblastic maturation of hematopoietic cells. Plasma homocysteine levels are elevated in deficiencies of both cobalamin and folate, but cobalamin also acts as a coenzyme for a separate reaction that converts L-methylmalonyl coenzyme A (CoA) to succinyl CoA. Defects in this reaction increase tissue levels of methylmalonyl CoA and its precursor propionyl CoA. The result is defective neuronal lipid synthesis. Impaired conversion of homocysteine to methionine also may be responsible for the neurologic complications; the methionine that should be formed by this reaction is needed to produce choline and choline-containing phospholipids and, presumably, the lack of these compounds is responsible for the neuropathy. The major dietary sources of cobalamin are meat and dairy products. The cobalamin ingested forms a stable complex with a binding-protein intrinsic factor in the stomach; cobalamin is then released by pancreatic proteases in the upper small intestine. Cobalamin is absorbed in the distal ileal mucosa and then is bound to the cobalamin transport protein to be distributed to the liver, bone marrow, and other cells. Stores of cobalamin are enough to support an adult for 3 to 6 years, even with complete absence of cobalamin absorption. The concentration of vitamin B_{12} in serum of plasma reflects both the B_{12} intake and the stores that are in the liver and other organs.

ALTERATIONS IN OF VITAMIN B_{12} METABOLISM IN KIDNEY FAILURE. Serum vitamin B_{12} values are higher in patients with uremia who have not undergone dialysis than in healthy adults, whereas serum vitamin B_{12} values in patients who have undergone peritoneal dialysis, HD, or renal transplants are not significantly different. Fortunately, EPO does not affect the vitamin B_{12} status of patients undergoing dialysis, and because vitamin B_{12} is largely protein bound, losses during dialysis are small compared with those of other water-soluble vitamins. *Helicobacter pylori*-positive patients undergoing HD may present with lower vitamin B_{12} levels and macrocytosis. Elevated serum homocysteine levels in patients undergoing dialysis are not affected by oral vitamin B_{12} supplements, but high-dose intravenous administration combined with oral folic acid supplements has achieved some success in lowering homocysteine levels. The recommended dietary intake for vitamin B_{12} in patients with kidney disease is 100% of RDA, and patients with an established vitamin B_{12} deficiency should receive the same therapeutic doses as patients without kidney disease.

Vitamin C (Ascorbic Acid)

Vitamin C functions as an antioxidant, with its best-understood function being the hydroxylation of proline when collagen is formed. Vitamin C also protects the folic acid pool by preventing oxidation of tetrahydrofolate; it regulates iron distribution and storage, probably by influencing the valence of stored iron; and it maintains a normal ratio of ferritin to hemosiderin. Vitamin C is present in vegetables and in milk and meats. Some 70% to 90% of dietary ascorbic acid (30 to 180 mg per day) is absorbed, but higher intakes cause a proportionate decrease in intestinal absorption plus an increase in urinary ascorbate excretion. The classic manifestation of severe vitamin C disease is scurvy, whereas a subclinical deficiency may contribute to anemia, delayed wound healing, and periodontal disease. Ascorbic acid levels in leukocyte- and platelet-rich layers of blood are more useful than plasma levels to diagnose vitamin C deficiency.

ALTERATIONS OF VITAMIN C METABOLISM IN RENAL FAILURE.   Predialysis patients and those undergoing renal transplant have low to normal plasma ascorbate levels, and urinary excretion of ascorbate increases with water diuresis, independent of sodium excretion. Ascorbic acid is readily dialyzed, so unsupplemented patients undergoing HD will have subnormal plasma levels of ascorbic acid. Patients treated with CPD have normal to low plasma vitamin C levels. Lately, attention has been focused on the role of oxidative stress in contributing to excess morbidity and mortality in patients with ESRD. Reactive oxygen species are generated by univalent reduction of molecular oxygen as part of normal metabolism in mammalian cells. Vitamin C scavenges highly reactive superoxide anion and hydroxyl radicals, thereby exerting its antioxidant properties. Deficient vitamin C status in patients with ESRD is one of several factors thought to be responsible for enhanced oxidative stress in this population. So far, no evidence exists that therapeutic vitamin C supplements reduce oxidative stress and the risk of cardiovascular events in patients with ESRD.

SUPPLEMENTATION OF VITAMIN C.   Because of dialysis losses and a generally marginal dietary intake, a vitamin C supplement of 60 to 100 mg per day is routinely recommended for patients undergoing dialysis. Higher doses of vitamin C can raise the already high plasma oxalate levels in patients with kidney disease, and excess oxalate can hasten the loss of renal function in predialysis patients, while increasing the risk of myocardial infarction, shunt failure, and muscle weakness related to deposition of oxalate crystals in soft tissue. Large doses of vitamin C (more than 2 g per day) in subjects with normal renal function have been reported to cause acute renal failure secondary to calcium oxalate deposition in the interstitium and renal tubules.

Biotin, Niacin, and Pantothenic Acid

Biotin is a coenzyme in bicarbonate-dependent carboxylation reactions. Biotin is produced by intestinal microorganisms, so biotin deficiency is rare except after prolonged consumption of raw egg white (egg whites bind biotin in the gut and prevent its absorption) or after parenteral nutrition without biotin supplements. Niacin (nicotinic acid) is an essential component of nicotinamide adenine dinucleotide and nicotinamide adenine dinucleotide phosphate, coenzymes in many oxidation–reduction reactions. Niacin also can be synthesized from the essential amino acid, tryptophan. Niacin deficiency causes pellagra, a chronic wasting disease typically associated with diarrhea, dermatitis, and dementia. In renal transplant patients, niacin supplements, containing slow- or sustained-release nicotinic acid, can substantially decrease total cholesterol and low-density lipoprotein cholesterol levels, while increasing high-density lipoprotein cholesterol. Although flushing developed in one study in 67% of patients treated in this fashion, this side effect is generally not sufficient to discontinue the vitamin.

Pantothenic acid functions as a component of CoA and phosphopantetheine, involved in the metabolism of fatty acids, steroid hormones, cholesterol, and certain amino acids. Little is known about the relations among serum levels and the requirements for supplemental biotin, niacin, or pantothenic acid in predialysis patients or those undergoing dialysis. Until further information is available for these vitamins, a recommended supplement containing the RDA for these vitamins should be given.

Fat-Soluble Vitamins

Vitamin A (Retinol)

Vitamin A can be ingested or synthesized within the body from plant carotenes, mainly the β-carotenes. Milk, liver, and kidney are the major sources of preformed vitamin A, which is present largely in the form of fatty acid esters. Vitamin A is absorbed from the small intestine and transported in chylomicrons to the liver, where it is stored. In the liver, retinyl esters are hydrolyzed to produce free retinol, which is bound to retinol-binding protein and transported to peripheral tissues. Vitamin A is required for normal vision and gene expression, reproduction, embryonic development, growth, and immune function. Retinoids also perform essential functions during growth of branching ureteric buds and the renal vasculature; in experimental animals, a mild fetal vitamin A deficiency is associated with a reduced number of nephrons. β-Carotene also blocks oral carcinogenesis in animals and causes oral precancerous lesions to regress in humans. Conversely, a β-carotene supplement does not prevent the development or progression of cancer or other diseases in well-nourished adults. In fact, supplemental β-carotene taken by cigarette smokers or by those exposed to asbestos appears to increase, rather than to reduce, the incidence of lung cancer and death from cardiovascular disease.

ALTERATIONS OF FAT-SOLUBLE VITAMINS METABOLISM IN RENAL FAILURE. Serum vitamin A levels are high in predialysis patients and in those undergoing dialysis or transplant. In acute renal failure, however, serum vitamin A levels are substantially lower than those of healthy adults, despite normal retinol-binding protein levels. This difference is relevant because the major factor that causes serum vitamin A levels to increase in CKD is an increase in retinol-binding protein. Despite high serum levels of vitamin A, overt toxicity is uncommon in CKD, although its features (anemia, hypercalcemia, and hypertriglyceridemia) may be attributed to other effects of uremia. Vitamin A supplements should not be given to patients with renal disease, unless chronic malabsorption syndrome is present.

Vitamin E (Tocopherol)

Of the eight naturally occurring forms of vitamin E, α-tocopherol is the most widely distributed and active form. Absorbed vitamin E in chylomicrons is taken up by the liver and resecreted in very low-density lipoproteins (VLDL). Approximately three fourths of absorbed vitamin E is excreted in the bile, while the remaining amount is excreted in the urine as glucuronides. Synthetic forms of vitamin E, present as esters of α-tocopherol, are in fortified foods and in vitamin supplements. Vitamin E is stored in all tissues and functions as an antioxidant by preventing lipid peroxidation. In atherosclerotic cardiovascular disease, oxidation of low-density lipoproteins (LDL) appears to be a crucial pathogenetic step, and low plasma vitamin E levels are associated with the development of atherosclerosis. A significant inverse correlation exists between serum vitamin E levels and mortality from coronary artery disease in patients with no kidney disease. In patients undergoing HD, free radicals are produced by dialysis membrane–induced activation of complement and leukocytes, increasing the risk of atherosclerosis. Serum vitamin E levels in patients undergoing HD are highly variable, but erythrocyte and LDL vitamin E levels are low and can be corrected with vitamin E supplementation. An oral vitamin E supplement given for 12 weeks was found to decrease the oxidative susceptibility of LDL both in patients undergoing HD and in those undergoing peritoneal dialysis. Despite these data, the effect of vitamin E supplementation in patients with a high risk of cardiovascular disease has been disappointing. Vitamin E supplementation in patients with mild CKD (serum creatinine levels approximately 1.4 to 2.3 mg per dL) in the Heart Outcomes Prevention Evaluation (HOPE) study had no effect on cardiovascular outcomes compared to placebo. Although vitamin E is considered to be safe, it may cause an increased risk of deep vein thrombosis and a vitamin K–responsive hemorrhagic condition, particularly in patients taking an oral anticoagulant. Until more definitive evidence is available, routine prescription of vitamin E is not recommended. Another potential role for vitamin E is to incorporate it on dialysis membranes to function as an antioxidant. Early reports suggest that this technique can improve leukocyte function and reduce markers of oxidative stress, but no data are available on clinical outcome.

CONCLUSIONS

In uremia, substantial changes occur in the concentrations of trace elements and vitamins in blood and tissue. These derangements are caused by decreased elimination and impaired protein binding of micronutrients. In addition, an inadequate diet or altered gastrointestinal absorption in patients with advanced uremia can limit the absorption of trace elements and vitamins. Dialysis can remove micronutrients, depending on their water solubility, membrane permeability, and the gradient between the fraction of an element in serum and its concentration in the dialysate. A major risk of giving supplements is that they can be removed inadequately, leading to accumulation and toxicity. Daily requirements for most trace elements and vitamins in patients with renal disease do not necessarily differ from those in the healthy population (see Table 10-5). Trace elements should not be given routinely to patients with renal failure, but a deficiency of zinc or selenium can cause symptoms. Iron deficiency is a common cause of anemia that does not respond to EPO: oral iron may correct this problem in the early phases of CKD, but parenteral administration is often necessary in advanced kidney failure. Water-soluble vitamins can be lost during dialysis, but the vitamin requirements of patients with CKD are not different from those of healthy adults. Pharmacologic doses of folic acid are recommended to reduce plasma homocysteine levels, but whether this supplement decreases the cardiovascular risk in patients with CKD is yet to be established. A vitamin C level of more than 100 mg per day can lead to tissue deposition of oxalate crystals, which hastens renal insufficiency and increases the risk of myocardial infarction, shunt failure, and muscle

Table 10-5. Comparison of the RDAs for micronutrients in healthy subjects and the measured intake by patients undergoing hemodialysis with recommended intake as the percent of RDA for patients with end-stage renal disease (ESRD)

Micronutrient	RDA in Healthy Population	Observed Intake in Patients undergoing HD[a]	Recommended Supplement as % of RDA
Zinc	8 mg in women 11 mg in men	N/A	None
Selenium	55 µg	N/A	None
Copper	900 µg	N/A	None
Thiamine	1.1 mg in women 1.2 mg in men	0.78–2.36 mg	100
Riboflavin	1.1 mg in women 1.3 mg in men	0.69–2.29 mg	100
Folic acid[b]	400 µg	71–378 µg	200–1,000
Vitamin B$_6$	1.3 mg	0.64–2.14 mg	100
Vitamin B$_{12}$	2.4 µg	1.2–7.5 µg	100
Vitamin C	75 mg for women 90 mg for men	14.6–125.4 mg	120
Vitamin A	700 µg for women 900 µg for men	285–1,385 µg	None
Vitamin E[c]	15 mg	N/A	None

ESRD, end-stage renal disease; HD, hemodialysis; RDA, recommended dietary allowance.
[a] From Rocco MV, Makoff R. Appropriate vitamin therapy for dialysis patients. *Semin Dialysis* 1997;10:272–277, with permission.
[b] Expressed as dietary folate equivalent.
[c] Represents α-tocopherol form only.

weakness in patients undergoing dialysis. Plasma levels of vitamin A and retinol-binding protein are increased in patients with CKD, so multivitamin preparations that contain vitamin A should be avoided. No evidence exists that vitamin E reduces the risk of cardiovascular events, and routine supplementation is not recommended. Patients with kidney disease who are eating an inadequate diet should take a multivitamin preparation that is formulated specifically for patients with kidney disease.

SELECTED READINGS

Bohm V, Tiroke K, Schneider S, et al. Vitamin C status of patients with chronic renal failure, dialysis patients and patients after renal transplantation. *Int J Vitam Nutr Res* 1997;67:262–266.

Druml W, Schwarzenhofer M, Apsner R, et al. Fat-soluble vitamins in patients with acute renal failure. *Miner Electrolyte Metab* 1998;24:220–226.

Fishbane S, Maeska JK. Iron management in end-stage renal disease. *Am J Kidney Dis* 1997;29:319–333.

Food and Nutrition Board: Institute of Medicine. *Dietary reference intakes: applications in dietary assessment: a report of the subcommittees on interpretation and uses of dietary reference intakes and the upper reference level of nutrients, and the standing committee on the scientific evaluation of dietary reference intakes.* Washington, DC: National Academy Press, 2000.

Gallieni M, Brancaccio D, Cozzolino M, et al. Trace elements in renal failure: are they clinically important? *Nephrol Dial Transplant* 1996;11:1232–1235.

Hung SC, Hung SH, Tarng DC, et al. Thiamine deficiency and unexplained encephalopathy in hemodialysis and peritoneal dialysis patients. *Am J Kidney Dis* 2001;38:941–947.

Ihara M, Ito T, Yanagihara C, et al. Wernicke's encephalopathy associated with hemodialysis: report of two cases and review of literature. *Clin Neurol Neurosurg* 1999;101:118–121.

Kalantar-Zadeh K, Kopple JD. Trace elements and vitamins in maintenance dialysis patients. *Adv Ren Replace Ther* 2003;10:170–182.

Kausz AT, Antonsen JE, Hercz G, et al. Screening plasma aluminum levels in relation to aluminum bone disease among asymptomatic dialysis patients. *Am J Kidney Dis* 1999;34:688–693.

Kletzmayr J, Horl WH. Iron overload and cardiovascular complications in dialysis patients. *Nephrol Dial Transplant* 2002;17(Suppl. 2): 25–29.

Mann JF, Lonn EM, Yi Q, et al. Effects of vitamin E on cardiovascular outcomes in people with mild-to-moderate renal insufficiency: results of the HOPE study. *Kidney Int* 2004;65:1375–1380.

Mydlik M, Derzsiova K, Zemberova E. Metabolism of vitamin B_6 and its requirement in chronic renal failure. *Kidney Int* 1997;62: S56–S59.

National Kidney Foundation. K/DOQI: clinical practice guidelines for anemia of chronic kidney disease, 2000. *Am J Kidney Dis* 2000; 37:S182–S238.

Rocco MV, Makoff R. Appropriate vitamin therapy for dialysis patients. *Semin Dial* 1997;10:272–277.

Roth HP, Kirchgessner M. Diagnosis of zinc deficiency. *Z Gerontol Geriatr* 1999;32(Suppl. 1):155–163.

Rovelli E, Luciani L, Pagani C. Correlation between serum aluminum concentration and signs of encephalopathy in a large population of patients dialyzed with aluminum-free fluids. *Clin Nephrol* 1998;29: 294–298.

Westhuzen J. Folate supplementation in the dialysis patient: fragmentary evidence and tentative recommendations. *Nephrol Dial Transplant* 1998;13:2748–2750.

Zima T, Tesar V, Mestek O, et al. Trace elements in end-stage renal disease, 2: clinical implication of trace elements. *Blood Purif* 1999;17: 187–198.

Nutritional Requirements in Hemodialysis

Mark C. Boxall and Timothy H. J. Goodship

MALNUTRITION IN HEMODIALYSIS: DEFINITION AND EXTENT OF THE PROBLEM

Malnutrition, in patients undergoing hemodialysis (HD), has no universally accepted definition; a major problem has been to establish cut off points in the spectrum of malnutrition. The malnutrition advisory group of the British Association of Parenteral and Enteral Nutrition (BAPEN) defines malnutrition as "a state of nutrition in which a deficiency or excess (or imbalance) of energy, protein, and other nutrients causes measurable adverse effects on tissue/body form and function, and clinical outcome." In this chapter, we have narrowed the definition to "a state in which there is evidence that body protein stores are depleted." Conceptually, body protein can be divided into visceral (liver derived) and somatic (muscle).

The body does not store protein in the same way that fat or carbohydrate is stored. The prevalence of depleted protein stores in reported series of patients treated with HD therapy ranges from 10% to 50%. This variability probably reflects not only differences in the patient population but also the means used to detect and determine the abnormality. Two distinct forms of malnutrition are seen in patients undergoing HD (see Table 11-1). Type 1 is the "classic" form and is characterized by a low dietary intake, loss of lean body mass, and usually a normal serum albumin concentration; type 2 is associated with inflammation and atherosclerosis and is characterized by a low serum albumin concentration, often despite a normal dietary intake.

IDENTIFYING DEPLETED PROTEIN STORES IN PATIENTS UNDERGOING HEMODIALYSIS

A full evaluation includes an assessment of dietary intake (e.g., weighed dietary inventory, diet diaries, dietary recall, and urea kinetic modeling), somatic protein "stores" (e.g., anthropometry, total body potassium, total body nitrogen, bioelectrical impedance, dual x-ray absorptiometry, and creatinine kinetics), visceral protein "stores" (e.g., total protein, albumin, prealbumin, and transferrin), and nitrogen metabolism (e.g., nitrogen balance and urea kinetic modeling). For many of these indicators, no absolute values are available to assist in making the diagnosis. Moreover, many indicators are not suitable for routine clinical practice. An alternative approach is to use a simple screening tool that produces reproducible results and then undertake a full assessment in susceptible patients. As a minimum requirement, screening should include subjective global assessment (SGA) and the measurement of

Table 11-1. Characteristics of types 1 and 2 malnutrition in patients undergoing hemodialysis (HD)

	Type 1	Type 2
Albumin	Normal	Low
Dietary protein intake	Low	Normal
Lean body mass	Low	Normal
CRP	Normal	Elevated

CRP, C-reactive protein.
From Stenvinkel P, Heimburger O, Lindholm B, et al. Are there two types of malnutrition in chronic renal failure? Evidence for relationships between malnutrition, inflammation and atherosclerosis (MIA syndrome). *Nephrol Dial Transplant* 2000;15:953–960, with permission.

height, weight, and serum albumin. SGA has been widely used in surveys of patients treated with HD therapy. A score is derived from subjective and objective aspects of the medical history and physical examination and allows patients to be categorized as having either normal, mild, moderate, or severe malnutrition. Body mass index (BMI) should be calculated (weight in kilograms divided by the square of the height in meters) and unintentional loss of edema-free weight recorded. A diagnosis of depleted protein stores should be considered if any one of the following criteria are met:

- SGA scores of 1 to 2 (severe) or 3 to 5 (mild to moderate) loss of protein stores
- BMI scores of 18.5 or less
- unintentional loss of edema-free weight of 10% or more in the previous 6 months
- albumin level of 35 g per L or less (bromocresol green) or 30 g per L (bromocresol purple)

BMI is a simple, accurate, and reproducible calculation based on height and weight and is automatically provided in most renal computer systems. In the United Kingdom, the cut off in the normal population is defined as a Z-score of 2 (2 standard deviation scores below the median), and unintentional loss of edema-free weight of greater than 10% in 6 months is associated with functional abnormalities and poor clinical outcome. In patients with end-stage renal failure, hypoalbuminemia is a powerful predictor of morbidity and mortality. The use of the above criteria would identify patients treated with HD therapy with both types 1 and 2 malnutrition.

NUTRITIONAL REQUIREMENTS IN HEMODIALYSIS

The measurement of nitrogen balance is the classic method by which dietary protein requirements are assessed. In healthy subjects, short- and long-term studies suggest that nitrogen balance is neutral with a dietary protein intake of 0.6 g/kg b.w./d. This outcome means that obligatory nitrogen losses are equivalent to 0.6 g/kg protein/d. Taking into account the variability of these measurements, the World Health Organization (WHO) recommends a safe level of intake to be 0.75 g/kg b.w./d. In patients

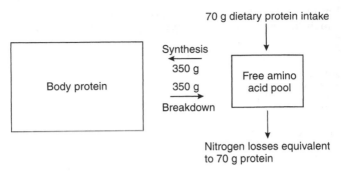

70 g dietary protein intake

Synthesis

350 g

350 g

Breakdown

Body protein

Free amino acid pool

Nitrogen losses equivalent to 70 g protein

Figure 11-1. **Protein turnover in a 70 kg subject consuming 1 g per kg dietary protein.**

undergoing HD, the number of nitrogen balance studies conducted is limited, but these studies suggest that a significantly higher intake of around 1.2 g/kg b.w./d is required, indicating that obligatory nitrogen losses are substantially greater in these patients. These studies also show that nitrogen balance is less positive on dialysis days. To understand the possible reasons for this outcome, a grasp of the relation between protein turnover and nitrogen balance is necessary. Figure 11-1 shows a model of whole-body protein metabolism in a healthy 70 kg man consuming 1 g/kg b.w./d of dietary protein. If the subject is in a stable state without any change in lean body mass, then on a daily basis, nitrogen losses from the free amino acid pool are equivalent to 70 g of protein. However, the turnover between the free amino acid pool and the body protein pool is on average 5 times greater than the dietary intake. In the patient undergoing HD, this system can be perturbed to increase nitrogen losses either through an imbalance between whole-body protein synthesis and catabolism or by increased losses of amino acids or protein.

Energy requirements of healthy subjects range between 35 and 40 kcal/kg b.w./d, depending upon physical activity. Resting energy expenditure in patients undergoing HD, measured with indirect calorimetry, is not different from that of healthy subjects, but whole-room calorimetry has shown that energy expenditure is increased on nondialysis days. Several studies have shown that the energy intake of many patients undergoing HD is below 35 kcal/kg/d, although these data represent serious underestimates of energy intake. Regardless, nitrogen balance can be substantially improved by increasing energy intake; the recommended intake in patients undergoing HD is 35 kcal/kg b.w./d or more.

CATABOLIC FACTORS IN HEMODIALYSIS

Increased catabolism is a potential cause of loss of lean body mass in patients undergoing HD (see Table 11-2). Factors that predispose patients to this condition are detailed in the following sections.

**Table 11-2.   Potential causes of loss of lean
body mass in patients undergoing hemodialysis (HD)**

Catabolic Factors	Blood–membrane interactions
	Dialysate amino acid, protein, and
	glucose losses
	Acidosis
	Inflammation
Anorexia	

Blood–Membrane Interactions

That dialysis might be a catabolic factor is suggested by the negative nitrogen balance seen on dialysis days. Blood–membrane interactions are known to result in complement activation and the release of cytokines from macrophages. Studies in healthy subjects undergoing "sham" HD have shown that amino acid efflux from the leg was increased in subjects dialyzed with "bioincompatible" cuprophane membranes; in contrast, no increase occurred in amino acid efflux when "biocompatible" polysulfone or cellulose-acetate membranes were used. Using stable isotopes, it has been shown that dialysis acutely suppresses whole-body protein synthesis and increases whole body muscle and skeletal muscle protein breakdown. This effect is accompanied by a decrease in both total muscle ribosome concentration and in the percentage of polyribosomes after dialysis. This outcome reflects a decreased capacity for protein synthesis. Substantial evidence exists, therefore, that dialysis with complement activating membranes exerts an acute catabolic effect by both decreasing protein synthesis and increasing protein breakdown. Both these responses are probably mediated by cytokines, such as interleukin-1 and tumor necrosis factor-α. Whether these changes affect the nutritional status of patients undergoing HD in the long term has been the subject of two large randomized prospective trials that gave conflicting results. In one study, 159 patients were randomized to either a low-flux bioincompatible membrane or a low-flux biocompatible membrane. Over an 18-month period, the use of the biocompatible membrane was associated with a favorable effect on weight, albumin, and IGF-1 levels. In the other study, 380 patients were randomized to one of four dialysis regimens: low-flux cuprophane HD, low-flux polysulfone HD, high-flux polysulfone HD, and high-flux polysulfone hemofiltration. Over a 24-month period, no difference in nutritional status between the groups was observed.

Dialysate Amino Acid, Protein, and Glucose Losses

Amino acid losses during dialysis range from 2 to 8 g of free amino acids and 2 to 5 g of peptides per treatment. Losses are not significantly greater with high-flux polysulfone membranes than with cuprophane. However, albumin losses are increased when polysulfone membranes are reused after processing with bleach. The extent to which amino acids and peptides are adsorbed to different membranes is not known. Glucose losses into the dialysate during a single HD treatment are reported to be approximately

25 g. These losses are small but assume increasing importance when dietary intake is compromised.

Acidosis

That acidosis in healthy subjects increases protein degradation and amino acid oxidation is well established. Acidosis causes this effect by activating the ATP-dependent ubiquitin-proteasome proteolytic pathway in a glucocorticoid-dependent manner and increasing the amount and activity of the branched-chain keto acid dehydrogenase. Several studies in patients undergoing HD have shown that correcting acidosis decreases protein breakdown. The importance of this observation has been confounded by cross sectional studies that suggest that acidosis in patients undergoing HD is not associated with evidence of malnutrition. How can these observations be reconciled? Hydrogen ions produced by the metabolism of dietary derived amino acids are an important determinant of acid–base balance. Perhaps the catabolic effects of acidosis in some patients can be counterbalanced by the anabolic effects of raising dietary protein intake. On the other hand, some studies show an improvement in muscle mass with long-term correction of acidosis. Moreover, a variety of factors affect the measurement of serum bicarbonate; underfilling of vacutainers, premature uncapping of vacutainers, and delay in analysis all lead to a falsely low serum bicarbonate concentration. For these reasons, using central laboratories located at a distance from the dialysis unit has been shown to lead to spurious reports of acidosis.

What constitutes adequate correction of acidosis in patients undergoing HD? The average of the post and predialysis bicarbonate concentration has been shown to accurately predict the time-averaged (area under the curve) interdialytic concentration. A pragmatic approach would be to maintain this average within the normal range.

Inflammation

Many patients undergoing HD show evidence of chronic inflammation, with intermittent or persistently elevated levels of the acute phase proteins; C-reactive protein (CRP) is most widely used in clinical practice. An elevated CRP is often accompanied by decreased levels of serum albumin, which acts as an inverse acute-phase protein. The decrease in serum albumin levels is secondary to impaired albumin synthesis. In this context, hypoalbuminemia is primarily an inflammatory marker, rather than an index of poor dietary intake, although the two may coexist. The acute phase response is driven by proinflammatory cytokines, such as IL-1, IL-6, and TNF-α. The source of the inflammation may include:

- infection—multiple sources, especially in diabetics
- cardiovascular disease—heart failure and atherosclerosis
- dialysis related factors—water purity, biocompatibility, reuse, and access infection

- vasculitis
- malignancy

ANOREXIA

Many reports conclude that a major proportion of patients treated with HD therapy consume less protein and energy than is recommended. Factors that may contribute to anorexia include:

- underdialysis
- comorbidity
- medication
- psychosocial factors

Advanced chronic renal failure is associated with appetite suppression, and HD can improve this condition. Moreover, nutritional status improves after dialysis is initiated. Whether increasing the dose of dialysis within the recommended range will improve dietary intake is uncertain, but daily nocturnal dialysis is believed to be associated with improved nutritional status. The relation between Kt/V and the protein equivalent of nitrogen appearance (PNA) is confounded by mathematical coupling, but an assessment of dialysis adequacy should be part of the routine investigation of the anorexic patient undergoing HD.

MANAGEMENT AND TREATMENT OF UNDERNUTRITION

If a diagnosis of undernutrition is suspected on screening, then a full nutritional assessment should be undertaken by a clinician and renal dietitian to elucidate the underlying cause. The evaluation should include a full medical history, an assessment of dietary intake (dietary record or recall and measurement of the PNA), measurements of CRP and serum bicarbonate levels, and measurements of dialysis adequacy, residual renal function, or both.

Strategies for treating malnutrition in HD patients are shown in Table 11-3. If a specific cause for malnutrition is identified, it should be corrected. If dietary protein and energy intake is low,

Table 11-3. Strategies for treating
malnutrition in patients undergoing hemodialysis (HD)

Increase nutrient intake	Dietary counseling
	Oral supplements
	Nasogastric feeding
	Percutaneous endoscopic gastrostomy feeding
	Intradialytic parenteral nutrition
Correct catabolic factors	Increase dialysate bicarbonate and/or give oral sodium bicarbonate
	Use biocompatible membrane and ultrapure water
	Treat occult infection
Correct anorexia	Increase dialysis dose
	Treat psychosocial factors

then attempts should be made to increase or supplement the diet. Appropriate measures, in addition to dietary counseling, include:

- oral supplements
- nasogastric (NG) and percutaneous endoscopic gastrostomy (PEG) feeding
- intradialytic parenteral nutrition (IDPN)

Oral Supplements

The acute response to oral supplements is normal in patients undergoing HD, but few long-term studies have examined the efficacy of oral supplements in treating malnutrition; however, for most patients, oral supplements are the first line of therapy. Measurements of PNA can be used to assess compliance. Consuming a protein- and energy-enriched meal has recently been shown to improve the balance between whole-body protein synthesis and breakdown during dialysis. The long-term effects of this strategy are unknown.

Nasogastric and Percutaneous Endoscopic Gastrostomy Feeding

Nasogastric and PEG feeding have been more widely used in children than in adults. PEG feeding, although initially more invasive, is more acceptable to the patient and is more suited to an extended period of supplementation.

Intradialytic Parenteral Nutrition

IDPN is often used if a trial of oral supplements has failed. Typical regimens consist of a mixture of lipids, glucose, and amino acids or peptides. The total volume given at each dialysis is approximately 1,000 mL, providing 2,000 to 7,000 kJ (500 to 1,750 kcal) and 45 to 60 g protein. Although patient adherence is achieved with this technique, the amount of supplemental protein and calories that is provided is less than that achieved with PEG feeding. Acute isotope studies have shown that IDPN results in a substantial increase in whole-body protein and forearm muscle protein synthesis in association with a decrease in whole-body protein breakdown. However, as soon as the infusion is stopped, protein degradation rises and remains high, even when the HD session is finished. The anabolic effects of IDPN during dialysis seem to be augmented by exercise. Prospective studies have shown an improvement in protein stores plus a concomitant increase in patient survival.

Growth Hormone and Insulin-like Growth Factor I

Resistance to the actions of both growth hormone (GH) and IGF-1 occurs frequently in patients with chronic renal failure. Availability of recombinant forms of both hormones has provided an attractive means to overcome this resistance and promote anabolism. Most studies have examined the use of GH and found that lean body mass increases as a result of increased muscle protein synthesis. This result is mediated by endogenous IGF-1, which increases to levels occurring clinically in patients with acromegaly. No data exists as to whether such increases in lean body mass are associated with a decrease in morbidity and mortality. The use of GH would seem most appropriate in those patients with a loss of lean body mass rather than hypoalbuminemia, especially if the loss is resistant to all other forms of treatment.

Overweight Patients Undergoing Hemodialysis

Overweight is graded by the WHO based on the BMI: grade 1 overweight is a BMI of 25.00 to 29.99, grade 2 is a BMI of 30.00 to 39.99, and grade 3 is a BMI of 40 or more. Within the general population, a gain in weight sufficient to become overweight and persistently being overweight are both associated with increased morbidity and mortality. However, no long-term intervention studies have been conducted to show that sustained weight loss will decrease morbidity and mortality. For patients treated with HD therapy, the lowest mortality rates occur in those patients with the highest BMI; an explanation for this occurrence might be that being overweight is accompanied by better nutrition. Certainly, those patients with the highest BMI have the highest albumin and prealbumin levels. A pragmatic approach would be to give all patients undergoing HD dietary advice to avoid weight gain to a BMI that exceeds 30.

Dietary Sodium Intake in Patients Undergoing Hemodialysis

The reference nutrient intake (2 standard deviations above the estimated average requirement) for sodium intake in adults in the United Kingdom is 70 mmol per day. The average intake of the population is substantially greater than this quantity. Although the beneficial effects of dietary sodium restriction on hypertension have been disputed, substantial evidence exists to suggest that a reduction in dietary sodium intake in the general population results in a greater reduction in blood pressure than that seen with a "healthy" diet. Similar results have been obtained in patients undergoing HD with a low sodium dialysate. Therefore, counseling patients to limit dietary salt intake to less than 6 g per day (equivalent approximately to 100 mmol of sodium) would seem wise.

SELECTED READINGS

Caglar K, Peng Y, Pupim LB, et al. Inflammatory signals associated with hemodialysis. *Kidney Int* 2002;62:1408–1416.

Galland R, Traeger J, Arkouche W, et al. Short daily hemodialysis rapidly improves nutritional status in hemodialysis patients. *Kidney Int* 2001;60:1555–1560.

Garibotto G, Barreca A, Russo R, et al. Effects of recombinant human growth hormone on muscle protein turnover in malnourished hemodialysis patients. *J Clin Invest* 1997;99:97–105.

Graham KA, Hoenich NA, Goodship THJ. Pre and interdialytic acid-base balance in hemodialysis patients. *Int J Artif Organs* 2001;24:192–196.

Greenland P. Beating high blood pressure with low-sodium DASH. *N Engl J Med* 2001;344:53–55.

Gutierrez A, Bergstrom J, Alvestrand A. Protein catabolism in sham-hemodialysis: the effect of different membranes. *Clin Nephrol* 1992;38:20–29.

Iglesias P, Diez JJ, Fernandez-Reyes MJ, et al. Recombinant human growth hormone therapy in malnourished dialysis patients: a randomized controlled study. *Am J Kidney Dis* 1998;32:454–463.

Ikizler TA, Flakoll PJ, Parker RA, et al. Amino acid and albumin losses during hemodialysis. *Kidney Int* 1994;46:830–837.

Ikizler TA, Pupim LB, Brouillette JR, et al. Hemodialysis stimulates muscle and whole body protein loss and alters substrate oxidation. *Am J Physiol Endocrinol Metab* 2002;282:E107–E116.

Jensen PB, Hansen TB, Frystyk J, et al. Growth hormone, insulin-like growth factors and their binding proteins in adult hemodialysis patients treated with recombinant human growth hormone. *Clin Nephrol* 1999;52:103–109.

Kalantar-Zadeh K, Block G, Humphreys MH, et al. Reverse epidemiology of cardiovascular risk factors in maintenance dialysis patients. *Kidney Int* 2003;63:793–808.

Kalantar-Zadeh K, Ikizler TA, Block G, et al. Malnutrition-inflammation complex syndrome in dialysis patients: causes and consequences. *Am J Kidney Dis* 2003;42:864–881.

Kloppenburg WD, De Jong PE, Huisman RM. The contradiction of stable body mass despite low reported dietary energy intakes in chronic hemodialysis patients. *Nephrol Dial Transplant* 2002;17: 1628–1633.

Krautzig S, Janssen U, Koch KM, et al. Dietary salt restriction and reduction of dialysate sodium to control hypertension in maintenance hemodialysis patients. *Nephrol Dial Transplant* 1998;13: 552–553.

Kopple JD. The National Kidney Foundation K/DOQI clinical practice guidelines for dietary protein intake for chronic dialysis patients. *Am J Kidney Dis* 2001;38:S68–S73.

Lofberg E, Essen P, McNurlan M, et al. Effect of hemodialysis on protein synthesis. *Clin Nephrol* 2000;54:284–294.

Mehrotra R, Berman N, Alistwani A, et al. Improvement of nutritional status after initiation of maintenance hemodialysis. *Am J Kidney Dis* 2002;40:133–142.

Pupim LB, Flakoll PJ, Brouillette JR, et al. Intradialytic parenteral nutrition improves protein and energy homeostasis in chronic hemodialysis patients. *J Clin Invest* 2002;110(4):483–492.

Pupim LB, Flakoll PJ, Levenhagen DK, et al. Exercise augments the acute anabolic effects of intradialytic parenteral nutrition in chronic hemodialysis patients. *Am J Physiol Endocrinol Metab* 2004;286:E589–E597.

Qureshi AR, Alvestrand A, Danielsson A, et al. Factors predicting malnutrition in hemodialysis patients: a cross-sectional study. *Kidney Int* 1998;53:773–782.

Sacks FM, Svetkey LP, Vollmer WM, et al. DASH-Sodium Collaborative Research Group. Effects on blood pressure of reduced dietary sodium and the Dietary Approaches to Stop Hypertension (DASH) diet. *N Engl J Med* 2001;344:3–10.

Stenvinkel P, Heimburger O, Lindholm B, et al. Are there two types of malnutrition in chronic renal failure? Evidence for relationships between malnutrition, inflammation and atherosclerosis (MIA syndrome). *Nephrol Dial Transplant* 2000;15:953–960.

Veeneman JM, Kingma HA, Boer TS, et al. Protein intake during hemodialysis maintains a positive whole body protein balance in chronic hemodialysis patients. *Am J Physiol Endocrinol Metab* 2003;284:E954–E965.

Veeneman JM, Kingma HA, Boer TS, et al. The metabolic response to ingested protein is normal in long-term hemodialysis patients. *Am J Kidney Dis* 2004;43:330–341.

World Health Organization. *Energy and protein requirements: report of a joint FAO/WHO/UNU expert consultation.* Geneva: World Health Organization, 1985:71–112. Technical Report Series.

Nutrition and Peritoneal Dialysis

Talat Alp Ikizler

CLINICAL IMPORTANCE OF NUTRITIONAL STATUS IN PATIENTS UNDERGOING PERITONEAL DIALYSIS

Multiple studies indicate that the nutritional status of patients undergoing peritoneal dialysis (PD) is an important predictor of their clinical outcome. The CANUSA study, a multicenter, international prospective cohort study, examined dialysis adequacy and nutrition in 689 patients undergoing continuous ambulatory peritoneal dialysis (CAPD). The investigators found that low serum albumin concentrations; low subjective global assessment (SGA) scores; and low, normalized protein intakes were important independent nutritional risk factors for death in patients treated with PD therapy. In an Australian study in which patients were treated with CAPD therapy, total body nitrogen, a sophisticated measure of nutritional status, was reported to be lower in patients who died or experienced major morbidity than in those who were alive and stable. These data indicate that poor nutritional status, as assessed by multiple nutritional markers, predisposes patients undergoing PD to an increased risk for hospitalization or death.

The prevalence of poor nutritional status in patients undergoing PD is also high, ranging from 20% to 50%, using various markers of nutritional status. In a large multicenter study of 224 patients treated with CAPD therapy, 8% of the patients were severely malnourished, 33% of the patients were mildly to moderately malnourished, and the remainder (59%) did not have evidence of poor nutritional status (principally, a low serum albumin value).

ASSESSMENT AND MONITORING OF NUTRITIONAL STATUS IN PATIENTS UNDERGOING PERITONEAL DIALYSIS

Assessment of protein and energy nutritional status is a broad and complex topic that involves indirect measures of visceral protein concentrations, somatic protein stores, and energy expenditure and requirements and measurements of protein and energy homeostasis. Although this topic is covered in detail in Chapter 14, some basic concepts must be discussed here as they relate to patients treated with PD therapy; assessment and monitoring of protein and energy nutritional status are crucial to prevent, diagnose, and treat the unique type of malnutrition observed in this patient population (see Fig. 12-1).

Poor nutritional status is a condition associated and interrelated with many diseases; this condition can be secondary to, or causative of, an underlying disease. Therefore, a clinically meaningful assessment of protein and energy nutritional status should not only assess the risk for the morbidity and mortality

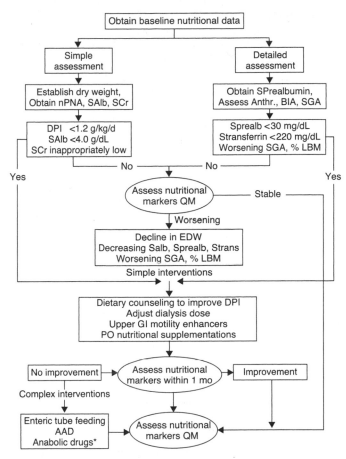

Figure 12-1. A proposed algorithm for the assessment and management of nutritional status in patients undergoing peritoneal dialysis (PD). nPNA, normalized protein nitrogen appearance rate; DPI, dietary protein intake; Salb, serum albumin; SPrealb, serum prealbumin; SCr, serum creatinine; Anthr, anthropometric measurements; BIA; bioelectric impedance analysis; SGA, subjective global assessment; LBM, lean body mass; QM, every month; EDW, estimated dry weight; GI, gastrointestinal; AAD, amino acid dialysate. * Mostly experimental.

that results from poor a nutritional state but should also distinguish the causes and consequences of both the poor nutritional state and the underlying diseases. A meaningful method should also determine whether patients could benefit from nutritional interventions.

Serum Albumin

Serum albumin, measured by a convenient, readily available laboratory test, is by far the most extensively studied serum protein. The concentration of serum albumin is the net result of its synthesis, breakdown, volume of distribution, and exchange between intra- and extravascular spaces, as well as losses. Albumin is a highly water-soluble protein synthesized in the liver and has a half-life of approximately 20 days. Albumin is primarily (two thirds) in the extracellular space. Inadequate dietary protein intake (DPI) is characterized by a decrease in the rate of albumin synthesis, which in the short term may have little effect on serum albumin levels, because albumin has a low turnover rate and a large pool size. Studies have shown that long-term protein and energy restriction in healthy subjects and patients with anorexia nervosa leads to substantial decrease in body weight but rarely decreases serum albumin concentration. In addition to inadequate protein intake, hypoalbuminemia can also occur with underlying conditions such as hepatic and inflammatory disorders that decrease albumin synthesis and increase albumin breakdown. We believe that serum albumin levels below 3.0 g per dL are usually the result of some cause other than low nutrient intake alone. Longitudinal studies that evaluate the validity of serum albumin as a nutritional marker in the presence of inflammation and changes in volume status are limited; available data on patients undergoing PD should be interpreted in this context.

Serum Prealbumin

Prealbumin, compared with serum albumin, has some advantages in nutritional assessment, because prealbumin is less abundant in the body and has a half-life of 2 to 3 days, making it a more sensitive marker than albumin of subtle changes in visceral protein stores. In addition, serum prealbumin concentration is not affected by hydration status. A low nutrient intake decreases serum prealbumin levels, and these levels can be restored by refeeding, characteristics of a useful tool to monitor nutritional supplementation. Unfortunately, serum prealbumin has the same inflammatory responses profile as serum albumin, and serum prealbumin level tends to increase as renal function decreases, so it may not be a reliable tool to assess protein stores in patients with progressive renal disease. However, in patients undergoing PD who have relatively stable renal function, serum prealbumin may be a useful tool, and a level below 29 mg per dL is recommended to indicate an abnormal nutritional state. Note that this value is within the normal range (i.e., 10 to 40 mg per dL) for populations with normal renal function.

Serum Transferrin

The primary function of serum transferrin is to transport iron in the plasma. It has a half-life of 8 to 10 days and a small body pool, making it sensitive to nutritional changes. Improvements in serum transferrin levels have also been observed with nutritional supplements. In patients undergoing PD, an assessment of serum transferrin as a marker of protein stores is problematic for two reasons: iron metabolism is altered by renal failure; and as with all the visceral proteins, conditions associated with inflammatory response or liver failure affect serum transferrin concentrations. Therefore, serum transferrin is not a recommended tool for monitoring nutritional status in patients with end-stage renal disease (ESRD).

C-Reactive Protein

C-reactive protein (CRP) is a positive acute phase reactant (APR) that correlates negatively with concentrations of visceral proteins. CRP is not a direct nutritional marker, but in the face of low levels of serum albumin or prealbumin (negative APRs), potential causes of protein depletion that are not related to the diet should be evaluated. If CRP levels are high, sources of infection, inflammation, or both should be investigated and, if possible, resolved.

Anthropometry

Anthropometric measurements have been used for decades and include height and weight, calculated body mass index (BMI), skinfold thickness, biceps and subscapular skinfolds, midarm circumference, and calculated midarm muscle circumference, diameter, or area (Chapter 14). Because almost 50% of the body's fat mass is found in the subcutaneous layer, these measurements can provide a reasonable index of total body fat. These measurements have the advantage of being inexpensive, easy to perform at the bedside, and simple to compare with well-established norms for healthy populations based on the Third National Health and Nutrition Examination Survey (NHANES III) data. However, they may have limitations for specific patient populations, such as the well-nourished patient with ESRD, because of the severely limited database and lack of correction for hydration status or the effects of chronic illness. In general, anthropometry is insensitive for detecting subtle changes in body composition, but it can be useful when available serially for a patient and when used in conjunction with other nutritional indices.

Bioelectric Impedance Analysis

Bioelectric Impedance Analysis (BIA) is a technique that has proven to be safe, generally accepted by patients, and easy to use. BIA is used for determining fluid management and for evaluating nutritional assessment. The accuracy of BIA in assessing the body composition of patients undergoing PD is subject to some important limitations. Many patients who receive PD treatment exhibit abnormal fluid balance, which can result in inaccurate estimations of lean body mass (LBM) and fat mass. For accurate results, BIA should be conducted when the patient is in an edema-free or near–edema-free state and should be performed with the peritoneal cavity drained of dialysate. In addition, the software packages provide calculations for comparing BIA results to those for healthy individuals, so they are inaccurate for comparing values obtained from well-nourished patients with specific diseases.

Dual-energy X-ray Absorptiometry

Dual-energy X-ray absorptiometry (DEXA) can be performed in 6 to 15 minutes with minimal radiation exposure (less than 5 mrem) and minor discomfort to the patient. Because of the minimal radiation exposure, serial measurements can be safely obtained. DEXA is a simple technique, has excellent precision, and can provide regional body composition. DEXA has been shown to be quite sensitive for detecting small changes in body composition, which makes it a very useful tool. As with most other methods, the hydration status of the patient must be considered for each evaluation, an important consideration for patients undergoing PD.

Subjective Global Assessment

SGA is a simple method that draws on the experience of a clinician to make an overall assessment of nutritional status in a standardized way. An overall SGA rating is assigned to the patient; scores range from a rating of 1 or 2 for severe malnutrition, indicating significant physical signs in most categories; 3 to 5 for mild to moderate malnutrition, indicating no clear evidence of normal status or of severe malnutrition; and 6 or 7 for very mild malnutrition to well nourished. The direct relation of SGA to various components of nutritional status has not been determined, and its reliability and validity remain somewhat controversial. Indeed, the very nature of this assessment is subjective, and scores can vary from practitioner to practitioner; however, reliability between trained observers reportedly is good. SGA does not replace formal nutrition assessment methods but can be used as a screening tool to determine the aggressiveness of nutritional intervention and to prioritize patient care. Research has shown that SGA is not a sensitive test or reliable predictor of the degree of malnutrition, although it can differentiate between severely malnourished patients and those with normal nutrition.

Dietary Assessment

Symptoms of nausea, vomiting, and anorexia, as well as recent changes in body weight, should be carefully evaluated to ascertain their cause. A patient's recall of the diet can provide information on the intake of protein, fats, and carbohydrates. Four-day dietary recalls are needed to provide reliable data; food frequency questionnaires may also provide useful information (Chapter 14).

Protein Equivalent of Total Nitrogen Appearance Rate

Ingested proteins are metabolized to several nitrogenous products (e.g., urea, amino acids, or creatinine). In the steady state (without catabolism or anabolism), nitrogenous waste products are removed from the body by urine, dialysate, stool, skin, and blood and are equal to the protein intake (6.25 g protein produces 1 g nitrogen). A strong relation exists between urea appearance rate (which can be calculated from urea dialysate and urine concentrations) and total nitrogen appearance, so PNA can be calculated from the urea appearance rate. Because protein losses must be considered in patients undergoing PD, PNA should be calculated by using the following equation:

$$PNA \text{ (g/24 h)} = [0.195 \times urea\ appearance\ (mmol/24\ h)] + 15.1$$
$$+ total\ protein\ losses\ (g/d)$$

PNA is usually normalized to g/kg b.w./d (nPNA) and was formerly called *protein catabolic rate* (*PCR*), but this term is not appropriate, because the true PCR is several times higher than the PNA (Chapter 6). In metabolically stable patients, nPNA reflects DPI, and the use of this parameter to assess nutritional status has several weaknesses. First, factors besides dietary protein influence generation of urea (urea appearance rate); for example, therapy of acidosis results in decreased urea excretion and therefore decreased PNA, even if DPI is held constant. This factor may explain why in several studies, only a weak correlation was seen between daily protein intake and PNA. Therefore, urea kinetics should be used to estimate protein intake only if a patient's protein metabolism is in the steady state. In catabolic situations, the PNA is increased out of proportion to DPI. In anabolic situations, the reverse occurs. Second, the reported relation between Kt/V and PNA may be caused by mathematical coupling, because both parameters are influenced by the amount of urea excreted in dialysate and urine. Third, because PNA reflects dietary protein, it is only an indirect marker of nutritional status, which might explain why PNA, unlike SGA and LBM, has not been correlated with mortality in most studies. Fourth, a controversy exists about the kind of weight that is appropriate for normalization of PNA. Using actual body weight for normalizing PNA yields considerably higher values in smaller, malnourished patients than those calculated in larger patients with good nutritional status. Therefore, several authors use ideal body weight or "desirable body weight" to normalize PNA.

FACTORS INFLUENCING NUTRITIONAL STATUS IN PATIENTS UNDERGOING PERITONEAL DIALYSIS

In spite of the strikingly increased prevalence of poor nutritional status and the important relation between nutritional status and clinical outcome in patients undergoing PD, whether PD treatment *per se* is the sole cause of these findings is not clear. Similar observations of an increased prevalence of poor nutritional status with an increased risk of morbidity and mortality can also be made for patients undergoing chronic hemodialysis, indicating that the underlying metabolic and hormonal derangements, the related advanced uremia, and other comorbid conditions play a critical role in this process. Multiple factors that influence the nutritional status of patients undergoing PD are listed in Table 12-1.

Altered Amino Acid and Protein Metabolism

Patients who receive chronic dialysis treatment have well-defined abnormalities in their plasma and, to a lesser extent, in their muscle amino acid profiles. Commonly, essential amino acid concentrations are low, and nonessential amino acid concentrations are high. Multiple factors are associated with this abnormal profile. The progressive loss of renal tissue, where several amino acids are metabolized, is an important factor that alters the plasma and muscle amino acid concentrations. Specifically, glycine and phenylalanine concentrations are elevated, and serine, tyrosine,

**Table 12-1.   Factors influencing the nutritional
status of patients undergoing peritoneal dialysis (PD)**

Increased protein and energy requirements
　　Loss of nutrients (amino acids, proteins, or both) during dialysis
　　Increased resting energy expenditure

Decreased protein and calorie intake
　　Overzealous dietary restriction
　　Anorexia
　　　　Advanced uremia
　　　　Suppression of oral intake by peritoneal dialysate glucose load
　　Frequent hospitalizations
　　Inadequate dialysis dose
　　Comorbidities (diabetes mellitus, GI diseases, ongoing
　　　　inflammatory response)
　　Multiple medications
　　Monetary restrictions
　　Depression
　　Altered sense of taste

Increased catabolism/decreased anabolism
　　Dialysis induced catabolism
　　　　Amino acid losses
　　　　Induction of inflammatory cascade
　　Amino acid abnormalities
　　Metabolic acidosis
　　Hormonal derangements
　　　　Hyperparathyroidism
　　　　Insulin and growth hormone resistance

GI, gastrointestinal.

and histidine concentrations are decreased. Plasma and muscle
concentrations of valine, leucine, and isoleucine (branched-chain
amino acids) are reduced in patients undergoing chronic dialysis, with valine displaying the greatest reduction. In contrast,
plasma levels of citrulline, cystine, aspartate, methionine, and
both 1- and 3-methylhistidine are increased. Although decreased
dietary protein is potentially a factor that yields an abnormal essential amino acid profile, certain abnormalities can occur when
nutrient intake is adequate, indicating that the uremic milieu
and associated metabolic abnormalities have additional effects
on amino acid profiles. Indeed, metabolic acidosis, commonly
seen in uremic patients, plays an important role in the increased
oxidation of branched-chain amino acids (see subsequent text).
Further, peritoneal loss of amino acids (5 to 12 g per day) is another factor contributing to abnormal amino acid profile in patients undergoing PD.
　　Patients undergoing PD are also at risk for substantially altered protein homeostasis, potentially leading to a net protein
catabolic state. In vitro data and animal studies suggest that abnormal metabolic conditions, such as uremia (and diabetes), are
associated with an increased rate of muscle protein breakdown.

If accompanied by decreased dietary nutrient intake, this condition would lead to a net negative protein balance and a potential loss of LBM. Nevertheless, several studies show a concomitant decrease in both protein synthesis and degradation in patients with advanced uremia, resulting in a net nitrogen balance that is not different from that in matched healthy controls, albeit at a significantly lower protein turnover rate. This result is a physiologically expected adaptation, as the rate of protein turnover is directly related to the production of certain end products, known as uremic toxins, that accumulate in advanced uremia.

Overall, these observations can be interpreted to indicate that advanced uremia may lead to a syndrome of metabolic abnormalities that result in a low protein turnover state but do not necessarily cause major abnormalities in net whole-body protein balance. A decreased dietary protein and energy intake, regardless of the cause (i.e., anorexia of uremia or prescription of low DPI), can be compensated to some extent with an adjustment in the protein and essential amino acid degradation, with no important effect on net balance. However, when accelerated protein degradation occurs because of increased metabolic needs (acute illness and stress conditions), metabolic derangements (metabolic acidosis, diabetes, inflammation), or both, patients with uremia likely cannot initiate the appropriate compensatory mechanisms, such as increased protein synthesis or suppression of protein breakdown. This lack of response can be caused by inadequate dietary intake, a deficiency in incorporating the available nutrients, or a defect in suppressing protein catabolic mediators. The clinical importance of these derangements can be witnessed in the increased prevalence of accelerated loss of LBM in patients undergoing chronic dialysis who have uncontrolled diabetes or an ongoing inflammatory response.

Dyslipidemia and Obesity in Patients Undergoing Peritoneal Dialysis

Dyslipidemia is quite common in patients undergoing PD and is often multifactorial (see Chapter 4). Abnormalities in lipid profiles can be detected in patients once renal function begins to deteriorate. The presence of nephrotic syndrome (related to the level of residual renal function) or other comorbidities, such as diabetes mellitus and liver disease, as well as the use of medications that alter lipid metabolism, all contribute to the dyslipidemia seen in patients undergoing PD. Patients who receive CAPD therapy exhibit higher concentrations of serum cholesterol, triglyceride, low-density lipoprotein (LDL) cholesterol, Lp(a), and apoB, even though the mechanisms that alter the lipid metabolism are similar to those present in patients undergoing chronic hemodialysis. This difference could be related to increased protein losses through the peritoneum plus the glucose absorbed from the dialysate.

Longitudinal studies examining body composition in patients undergoing PD show that a tendency toward increased body weight is primarily because of an increase in fat mass. Obesity is an important risk factor for morbidity and mortality in the general population; but on the basis of epidemiologic studies, obesity seems to confer a considerable survival advantage in the population receiving chronic dialysis therapy. However, a recent report from the United States Renal Data System suggested that this association is valid only for patients undergoing chronic hemodialysis not for patients undergoing PD. The fat-free mass component of the body composition of obese patients undergoing chronic hemodialysis seems to provide a survival advantage, and the adipose tissue contributes strongly to the inflammatory response observed in obese individuals. Overall, the available evidence suggests that the risk and benefit ratio of obesity, especially if associated with increased fat mass, should be critically reexamined in patients undergoing PD.

Metabolic Acidosis

Extensive research has shown conclusively that metabolic acidosis, through activation of the ubiquitin-proteasome pathway by a glucocorticoid-dependent mechanism, induces protein breakdown, accelerates amino acid oxidation, and decreases muscle protein synthesis, which would ultimately result in loss of LBM. Importantly, correcting acidosis has been shown to improve nutritional status and to prevent acidosis-related muscle wasting in patients undergoing PD. Notably, patients undergoing PD are usually less acidotic than patients undergoing hemodialysis. The use of recently available bicarbonate-based PD solutions enables acidosis to be normalized in most, if not all, patients undergoing PD. A minimum serum bicarbonate level of 22 mmol per L is suggested for patients undergoing PD.

Hormonal Derangements

Insulin is a major anabolic hormone that stimulates muscle protein synthesis and suppresses protein degradation. Uremia is also characterized by resistance to insulin; although the insulin binding to its receptor in patients with chronic kidney disease (CKD) and ESRD is normal, a postreceptor defect in tissue insulin responsiveness can occur, causing insulin resistance and glucose intolerance. Similar abnormalities can be observed with decreased food intake, as well as with experimental metabolic acidosis. Metabolic acidosis also causes impaired function, resistance to several anabolic hormones, or both, including insulin, growth hormone (GH), and thyroid hormone. Abnormalities in GH and the insulin-like growth factor-1 (IGF-1) axis are thought to constitute an important factor in the development of malnutrition in patients with uremia. GH is the major promoter of growth in children and exerts several anabolic actions in adults, such as enhanced protein synthesis, increased fat mobilization, and increased gluconeogenesis. IGF-1 is the major mediator of these actions. Evidence suggests that uremia is associated with the development of resistance to GH action at cellular levels. In animal experiments, uremia is characterized by reduced levels of the mRNAs that encode the hepatic GH receptor and hepatic IGF-1, plus a defect in GH signal transduction. This blunted response would be expected to attenuate the anabolic actions of these hormones. These observations have led to experimental therapies to examine the anabolic effects of administering pharmacologic doses of recombinant human GH (rhGH) and recombinant human IGF-1 (rhIGF-1).

Inflammation as a Catabolic Factor in Patients Undergoing Peritoneal Dialysis

Recent studies have pointed out that patients with ESRD, including patients receiving PD therapy, have a high prevalence of elevated levels of inflammatory markers. The etiology of chronic inflammation in patients undergoing PD is multifactorial and includes decreased clearance of cytokines and accumulation of uremic toxins (middle molecules, parathyroid hormone, and leptin) caused by decreased renal function; certain factors associated with dialysis, such as endotoxin transfer from the dialysate, peritoneal dialysate bioincompatibility, and PD catheters; and comorbidities that include chronic infections (periodontal disease, peritonitis), diabetes mellitus, atherosclerosis, and congestive heart failure. Inflammation, more correctly termed the *systemic inflammatory response syndrome*, is a complex combination of physiologic, immunologic, and metabolic effects that occur in response to a variety of stimulators resulting from tissue injury or disease processes. Certain cytokines, such as interleukin-1 (IL-1), interleukin-6 (IL-6), and tumor necrosis factor-alpha (TNF-α), are the primary mediators of these effects. Because the predominant metabolic effects of these cytokines are catabolic, limiting the biological activities of the host by eliciting a strong anti-inflammatory response is important. However, in conditions in which the inflammatory response is ongoing and cannot be controlled effectively, such as in chronic diseases, adverse effects generally result.

The metabolic and nutritional effects of chronic inflammation are many and include anorexia, increased skeletal muscle protein breakdown, increased whole-body protein catabolism, cytokine-mediated hypermetabolism, and disruption of the GH and IGF-1 axis, leading to decreased anabolism. These effects closely mimic the metabolic abnormalities associated with uremic malnutrition that is observed in patients undergoing dialysis. These findings suggest that the chronic inflammation observed in patients undergoing PD may be a causative factor in their worsening nutritional status.

Leptin

Serum leptin levels are substantially higher in patients undergoing PD than in healthy subjects. An important positive relation exists between leptin and both BMI and body fat mass, but no correlation exists between serum leptin and daily protein intake, daily energy intake, or normalized PCR. In one report, patients undergoing PD with a loss of LBM had significantly higher serum CRP levels and higher serum leptin levels than those with no change in nutritional status. The removal rate of leptin through the peritoneal membrane is comparable to that of β_2-microglobulin, but the dialysate-to-plasma ratio of leptin is higher than expected from its molecular weight. The serum leptin level and dialysate-to-plasma ratio of β_2-microglobulin are also related to abdominal visceral fat. These results suggest that leptin found in the peritoneal dialysate is derived from plasma as well as from visceral fat tissue.

Dialysis-Related Factors

Dialysis Adequacy

The association between inadequate dialysis and decreased nutrient intake has long been recognized. In the CANUSA study, estimates of nutritional status and dialysis adequacy were positively correlated, and this relation is reported to have been primarily driven by the loss of residual renal function. However, the optimal dosage for dialysis, after which no further improvement in nutritional status is observed, has not been established.

Loss and Gain of Nutrients from the Peritoneal Dialysate

The average loss of amino acids into the dialysate ranges between 1.2 and 3.4 g per 24 hours in patients undergoing PD. In addition, substantial amounts of proteins are lost into the dialysate, ranging between 5 and 15 g per 24 hours in different studies. A major portion of these proteins is albumin (50% to 65%). Notably, amino acid and protein losses increase substantially during episodes of peritonitis. The protein losses in the dialysate can lead to several metabolic disturbances in patients undergoing PD, most notably in the lipid profiles. Furthermore, patients undergoing PD tend to have higher prevalence of hypoalbuminemia, which is closely associated with the dialysate losses. Although patients undergoing PD generally have a negative protein balance because of dialysate losses, they absorb about 60% of the daily dialysate glucose, resulting in glucose absorption of about 100 to 200 g of glucose every 24 hours. This amount should be taken into account when prescribing a dietary regimen to patients undergoing PD (see subsequent text). The large influx of glucose from the dialysate can potentially suppress appetite in these patients.

Reduced Appetite because of the Dialysate Fill

Patients undergoing CAPD experience less hunger and desire to eat, compared with patients undergoing hemodialysis or healthy subjects. In a study examining hunger, fullness, and food preferences in patients undergoing chronic dialysis, patients undergoing PD consumed approximately 8% less food with dialysate in the abdomen than without dialysate. Patients undergoing PD also had a significantly lower food intake than healthy controls or patients undergoing chronic hemodialysis. The feeling of fullness from dialysate in the abdomen, as well as the continuous glucose load, can conceivably suppress hunger and appetite.

Peritoneal Transport Rate

Patients undergoing PD who have high peritoneal transport rates display a higher incidence of poor nutritional status than patients with low peritoneal transport rates. These patients lose greater amounts of amino acids and protein into the dialysate and have lower serum albumin concentrations. High transporters are also at higher risk for death and technique failure than low transporters. There is no indication that the high transport rate directly worsens the nutritional status of patients undergoing PD, other than the observed abnormalities in plasma amino acid, protein, and lipid profiles.

Influence of Comorbid Conditions

Patients undergoing chronic dialysis have a high incidence and prevalence of comorbid conditions. Approximately 45% of patients undergoing PD have a primary diagnosis of diabetes mellitus, which, if uncontrolled, can lead to increased muscle protein breakdown and accelerated LBM loss. Diabetic gastroparesis is also the primary reason for delayed gastric emptying in patients undergoing PD. The population that receives PD therapy is relatively old, and a significant proportion has cardiovascular disease, which independently is associated with poor nutritional status. The recurrent peritonitis episodes can lead to decreased nutrient intake and increased losses of amino acids and proteins; they can also activate the systemic inflammatory response syndrome, which in itself is a major protein catabolic stimulus.

INTERVENTIONS TO MAINTAIN AND IMPROVE NUTRITIONAL STATUS IN PATIENTS UNDERGOING PERITONEAL DIALYSIS

General Measures

Certain general measures for preventing (or treating) a poor nutritional status should be considered for all patients undergoing PD. Considering the catabolic nature of uremia, chronic dialysis, and concurrent comorbid conditions, patients undergoing PD should be continuously encouraged to maintain an adequate protein and calorie intake. Some of these patients tend to continue their predialysis diets while receiving renal replacement therapy, so ensuring that the protein and energy intake of these patients is sufficient to meet their increased requirements during chronic dialysis is important. Frequent comprehensive dietary counseling by an experienced dietitian is critically important, as is the detection of early signs of uremic malnutrition. Such efforts should be made not only in outpatient settings but also when the patients are hospitalized, when protein and energy intakes frequently become deficient. Every effort should be made to correct the influential factors described in the preceding text that can lead to worsening of the nutritional status of patients undergoing PD. These measures include, but are not limited to, timely initiation of dialysis, optimal dose of dialysis, treatment of metabolic acidosis, and appropriate management of comorbid illnesses, such as diabetes mellitus, congestive heart failure, and infections. Table 12-2 provides a summary of recommended nutritional intake of various nutrients for patients undergoing PD.

Protein Intake in Patients Undergoing Peritoneal Dialysis

The minimal daily protein requirement is one that maintains a neutral nitrogen balance and prevents malnutrition; this amount has been estimated to be a daily protein intake of approximately 0.6 g per kg b.w. in healthy individuals, with a safe level of protein intake equivalent to the minimal requirement plus 2 standard deviations, or approximately 0.75 g/kg b.w./d. The optimal protein requirement for patients with ESRD has not been clearly established: several studies have indicated that some patients with CKD spontaneously restrict their DPI to levels below

Table 12-2.   Recommended daily nutritional intake in patients undergoing peritoneal dialysis. All intakes calculated on the basis of normalized body weight (i.e., the average body weight of normal persons of the same age, height, and sex as the patient)

Protein (g/kg b.w.)	1.2–1.3
Calories (kcal/kg)	30–35 (including dialysate glucose absorption)[a]
Cholesterol (mg)	300–400
Polyunsaturated/saturated fat ratio	2.0:1.0
Crude fiber (g)	25
Sodium (1 g = 43 mEq)	2–4 g + 1 g/LUO
Fluids (L/LUO)	1.0–2.5 L + 1 L/LUO (also depends on UF rate)
Potassium (1 g = 25 mEq)	4 g + 1 g/LUO
Calcium (g)	Diet + 1.2 (not to exceed 2 g, including calcium containing PO4 binders)
Phosphorus (g)	0.6–1.2
Magnesium (g)	0.2–0.3
Iron (mg)	10–15
Vitamin A	None
β carotene	None
Retinol	None
Thiamine (mg)	1.5
Riboflavin (mg)	1.8
Vitamin B_6 (mg)	10
Vitamin B_{12} (mg)	0.006
Niacin (mg)	20
Folic acid (mg)	>1.0
Pantothenic acid (mg)	10
Biotin (mg)	0.3
Vitamin C (mg)	60–100
Vitamin E (mg)	None (maybe indicated in some cases)

[a]Carbohydrate intake should be decreased in patients with hypertriglyc-eridemia, hyperglycemia, diabetes mellitus, and obesity. Calorie intake should be 30 kcal/kg for patients older than 60 years or who have decreased physical activity.
b.w., body weight; LUO, liters of urine output per day.

0.6 g/kg b.w./d when glomerular filtration rate is less than 10 mL per minute. Further, patients with CKD encounter catabolic stresses once they begin chronic dialysis. On the basis of these ob-servations, Kidney Disease Outcomes Quality Initiative (K/DOQI) recommendations were published. These recommendations are based on extensive literature review and opinions of the experts on the field, and a detailed review of these recommendations as well as their rationale can be found at: http://www.kidney.org/professionals/kdoqi/guidelines_updates/doqi_nut.html. The recom-mended DPI for clinically stable PD patients is 1.2 to 1.3 g/kg b.w./d, and a protein intake of 1.2 g/kg b.w./d or greater is almost always associated with neutral or positive nitrogen balance. It is also recommended that at least 50% of the dietary protein should be of high biological value (i.e., rich in essential amino acids, Chapter 14).

Dietary Calorie Intake in Peritoneal Dialysis Patients

For patients undergoing PD, the recommended total daily energy intake, including both diet and the energy intake derived from the glucose absorbed from peritoneal dialysate, is 35 kcal/kg b.w./d and does not differ from that of adults with CKD who participate in moderate exercise. These recommendations are approximately the same as those for healthy adults of the same age who are engaged in mild daily physical activity as indicated in the Recommended Dietary Allowances. Because nitrogen balance is correlated with total energy intake, a sufficient energy intake is required to increase protein anabolism, whereas a low energy intake results in reduced use of dietary proteins; protein is used as energy source as a substrate for gluconeogenesis. Notably, the required energy intake of patients undergoing PD depends on physical activity. Because older age may be associated with reduced physical activity and LBM, a daily energy intake of 30 kcal/kg b.w./d for older patients with more sedentary lifestyles is acceptable. Special consideration should be given to the actual caloric needs of patients undergoing PD, because extra calories will eventually lead to hyperglycemia, worsen already deranged lipid metabolism, and predispose patients to increased body weight and fat mass.

Complimentary Nutritional Supplementation

Owing to the magnitude of the catabolic processes that lead to uremic malnutrition, dietary counseling fails to optimize dietary intake only in certain subgroups of patients undergoing PD. For these patients, other forms of supplementation (including oral protein, amino acid tablets, and energy supplementation) such as enteral supplementation (with nasogastric tubes, percutaneous endoscopic gastrostomy tubes, or jejunostomy tubes) as well as the use of amino acid dialysate (AAD), can be considered.

Oral and Enteral Nutrition Supplementation

Only a limited number of studies evaluate the efficacy of oral nutritional supplementation in patients undergoing PD, and these studies have provided conflicting results; for example, in a study of 14 malnourished patients undergoing PD, more than 50% of the subjects were unable to comply with the food supplements because of nausea or intercurrent illnesses. Thus, the available data do not permit us to precisely define the role of oral food supplements in the management of patients undergoing continuous peritoneal dialysis (CPD).

Only anecdotal reports are available of use of gastrostomy or jejunostomy feedings in adult patients undergoing PD, but most reports of the nutritional efficacy of gastrostomy or jejunostomy feeding are limited to use in infants and older children. In practical terms, if a patient undergoing PD requires a gastrostomy, it is usually necessary to temporarily switch the patient to hemodialysis for a few weeks before resuming PD to prevent any complications, such as dialysate leaks, peritonitis, and exit-site infections.

Amino Acid Dialysate

In carefully conducted nitrogen balance and protein turnover studies, administering amino acid-based peritoneal dialysate solutions resulted in significantly improved net nitrogen and protein balance. On the other hand, large-scale clinical studies using this strategy as a nutritional intervention for malnourished patients undergoing PD have provided conflicting results. In a large prospective randomized study, nutritional benefit was reported, with increases in serum transferrin and total protein concentrations and a trend in plasma amino acid profiles toward normal levels, with one or two exchanges of the amino acid–containing dialysate. Significant improvements were observed in serum albumin and prealbumin concentrations in malnourished patients undergoing PD, particularly for those who had serum albumin concentrations in the lowest tertile. These results are consistent with reports suggesting that these interventions are most useful in patients undergoing chronic hemodialysis who are severely malnourished. Notably, an increase in the blood urea nitrogen (BUN) plus an exacerbation of some uremic symptoms, a decrease in serum potassium and uric acid levels, and a worsening of metabolic acidosis are potential complications of AADs. Overall, the available evidence suggests that treatment with amino acid–based peritoneal dialysate solutions may be useful for malnourished patients undergoing chronic PD and offers an alternative method of nutritional intervention in patients undergoing PD in whom oral or enteral intake cannot be maintained. No data are available to show that aggressive nutritional supplementation through the gastrointestinal (GI) tract is inferior to AAD in patients undergoing PD. Until a controlled study that compares various forms of nutritional supplementation in similar patient groups is completed, one should be cautious about choosing very costly nutritional interventions.

Experimental Nutritional Therapies

Anabolic Agents

The availability of recombinant forms of certain anabolic agents has made it possible to use pharmacologic doses of these agents to promote net anabolism in multiple patient populations. Several preliminary studies have suggested that rhGH administration in patients undergoing PD results in significant improvements in nitrogen balance, IGF-1 concentrations, and other responses that indicate a general anabolic effect. Recombinant human IGF-1 has also been proposed as an anabolic agent, but the side effects from this agent, at least as observed in patients with CKD, impede its widespread use. Interestingly, the combined use of rhGH and rhIGF-1 in healthy subjects has yielded the most efficient anabolic action with the fewest side effects. Whether long-term use of these agents in malnourished patients undergoing PD would result in improved nutritional parameters and better outcomes is not known.

Appetite Stimulants

Appetite stimulants such as megestrol acetate are treatment options, but very limited studies of patients with ESRD have been conducted. Although a variety of benefits have been suggested, adherence, appropriate dosing, and side effects are important issues that remain to be evaluated. Large-scale prospective studies are needed to assess whether these stimulants are of value as adjunctive nutritional therapy for patients undergoing dialysis.

Anti-inflammatory Interventions

With the understanding that chronic inflammation is an important catabolic factor, new strategies aimed at blocking the adverse effects of inflammation have been proposed in multiple patient populations. At present, few studies have been conducted in patients with ESRD that evaluated the use of anti-inflammatory interventions to ameliorate the adverse effects of chronic inflammation on nutritional status. The goal of anti-inflammatory therapy is selectively to block, inhibit, decrease production, or increase degradation of proinflammatory substances, while avoiding compromise of host defenses. Whether anti-inflammatory drugs would be helpful in improving uremic malnutrition is to be determined by potential future studies.

SELECTED READING

Abbott KC, Glanton CW, Trespalacios FC, et al. Body mass index, dialysis modality, and survival: analysis of the United States Renal Data System Dialysis Morbidity and Mortality Wave II Study. *Kidney Int* 2004;65(2):597–605.

Bergström J, Heimbürger O, Lindholm B. Calculation of the protein equivalent of total nitrogen appearance from urea appearance. Which formulas should be used? *Perit Dial Int* 1998;18:467–473.

Caglar K, Hakim RM, Ikizler TA. Approaches to the reversal of malnutrition, inflammation, and atherosclerosis in end-stage renal disease. *Nutr Rev* 2002;60:378–387.

Churchill DN, Taylor DW, Keshaviah PR. Adequacy of dialysis and nutrition in continuous peritoneal dialysis: association with clinical outcomes. *J Am Soc Nephrol* 1996;7:198–207.

Churchill DN, Thorpe KE, Nolph KD, et al. Increased peritoneal membrane transport is associated with decreased patient and technique survival for continuous peritoneal dialysis patients. *J Am Soc Nephrol* 1998;9:1285–1292.

Feriani M, Kirchgessner J, La Greca G, et al. Randomized long-term evaluation of bicarbonate-buffered CAPD solution. *Kidney Int* 1998;54:1731–1738.

Heimburger O, Stenvinkel P, Lindholm B. Nutritional effects and nutritional management of chronic peritoneal dialysis. In: Massry SG, Kopple JD, eds. *Nutritional management of renal disease*, 2nd ed. Philadelphia: Lippincott Williams & Wilkins, 2003:477–511.

Hylander B, Barkeling B, Rössner S. Eating behavior in continuous ambulatory peritoneal dialysis and hemodialysis patients. *Am J Kidney Dis* 1992;20:592–597.

Jones M, Hagen T, Boyle CA, et al. Treatment of malnutrition with 1.1% amino acid peritoneal dialysis solution: results of a multicenter outpatient study. *Am J Kidney Dis* 1998;32:761–769.

Kang DH, Yoon KI, Choi KB, et al. Relationship of peritoneal membrane transport characteristics to the nutritional status in CAPD patients. *Nephrol Dial Transplant* 1999;14:1715–1722.

Kaysen GA, Dubin JA, Muller H-G, et al. Inflammation and reduced albumin synthesis associated with stable decline in serum albumin in hemodialysis patients. *Kidney Int* 2004;65:1408–1415.

Kopple JD. National kidney foundation K/DOQI clinical practice guidelines for nutrition in chronic renal failure. *Am J Kidney Dis* 2001;37:S66–S70.

McCusker FX, Teehan BP, Thorpe KE, et al. How much peritoneal dialysis is required for the maintenance of a good nutritional state? *Kidney Int* 1996;50(Suppl. 56):S56–S61.

Mehrotra R, Kopple JD. Protein and energy nutrition among adult patients treated with chronic peritoneal dialysis. *Adv Ren Replace Ther* 2003;10(3):194–212.

Merkus MP, Jager KJ, Dekker FW, et al. Physical symptoms and quality of life in patients on chronic dialysis: results of the Netherlands Cooperative Study on Adequacy of Dialysis (NECOSAD). *Nephrol Dial Transplant* 1999;14:1163–1170.

Pupim LB, Ikizler TA. Uremic malnutrition: new insights into an old problem. *Semin Dial* 2003;16:224–232.

Pupim LB, Ikizler TA. Assessment and monitoring of uremic malnutrition. *J Ren Nutr* 2004;14:6–19.

Stein A, Moorhouse J, Iles-Smith H, et al. Role of an improvement in acid-base status and nutrition in CAPD patients. *Kidney Int* 1997;52:1089–1095.

Stenvinkel P, Heimbürger O, Paultre F, et al. Strong association between malnutrition, inflammation and atherosclerosis in chronic renal failure. *Kidney Int* 1999;55:1899–1911.

Stenvinkel P, Lindholm B, Lönnqvist F, et al. Increases in serum leptin levels during peritoneal dialysis are associated with inflammation and a decrease in lean body mass. *J Am Soc Nephrol* 2000; 11:1303–1309.

Tranaeus A. The Bicarbonate/Lactate Study Group. A long-term study of a bicarbonate/lactate-based peritoneal dialysis solution: clinical benefits. *Perit Dial Int* 2000;20:515–523.

Young GA, Kopple JD, Lindholm B, et al. Nutritional assessment of continuous ambulatory peritoneal dialysis patients: an international study. *Am J Kidney Dis* 1991;17:462–471.

13

Nutritional Requirements of Renal Transplant Patients

J. Andrew Bertolatus

Successful transplantation of a kidney into a patient with renal failure restores near-normal renal function and is expected to correct the nutritional abnormalities arising from renal insufficiency. In the minds of both patients and physicians, one of the major benefits of renal transplantation is an end to the dietary restrictions required for therapy during periods of progressive renal failure and dialysis. Typically, the recipients of renal transplants experience an improvement in general sense of well-being, along with a marked improvement in appetite and an increase in dry body weight. These patients, nevertheless, face many nutritional challenges because of the metabolic complications of pre-existing medical conditions and as a consequence of transplant-related immunosuppression. Adding to these challenges is the fact that during the posttransplantation follow-up period, many recipients never develop optimal renal function, whereas others experience declining renal function with the passage of time. Therefore, many recipients of transplants may require nutritional management, as appropriate for patients with chronic renal failure, even though these recipients do not require dialysis (see Chapter 6 and Chapter 14).

The implications of proper nutritional therapy for the recipients of renal transplants are far reaching. Immunosuppressive therapies used to maintain the renal allograft, especially glucocorticoids, calcineurin inhibitors (cyclosporine and tacrolimus), and sirolimus, are associated with metabolic side effects, including protein hypercatabolism, obesity, hyperlipidemia, glucose intolerance, hypertension, hyperkalemia, hypophosphatemia, hypomagnesemia, and interference with the metabolism and action of vitamin D. These metabolic effects of immunosuppression tend to interact with the aspects of nutrition and metabolism that are most likely to have affected patients during the period of renal failure: protein depletion, hyperlipidemia, hypertension, calcium malabsorption, and hyperparathyroidism. Many of these factors contribute to accelerated atherosclerosis and consequent cardiovascular disease, the major cause of death among recipients of renal transplants. Some authors have postulated that the fate of the graft itself may be affected by the amount of dietary protein, by virtue of the glomerular hyperfiltration response, or by the degree of hyperlipidemia. For these reasons, careful attention to the nutritional and metabolic state of the recipient of a renal transplant is warranted. Because metabolic problems tend to occur early after transplantation, a nutritional plan should be formulated at the time of transplantation, and the patient should be introduced to this plan in the immediate posttransplantation period. The plan should consider the following elements: maintenance of appropriate weight for height; dietary lipid composition; protein intake in the immediate posttransplantation period and during long-term therapy; and intake of calcium, phosphate, magnesium, and vitamin D. Patients with pre-existing diabetes will need continued attention to carbohydrate metabolism, as will those in whom steroid-induced diabetes develops after transplantation. Finally, some patients may need iron supplementation, sodium or potassium restriction, supplementation with water-soluble vitamins, or some combination of these approaches.

OBESITY

Obesity has arguably now become the most important nutritional disorder among recipients of renal transplants. Most of the recipients are overweight or obese at the time of transplantation. Data from the United Network for Organ Sharing (UNOS) show that in 2000 to 2001, approximately 34% of patients who had undergone transplantation were overweight [body mass index (BMI) 25 to 29.9], whereas 25% were obese (BMI of 30 or more). From 1987–1989 to 2001–2002, the percentage of obese recipients (at the time of transplantation) has increased from 11.6% to 25%, representing a 116% increase in the proportion of obese subjects. The proportions of overweight and obese individuals in the population undergoing transplantation, and the trends in those proportions over time by year of transplantation, reflect fairly closely what is observed in the general US population (see Fig. 13-1). Interestingly, the fraction of obese persons in the population

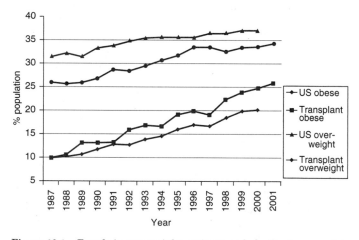

Figure 13-1. Trends in overweight patients and obesity in general populace compared to patients at the time of kidney transplantation. US population data obtained from the Behavioral Risk Factor Surveillance System, CDC. (From Friedman AN, Miskulin DC, Rosenberg IH, et al. Demographics and trends in overweight and obesity in patients at time of kidney transplantation. *Am J Kidney Dis* 2003;41:480–487, with permission.)

undergoing transplant is if anything greater, and increasing more rapidly over the last 10 years, than the fraction with obesity in the general population (Fig. 13-1). Such analyses support the concept, at least among the subpopulation of those with chronic kidney disease (CKD) who are selected to undergo renal transplantation, that excess weight and excessive energy intake may be replacing insufficient energy and protein intake as the most common nutritional problem. After transplantation, the tendency toward overweight and obesity worsens. By 1 year after transplantation, approximately 60% of recipients have gains in weight of 10% or more, and the percentage of recipients who are overweight more than doubles, to 43% in one study. Female patients and African Americans of either gender have greater weight gains than others. Whereas obesity may not be a risk factor for short-term posttransplant complications, it is clearly a risk factor for chronic graft loss (see Fig. 13-2). Potential mechanisms for the negative effect of obesity include a greater chance for mismatches

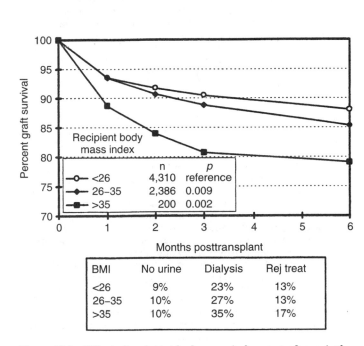

Figure 13-2.   Effect of recipient body mass index on graft survival. Recipients with body mass index [weight in kg/(height in cm)^2] greater than 26 had significantly reduced graft survival, with the effect being particularly large for those with body mass index greater than 36. The larger individuals also had a greater need for dialysis in the posttransplantation period. (From Cho YW, Terasaki PI, Cecka JM. New variables reported to the UNOS Registry and their impact on cadaveric renal transplant outcomes: a preliminary study. In: Cecka JM, Terasaki PI, eds. *Clinical transplants 1995*. Los Angeles: UCLA Tissue Typing Laboratory, 1996:405–415, with permission.)

in recipient and donor size, and hence for "nephron underdosing" and hyperfiltration; underdosing or perhaps impaired bioavailability of immunosuppressive agents; or the effect of hyperlipidemia to promote chronic graft dysfunction. Corticosteroids are often blamed for increased appetite with weight gain and the higher percentage of body fat after renal transplantation. Indeed, the high doses of steroids often administered in the first few weeks and months posttransplantation may be associated with increased body fat mass and redistribution of body fat, resulting in increased abdominal and visceral adipose tissue. Multiple mechanisms exist by which corticosteroids may cause these effects on adipose tissue, such as increased appetite and the induction of hepatic gluconeogenesis, leading to hyperglycemia and hyperinsulinemia. However, most transplant programs currently reduce steroid doses rapidly to minimal levels (e.g., prednisone 5 to 10 mg per day or every other day) by 2 to 3 months after transplantation. Many recipients are now completely withdrawn from steroid therapy, and a few receive little or no steroid therapy, even in the immediate posttransplant period (a practice known as "steroid avoidance"). In randomized studies, the use of steroid withdrawal and steroid avoidance protocols in some cases has afforded the opportunity to evaluate the contribution of steroids to posttransplantation obesity more rigorously. Importantly, a number of recent prospective studies suggest that steroid withdrawal does not have much effect on posttransplant weight gain, and that weight gain is not significantly related to steroid dose. Instead, some of these studies suggest that limited physical activity may be the most important factor in posttransplant obesity. These observations also suggest that greater emphasis on activity and exercise would be a more effective approach to preventing posttransplantation obesity.

Some recipients of renal transplants are now attempting to deal with posttransplantation weight gain by following low-carbohydrate diets (such as the Atkins diet and its variants), with or without consultation with health care professionals. Recent randomized studies in obese subjects demonstrate that over periods of 6 to 12 months, following a low-carbohydrate diet can be associated with modest weight loss and slight improvements in lipid status. However, no data exist concerning the safety and efficacy of these diets in individuals with CKD or in recipients of kidney transplants. Because of concern over the potential effect of a high protein intake on kidney function (discussed below), patients receiving renal transplants should probably be counseled not to pursue low-carbohydrate or high-protein diets for weight loss until further data are available concerning the use of these diets in recipients of renal transplants.

HYPERLIPIDEMIA

As the short-term graft survival after kidney transplantation has improved, and the number of life-threatening infections has decreased, atherosclerotic cardiovascular disease has emerged as the most important health risk and most common cause of death among recipients of renal transplants. A number of factors contribute to posttransplantation atherosclerosis: a history of nephrotic syndrome with hyperlipidemia and hypertension induced by the underlying renal disease; the effects of altered lipid metabolism during the dialysis period; and the metabolic effects of the transplant immunosuppressive therapy with glucocorticoids, calcineurin inhibitors (cyclosporine or tacrolimus), or sirolimus. Weight gain may be an independent factor that leads to hyperlipidemia. In one study, only those individuals experiencing weight gain during the first year after transplantation had significant increases in cholesterol and triglycerides. Serum lipid levels did not worsen in recipients who did not also gain weight, indicating that control of body weight by a combination of diet and exercise is critical in this patient population.

The prevalence of hyperlipidemia after renal transplantation has been variably reported to be between 16% and 60%. Some of this variability may be related to different patient populations and different immunosuppressive protocols, but much of the variability remains unexplained. Unlike patients with chronic renal failure or those treated with dialysis therapy, who frequently have isolated hypertriglyceridemia, recipients of renal transplants are more likely to have hypercholesterolemia, either isolated or in association with hypertriglyceridemia. Hypertriglyceridemia improves shortly after transplantation, only to be replaced by an increase in cholesterol. The increase in cholesterol is associated with an increase in low-density lipoprotein (LDL) cholesterol as well as an increase in high-density lipoprotein (HDL) cholesterol, from very low levels toward normal.

The immunosuppressive agents used, including prednisone, cyclosporine, tacrolimus, and sirolimus, contribute to posttransplantation lipid disorders. The mechanisms by which prednisone exerts its hypercholesterolemic effects have been somewhat clarified. Studies in animals and in humans indicate that the underlying cause of hyperlipidemia after glucocorticoid therapy is insulin resistance in peripheral tissues, with impaired synthesis of lipoprotein lipase, together with persistent responsiveness of the liver to the elevated plasma insulin levels, leading to enhanced lipoprotein synthesis.

Whereas the hyperlipidemic effects of glucocorticoids have been well described and investigated, the hyperlipidemic effects of cyclosporine and the magnitude of this effect remain controversial. Isolating the effects of cyclosporine from those of the other antirejection medications and metabolic derangements associated with renal disease is difficult, but a number of observations demonstrate an independent effect of cyclosporine on serum lipids. For example, patients with psoriasis who are treated with cyclosporine monotherapy for 4 weeks had increased LDL cholesterol and triglyceride levels, followed by return to baseline levels within 2 weeks. In another study, recipients of renal transplants receiving cyclosporine and azathioprine after successful withdrawal from prednisone had modest improvements in serum cholesterol levels, but these levels remained significantly above normal and pretransplantation levels. Investigators have reported improvement in lipid abnormalities among patients who have undergone renal transplantation treated with cyclosporine and prednisone after conversion to the azathioprine–prednisone regimen. Little is known about the etiology of hypercholesterolemia associated with cyclosporine. Proposed mechanisms include cyclosporine interference with the feedback mechanism that regulates LDL cholesterol synthesis by altering the binding kinetics of LDL and its receptor; inhibition of 26-hydroxylase and subsequent reduction in the synthesis of bile acids from cholesterol; decreased hepatic lipase and lipoprotein lipase activity, which could decrease the conversion of very–low-density lipoproteins (VLDL) to intermediate-density lipoprotein and LDL.

The calcineurin inhibitor tacrolimus (FK506) is now often used as an alternative to cyclosporine. Initially, most of the clinical experience with this drug was in recipients of liver transplants, who experience less weight gain and less marked elevations in serum cholesterol levels when on a tacrolimus-based regimen than during cyclosporine-based immunosuppression. In a large randomized trial comparing tacrolimus and cyclosporine in 412 recipients of renal transplants, patients who were treated with tacrolimus had significantly lower levels of total cholesterol, LDL cholesterol, and triglycerides. Mean total cholesterol levels in the cyclosporine and tacrolimus groups were 230 and 194 mg per dL, respectively, a difference that is likely to have substantial clinical importance. The use of tacrolimus instead of cyclosporine can be considered as part of the approach to patients with substantial pretransplant or posttransplant hypercholesterolemia.

Sirolimus (rapamycin) is a cyclophilin-binding immunosuppressive agent that does not act through calcineurin inhibition. Sirolimus has little or no nephrotoxicity and is generally used in combination with either cyclosporine or tacrolimus, often with the aim of using lower doses and levels of the calcineurin inhibitor than might have been used in the past. Sirolimus-containing regimens are associated with very low rates of rejection, but the agent causes a marked increase in the incidence of elevated triglycerides and (to a lesser degree) cholesterol. The effects on the lipid profile are more marked in the first few months than at the end of the first posttransplant year. Other antiatherogenic properties of the drug could offset the effect of the increased lipids on vascular biology. Nonetheless, the alterations in lipid status remain among the major concerns with the use of this drug.

Dietary factors likely contribute to posttransplant hyperlipidemia. In one study, recipients of renal transplants with hyperlipidemia averaged 129% of ideal body weight; the major weight gained occurred during the first 6 months after transplantation. Few reports have examined the effectiveness of diet therapy in controlling posttransplant hypercholesterolemia, and unfortunately none has investigated the long-term efficacy of dietary manipulations in this population. One group evaluated the effect over 1 year of a weight-reduction diet containing no more than 300 mg of cholesterol daily, eliminating simple sugars, and adding 30 mL of sunflower seed oil to increase polyunsaturated fat intake. The investigators reported a modest weight loss from 129% ideal body weight to 121% and a significant decrease in cholesterol from 356 to 294 mg per dL. Other investigators have reported similar findings. Unfortunately, in one of these studies, a survey showed that dietary treatment was considered undesirable by 48% of the patient population, and that of those who agreed to participate in dietary manipulation, none was totally adherent. Most recently, Moore et al. studied the effect of the American Heart Association (AHA) "step one" diet over an 8-week period on 17 stable posttransplant patients with hyperlipidemia. These investigators reported that most of these individuals were able to adhere to the diet and reduce their weight, leading to a modest reduction in the level of serum cholesterol from 262 to 241 mg per dL. However, they noted no decrease in LDL cholesterol and suggested that long-term adherence to this diet would likely diminish with time and that the altered lipid metabolism of transplantation may render dietary therapy alone ineffective.

Long-term control of hyperlipidemia after renal transplantation depends on some dietary intervention, and this treatment may also require pharmacotherapy. Because obesity is an important contributor to hyperlipidemia in patients receiving renal transplants, and because the greatest weight gain in this population is within the first 6 months, recipients of renal transplants should receive intensive counseling regarding calories and cholesterol before and after transplantation. The AHA "one-step" diet is a reasonable initial approach for patients receiving renal transplants. This diet, consisting of less than 300 mg of cholesterol per day (with a goal of less than 250 mg per day), 30% total calories as fat, 50% as carbohydrate, and 20% as protein, is an easily attainable diet and is familiar to nutritionists.

Guidelines for evaluation and treatment of dyslipidemias in patients who have undergone kidney transplantation, together with an excellent summary of research in this area, have recently been published by a work group of the National Kidney Foundation Kidney Disease Outcomes Quality Initiative (NKF-K/DOQI; see Selected Readings). One important recommendation in these guidelines is that renal transplantation *per se* be classified as a risk factor for coronary heart disease, independent of other "traditional" risk factors. Therefore, the authors recommend that attempts be made by lifestyle changes, drug intervention, or both to lower LDL cholesterol below 100 mg per dL.

PROTEIN METABOLISM

Posttransplantation Period

One of the principal metabolic effects of glucocorticoid hormones is to increase hepatic gluconeogenesis associated with increased catabolism of amino acids and proteins. Thus, the fact that large doses of steroids used early in the posttransplantation period, together with the stresses of surgery, are associated with evidence of markedly increased protein catabolism is not surprising. Protein hypercatabolism is further increased when rejection episodes are treated with high-dose intravenous methylprednisolone. Patients with chronic renal insufficiency who present for transplantation may have pre-existing protein malnutrition, especially if they are diabetic (see Chapters 6 and 7). Although the benign clinical course of such patients after transplant surgery is remarkable, protein catabolism combined with pre-existing protein depletion may add substantially to poor wound healing and susceptibility to infection. These problems are likely to be exaggerated in patients in whom the onset of function of the transplanted kidney is delayed, with dialysis needed early in the posttransplantation course.

Fortunately, several investigators have shown convincingly that preventing negative nitrogen balance is possible during the immediate posttransplantation period simply by increasing dietary protein. The studies of these investigators have shown that steroid therapy increases the protein catabolic and urea appearance rates to a degree, depending on the total corticosteroid dose but independently of dietary protein; patients who receive less than 1 g of dietary protein/kg b.w./d are invariably in negative nitrogen balance. An isocaloric increase in dietary protein does not result in a substantial increase in the protein catabolic rate. Rather, as illustrated in Figure 13-3, increases in dietary protein restore nitrogen balance. According to consensus among these investigators, neutral (or zero) net nitrogen balance occurs in patients treated with typical posttransplantation doses of steroid when daily protein intake is 1.3 to 1.5 g per kg. Given the protein depletion seen in many pretransplantation patients and the frequent need for pulse steroid therapy for rejection episodes, prescribing a protein intake at the upper end of this range would seem prudent. Higher levels

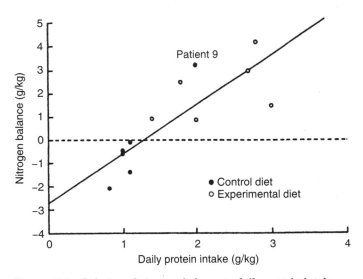

Figure 13-3. Relation of nitrogen balance to daily protein intake. Patients given the control diet were told to eat 1.0 g/kg protein/d, but patient 9 actually consumed 2.0 g/kg/d. Those on the experimental diet were told to eat 3.0 g/kg protein/d, but actual intake ranged from 1.4 to 3.0 g/kg/d. A direct relation exists between protein intake and nitrogen balance ($r = 0.83$; $p < 0.01$), with zero nitrogen balance at an intake of approximately 1.3 g/kg/d. (From Whittier FC, Evans DH, Dutton S. Nutrition in renal transplantation. *Am J Kidney Dis* 1985;6:405–411, with permission.)

are unlikely to be acceptable to patients accustomed to protein-restricted diets and will increase the tendency to accumulate waste products that arise from dietary protein.

The diet also must contain adequate calories to ensure that the dietary protein is used for anabolism; in general, an intake of 30 to 35 kcal/kg b.w./d is prescribed for the first several weeks after transplantation. Contrary to expectations, this dietary approach may not complicate the clinical course of the patient with delayed graft function; the higher protein intake should not increase the protein catabolic rate or the urea appearance rate further, so the need for dialysis should not be increased. Finally, a relatively high protein intake in the weeks after transplantation could minimize some of the steroid-induced side effects other than muscle wasting. Whittier et al. found that patients given a high-protein, low-carbohydrate diet had only a mild cushingoid appearance 4 weeks after transplantation, whereas patients with lower protein intakes had moderate to severe cushingoid changes.

Maintenance Prescription for Dietary Protein

Whereas a moderate increase in protein intake is clearly indicated early in the posttransplantation course (and probably during any subsequent therapy for acute rejection or recovery from surgical complications), the optimal dietary prescription is less well established for patients who have undergone renal transplantation treated with maintenance immunosuppression. This uncertainty results from the conflicting goals of optimizing protein nutrition and, at the same time, optimizing long-term renal function.

The argument for maintaining a relatively generous dietary protein intake during long-term therapy after successful renal transplantation rests on the evidence that a continued increase in protein catabolism occurs even in patients receiving glucocorticoids at relatively low maintenance dosages (equivalent to 0.15 to 0.20 mg prednisone/kg b.w./d). That steroids continue to cause protein wasting in these patients is evidenced by the high prevalence of steroid-induced side effects seen in long-term recipients of transplants, including truncal obesity with wasting of the musculature of the extremities, fragile and atrophied skin, and delayed wound healing.

The extent of muscle wasting in these patients has been documented by several authors. In one study, even with good renal allograft function and a diet containing 1.0 g of protein per kg and 25 to 35 kcal/kg b.w./d, 50% of patients with diabetes and 25% of the patients without diabetes had midarm muscle circumferences that were less than the fifth percentile of healthy control subjects. On average, body weights had increased from before transplantation, but the increase was mostly in adipose tissue. Another study was performed in stable patients receiving renal transplants at least 6 months after transplantation, at a time when the average serum creatinine level was 1.46 mg per dL and the dose of prednisone was 9.6 mg per day. All the patients had been fully rehabilitated and had returned to work or full activities, and none had any known musculoskeletal disease or neuropathy. Compared with matched healthy subjects, these patients had 20% less midthigh muscle area and 36% more midthigh fat, as measured quantitatively by computed tomography. These radiographic indices of reduced muscle mass correlated with a reduction in the peak torque and total work output from these muscles. Thus, even patients with excellent transplant renal function and excellent rehabilitation exhibit evidence of substantially reduced muscle mass. Evidence indicates that muscle atrophy and weakness in these patients could be reversed by physical training, at least in those patients receiving less than 0.20 mg of prednisone/kg b.w./d. Whether or not dietary intakes greater than 1.0 g of protein/kg b.w./d, especially when combined with exercise, might minimize muscle wasting and possibly the other evidences of protein depletion remains uncertain. Reduced muscle mass may contribute directly to increased body adipose tissue and obesity, if, as noted earlier, physical inactivity is a major factor in posttransplantation weight gain.

The argument to restrict protein stems from the hypothesis that excess protein intake induces a hyperfiltration injury through mechanisms analogous to those suggested for other patients with reduced renal function. Several small, short-term studies evaluated the effect of low-protein diets (approximately 0.6 g/kg b.w./d) in recipients of renal transplants who exhibited well-established progressive renal insufficiency and had renal biopsy specimens showing the typical findings of chronic allograft nephropathy ("chronic rejection"). In one study, a distinct change was observed in the slope of reciprocal serum creatinine (1/serum creatinine) values, and previously declining renal function stabilized (see Fig. 13-4) over a 6-month period after the low-protein diet was instituted. Notably, stabilization of serum creatinine in these patients might have resulted from a decrease in endogenous creatinine synthesis caused by progressive muscle wasting or from a decreased exogenous creatinine intake, rather than from preservation of renal function. No long-term studies have been conducted of the effect of low-protein diets on the course of renal function with radionuclide measurements of glomerular filtration rate (GFR). These short-term studies also included a number of nutritional assessments. Recipients of renal transplants receiving a protein intake of 0.55 to 0.6 g/kg b.w./d could have neutral nitrogen balance if their energy intake was maintained at or greater than 25 kcal/kg b.w./d. However, many of the patients found this intake difficult to achieve consistently. In addition, enthusiasm for dietary protein restriction to these relatively low levels has waned considerably since the results of the Modification of Diet in Renal Disease (MDRD) study showed little or no benefit of dietary protein restriction in preserving renal function in patients with CKD (see Chapter 9). With respect to the nutritional safety of these low-protein diets in the population of patients who have undergone transplantation, the results of these studies are inconclusive, perhaps because the studies have been of insufficient duration. However, low-protein diets did not cause loss of protein stores in patients participating in the MDRD study (Chapter 6). Other findings of these studies include the fact that the low-protein diet is associated with a reduction in proteinuria and decreased activity of the renin–angiotensin system.

Clearly, additional studies of protein metabolism are needed in patients receiving renal transplants before therapeutic decisions can be rendered from established and accepted fact rather than

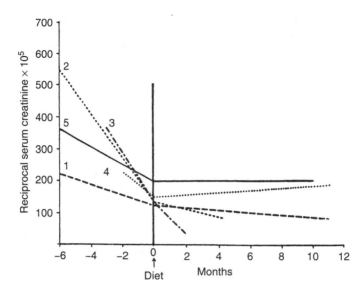

Figure 13-4. Changes in reciprocal of serum creatinine values in recipients of renal transplants with chronic graft rejection on introduction of dietary protein restriction to 0.6 g/kg b.w./d. Four of five patients had a significant change in the slope of 1/creatinine. This change may reflect either a slowing in the progression of renal failure or a reduction in creatinine excretion, possibly from reduction of dietary creatinine intake or loss of muscle mass. (From Feehally J, Harris KP, Bennett SE, et al. Is chronic renal transplant rejection a nonimmunologic phenomenon? *Lancet* 1986;2:486–488, with permission.)

from hypothesis and opinion. In the interim, a defensible approach for most patients is to prescribe a diet that contains approximately 1.0 g of protein/kg b.w./d of protein and to encourage regular exercise as a way to avoid muscle wasting.

GLUCOSE METABOLISM

An increasing fraction of patients presenting for renal transplantation, approximately 25% currently, have renal failure caused by diabetes mellitus, either type 1 or type 2. The posttransplantation nutritional care of these patients is considerably complicated by diabetes, and the treatment of diabetes is complicated by the insulin resistance induced by steroid therapy. Nutritional deficits tend to be more severe in patients with diabetes who have chronic renal failure. Because the nutritional problems of patients with diabetes and nephropathy are discussed in Chapter 7, treatment of these patients is not detailed here. However, the nutritional and other aspects of the medical care of patients with diabetes occupy a disproportionate share of the time physicians and dietitians spend caring for recipients of renal transplants.

In addition to the patients with diabetes who come for renal transplantation, other patients often develop clinical diabetes as a result of immunosuppressive therapy with glucocorticoids and calcineurin inhibitors (cyclosporine or tacrolimus). Not surprisingly, even recipients of renal transplants with overtly normal glucose tolerance have evidence of insulin resistance when studied by the insulin-clamp technique. The development of clinical diabetes seems to occur when relative insulin deficiency develops, such that insulin production is inadequate, relative to the degree of insulin resistance.

Posttransplantation diabetes is more common with tacrolimus-based immunosuppression for renal transplantation. In a randomized study of 412 patients, the incidence of posttransplant diabetes during the first posttransplant year (defined as the need for insulin therapy for 30 days or more) was 20% in patients receiving tacrolimus, as compared with 4% in those receiving cyclosporine-based immunosuppression. The diabetogenic effect of tacrolimus is dose dependent, so that with downward dose adjustment, the long-term prevalence of diabetes decreases and may eventually be similar to the rate observed in cyclosporine-treated patients.

In one of the larger reported surveys, Friedman et al. found that clinical diabetes developed in 15.7% of recipients of renal transplants who did not have diabetes previously; diabetes was defined as three consecutive, fasting blood glucose values greater than 150 mg per dL. More than 50% developed diabetes within 3 weeks of starting steroid therapy. Other factors were clearly important, however, as the average steroid dose of the recipients who developed diabetes was actually less than that of a matched group of recipients whose blood glucose values remained normal. The patients with diabetes and control patients without diabetes had similar body weights, a similar male–female ratio, similar serum creatinine values, and a similar incidence of diabetes in family members. The only significant difference between the two groups was that the group with diabetes had a higher proportion of African Americans. In more than 50% of the patients in whom diabetes develops, no specific therapy was needed. The other 50% of the group required dietary therapy and either an oral hypoglycemic agent or insulin. With time and a lower dose of prednisone, steroid-induced diabetes tended to improve. Only 33% of patients still had clinical diabetes after 6 months, and only 28% had diabetes after 1 year. Despite this apparently benign course, the 2-year survival rate of patients in whom posttransplantation diabetes developed was significantly lower than that of other patients (patients with diabetes, 67%; controls, 83%; p <0.05), primarily because of more frequent and severe infections. Thus, posttransplantation diabetes remains a major metabolic problem.

METABOLISM OF CALCIUM, PHOSPHORUS, AND VITAMIN D

Metabolic bone diseases, including osteonecrosis and osteopenia, are a major source of morbidity and mortality after successful renal transplantation. The incidence of osteonecrosis after renal transplantation has been variably reported to be from 3.5%

to 5.0% to almost 30%. Much of the variability depends on different methods for identifying cases, differences in the transplant populations, and varying immunosuppressive regimens. Julian et al. reported on the continuing problems of vertebral osteopenia in renal transplantation, related primarily to steroid therapy. The metabolism of calcium, phosphorus, and vitamin D in recipients of renal transplants is determined by a complex interplay of factors resulting from the patient's previous period of renal insufficiency, from the immunosuppressive therapy, and from incomplete restoration of normal renal function by the transplantation (see Table 13-1). In addition, recent observations suggest that some individuals have a genetic susceptibility to increased bone loss after transplantation, based on polymorphisms in the vitamin D receptor. Although all individuals (regardless of receptor genotype) lost bone density to the same degree in the first 3 months after transplantation, those with the "favorable" genotype showed significantly better recovery of bone density at the end of the first posttransplant year. Perhaps in the future, pretransplant testing for receptor genotype will identify those individuals with the highest risk for bone loss and therefore the greatest need for monitoring and intervention.

Pre-existing Hyperparathyroidism and Osteopenia

Factors that lead to metabolic bone disease in patients in the preuremic state and in patients undergoing dialysis are reviewed in Chapter 3. Many patients have marked hyperparathyroidism, and extensive osteopenia is often present. The restoration of near-normal renal mass after transplantation immediately leads to correction or overcorrection of phosphate excretion and to a restoration of vitamin D metabolism to produce its active form, calcitriol. These changes, as well as steroid-induced bone resorption, lead to an increase in serum calcium to normal or elevated levels.

Table 13-1. Factors affecting mineral metabolism in recipients of renal transplants

Prior renal insufficiency
    Hyperplastic, poorly suppressible parathyroid glands with hyperparathyroidism
    Pre-existing parathyroid bone disease, osteomalacia with depletion of bone mineral, or both
Effects of glucocorticoid immunosuppressive therapy
    Inhibition of osteoblast division, maturation, and function
    Inhibition of calcitriol-dependent absorption of calcium and phosphorus by the gut
    Increased urinary excretion of calcium and phosphorus
Effects of incomplete restoration of normal renal function
    Persistent hyperparathyroidism related to reduced glomerular filtration rate
    Parathyroid hormone-independent renal "leak" of phosphate
Other factors
    Vitamin D–receptor genotype

The expected effect of these changes on parathyroid gland function should be its complete suppression, but this effect does not usually occur. The persistent inappropriate secretion of parathyroid hormone is widely believed to be secondary to some degree of functional autonomy of the gland, either because of the large size of the gland from years of chronic stimulation or, rarely, because of the development of a parathyroid adenoma. Others argued that steroid use also participates in a maladaptive oversecretion of parathyroid hormone. The consequences of posttransplantation hyperparathyroidism are hypercalcemia, hypophosphatemia, and hyperphosphaturia, with persistent bone resorption and consequent osteopenia. The rate of reduction in bone density during the first 3 months after transplantation has recently been shown to be highly correlated with pretransplant parathyroid hormone levels.

Glucocorticoid Effects

Pre-existing bone disease notwithstanding, the single most important determinant of posttransplantation osteopenia and osteonecrosis is likely to be steroid use. The effects of glucocorticoids on bone metabolism are numerous, and although not completely understood, are believed to be mediated by the nuclear mechanisms that are dependent on the glucocorticoid receptor. Glucocorticoids exert direct inhibitory effects on osteoblast function, inhibiting a variety of cellular functions including cell growth, multiplication, and differentiation and synthesis of type I collagen and noncollagenous proteins. Whereas bone resorption (by osteoclasts) and formation (by osteoblasts) are normally sequentially linked, the alterations in osteoblast function favor net resorption of bone. Using osteocalcin as a marker of osteoblast numbers, several investigators demonstrated a reduction in bone formation that occurs rapidly after initiation of steroid treatment and is maintained even with small doses of steroid. Julian et al. showed that stable recipients of renal transplants who take low doses of glucocorticoids exhibit a halving of the rate of vertebral bone formation, leading to progressive vertebral bone loss even as their parathyroid hormone and vitamin D metabolism are returning to normal. This effect of glucocorticoid can be partially reversed with calcitriol therapy.

Glucocorticoids also impair end-organ responsiveness to vitamin D. Impaired active calcium absorption in the gut, a vitamin D–dependent process, has been observed in patients treated with steroids and is partially dose dependent. Because diffusional calcium absorption is unaltered, this effect can be minimized by increased dietary calcium and partially reversed by pharmacologic doses of calcitriol. Some investigators have reported decreased conversion of 25(OH)-vitamin D to active calcitriol in the renal tubules, but others have contradicted this finding, and calcitriol levels have variously been reported to be low, normal, or high in patients treated with glucocorticoids. Glucocorticoids also increase urinary excretion of both calcium and phosphate, which some investigators ascribe to steroid-induced secondary hyperparathyroidism; others postulate that steroids directly suppress renal tubular calcium resorption. Whether glucocorticoids have any direct effect on parathyroid hormone level remains controversial. The net effects of long-term glucocorticoid therapy favor osteopenia through impaired calcium absorption in the gut, impaired calcium and phosphate resorption by the renal tubule, and impaired bone formation by osteoblasts.

Persistently Reduced Renal Function

Finally, although the renal transplant may restore a substantial degree of renal function, transplantation rarely returns renal function completely to normal. Hyperparathyroidism tends to resolve incompletely even for years after successful transplantation, so reduced tubular resorption of phosphate, resulting in hypophosphatemia, is not uncommon. Persistent hyperparathyroidism could result in part from a moderate reduction in GFR, even in successful transplants, by the same mechanisms that produce hyperparathyroidism in early renal insufficiency. Because the renal tubular phosphate "leak" correlates poorly with parathyroid hormone levels and is not corrected with phosphate restriction, this leak could also be the result of tubular injury or steroid effects on the tubule, independent of the level of parathyroid hormone.

The result of all these factors is to produce, in the immediate posttransplantation period, modest hypercalcemia and hypophosphatemia in approximately 50% of subjects, with increased urinary losses of both calcium and phosphorus and a further reduction in bone mineral. With regression of the hyperparathyroidism and reduction of the glucocorticoid dose, hypercalcemia tends to regress, and serum calcium levels return to normal in two thirds of patients within 3 years. The remaining patients have few symptoms related to hypercalcemia, and parathyroidectomy is rarely necessary. Without treatment, hypophosphatemia persists in many patients with good transplant function. Despite restoration of near-normal renal function, skeletal mineralization often worsens, leading to osteoporosis in many patients and to osteonecrosis in a substantial fraction. The factors that are clearly associated with osteonecrosis include duration of uremia and dialysis, the degree of hyperparathyroidism before transplantation, and the total steroid dose.

To minimize the long-term metabolic bone complications after transplantation, careful attention must be paid to calcium and phosphate metabolism. In the presence of hypercalcemia, hypophosphatemia is usually managed by administering supplemental oral phosphorus (sodium phosphates, approximately 150 mg, 3 times daily). The diet should contain an adequate calcium and phosphorus content and be relatively free of phosphate binders, including magnesium-containing antacids, because these compounds also bind phosphates. Administration of calcitriol can ameliorate the renal phosphate leak and hyperparathyroidism and the depressed intestinal absorption of calcium and perhaps increase the rate of bone formation. One recent large, randomized, double-blind study showed that use of calcitriol (0.5 to 1 µg per day) could significantly reduce bone loss from the lumbar spine in patients during 1 year of corticosteroid therapy given for a variety of indications, not including organ transplantation. The benefit was not observed in patients receiving calcium supplements alone. However, calcitriol must be used judiciously, because it can cause hypercalcemia and hypercalciuria and lead to stone formation in the transplanted kidney. At least theoretically, hypercalcemia also may contribute to vascular calcifications, which occur at much higher frequency in the population of patients with end-stage renal disease.

MAGNESIUM

In up to 25% of cyclosporine-treated recipients of renal transplants, hypomagnesemia develops (serum magnesium <1.5 mg/dL), which is usually mild. Cyclosporine and tacrolimus induce renal magnesium wasting. Sirolimus, despite its lack of nephrotoxicity in general, is associated with renal magnesium loss in animals. Diuretics also may contribute to this problem. Consequences of hypomagnesemia may include muscle weakness, hypokalemia, hypocalcemia, and hyperlipidemia (elevated LDL). Serum magnesium levels should be monitored after renal transplantation, and oral supplementation prescribed if hypomagnesemia develops.

OTHER NUTRIENTS

The pathogenesis of hypertension in recipients of renal transplants is multifactorial, resulting from cyclosporine therapy, glucocorticoid therapy with activation of the renin–angiotensin system, acute and chronic rejection, renal artery stenosis, and other factors. A thorough discussion of this topic is beyond the scope of this chapter, but the issue is raised because cyclosporine-induced hypertension has been clearly shown to be sodium dependent and to be ameliorated by sodium restriction. Consequently, salt restriction should be part of the diet prescription for these patients. Tacrolimus may be associated with a lower incidence of posttransplantation hypertension than is cyclosporine, even though both agents increase renal salt reabsorption to the same degree. Although in the randomized trial comparing tacrolimus-based immunosuppression with cyclosporine-based immunosuppression, the incidence of hypertension during the first year was similar for the two regimens, the percentage of patients not taking any antihypertensive medications at the end of the year was significantly higher in the tacrolimus group (39% versus 30%, tacrolimus versus cyclosporine).

Cyclosporine- and tacrolimus-based immunosuppressive regimens also may be associated with hyperkalemia, even when the GFR is relatively high. The predominant mechanism of hyperkalemia seems to be a tubular defect in potassium secretion, with tubular insensitivity to mineralocorticoids. Other contributing factors may include suppression of the renin–aldosterone axis and altered distribution of potassium between the intra- and extracellular compartments. This effect is most often seen in the early posttransplantation period when doses of cyclosporine or tacrolimus are highest, but hyperkalemia may be sustained in some patients. An occasional patient may require restriction of dietary potassium intake. Because many good sources of calories and virtually all high-protein foods have a high potassium content, dietary potassium restriction conflicts directly with the prescription of a high-protein, high-calorie diet and may cause considerable malnutrition. β-Blockers, angiotensin-converting enzyme inhibitors, and angiotensin II–receptor blockers appear to act synergistically with cyclosporine or tacrolimus to reduce aldosterone levels and must be used with care in patients with hyperkalemia. Measures used to increase potassium excretion in other instances of type IV renal tubular acidosis, such as administration of sodium bicarbonate, diuretic therapy, or the use of ion-exchange resins (e.g., sodium polystyrene sulfonate), may permit some liberalization of dietary potassium.

Iron stores vary widely in patients with renal failure who present for transplantation and may be reduced in patients receiving hemodialysis therapy as a result of blood loss during dialysis. Iron absorption is normal in recipients of renal transplants, but the rapid expansion of the red cell mass after restoration of normal renal function may outstrip the iron absorption from foods, and some patients will require supplemental ferrous sulfate. Other patients may have excessive iron stores as a result of frequent transfusions and should not receive iron supplements. The extensive use of recombinant erythropoietin in patients receiving dialysis therapy over the past several years has lessened both the incidence of iron overload and the degree of posttransplantation expansion of red cell mass seen previously. Therefore, iron studies should be performed before oral supplements are prescribed.

Prescribing a supplement of water-soluble vitamins for recipients of transplants is a traditional therapy; however, unlike patients receiving dialysis therapy (see Chapters 10, 11, and 14), who can lose these vitamins during dialysis, recipients of renal transplants have little rationale for using these vitamins. Vitamin A levels are elevated in patients with chronic renal failure and in recipients of renal transplants. In these patients, the high levels of vitamin A are less likely to be toxic because they also have high circulating levels of retinol binding protein, which tightly binds the vitamin. For these reasons, vitamin A supplements should not be given. Vitamin C intakes and plasma levels are normal in recipients of renal transplant.

In the future, recommendations for vitamin supplementation in recipients of renal transplant may be influenced by the growing evidence that these patients, like predialysis patients with chronic renal failure and those receiving dialysis, have elevated plasma levels of homocysteine, which appears to be a significant risk factor for atherosclerotic complications. The prevalence and degree of hyperhomocysteinemia in the population of patients who have undergone transplantation seems to be similar to that observed in other populations of patients with end-stage renal disease. Observational studies in patients receiving renal transplantation show that elevated homocysteine levels are associated with a greater apparent risk for cardiovascular complications, similar to that observed in the general population, but a causal relationship has not been convincingly demonstrated. Evidence to date suggests that supplementation with a regimen of folic acid (5 to 15 mg per day), vitamin B_6, and vitamin B_{12} can reduce homocysteine levels in this population, but whether the reduction is associated with any decrease in risk for cardiovascular morbidity or mortality is yet unknown. Unfortunately, a recent, large, prospective randomized study in the general (nontransplant) population [the Vitamin Intervention for Stroke Prevention (VISP) trial] did not show any significant risk reduction for vascular outcomes in association with an intervention to lower homocysteine levels using high doses of folic acid and vitamins B_6 and B_{12}.

**Table 13-2.   Recommended
nutrition for recipients of renal transplants**

First month after transplantation and during therapy
for acute rejection

Protein	1.3–1.5 g/kg b.w./d
Calories	30–35 kcal/kg b.w./d

After first month

Protein	1.0 g/kg b.w./d
Calories	Sufficient to achieve and maintain optimal weight for height

At all times

Carbohydrates	50% of calories
Fats	Not >30% of calories
Cholesterol	Not >300 mg/d
Polyunsaturated–saturated fats ratio	>1
Calcium	1,200 mg/d
Phosphorus	1,200 mg/d
Ferrous sulfate	300 mg/d if iron stores are reduced
Sodium	No added salt diet (3–4 g/d sodium chloride) if patient is taking cyclosporine; generally no salt restriction needed otherwise

CONCLUDING COMMENTS

Recommended diets for the immediate posttransplantation period and for long-term therapy are summarized in Table 13-2. A
recurrent theme in the preceding discussion of nutritional and
metabolic abnormalities in recipients of renal transplants is the
adverse effects of glucocorticoid immunosuppressive therapy.
Given all the problems that these steroids cause, the fact that
several studies have been undertaken to see whether they can be
eliminated or given at reduced dosages is not surprising. In
smaller studies, patients removed from steroid therapy 6 months
or more after transplantation seem to do very well, but a large
multicenter Canadian study suggested that excess late graft losses might occur when steroids are stopped completely. Even with
use of cyclosporine and mycophenolate mofetil,the risk increases
for late rejection after steroid discontinuation, although the risk
seems to be primarily in African American patients. In some centers, steroid elimination or avoidance is routine; even those centers in which steroids are not discontinued show a trend toward
administering lower doses on alternate days.

SELECTED READINGS

Arnadottir, M, Hultberg B, Vladov V, et al. Hyperhomocysteinemia in
cyclosporine-treated renal transplant recipients. *Transplantation*
1996;61:509–512.

Bantle JP, Nath KA, Sutherland DE, et al. Effects of cyclosporine on the renin-angiotensin-aldosterone system and potassium excretion in renal transplant recipients. *Arch Int Med* 1985;145:505–508.

Bostom AG. Homocysteine: "expensive creatinine" or important modifiable risk factor for arteriosclerotic outcomes in renal transplant recipients? [Editorial]. *J Am Soc Nephrol* 2000;11:134–137.

Canzanello VJ, Textor SC, Taler SJ, et al. Renal sodium handling with cyclosporin A and FK506 after orthotopic liver transplantation. *J Am Soc Nephrol* 1995;5:1910–1917.

Cho YW, Terasaki PI, Cecka JM. New variables reported to the UNOS Registry and their impact on cadaveric renal transplant outcomes: a preliminary study. In: Cecka JM, Terasaki PI, eds. *Clinical transplants 1995*. Los Angeles: UCLA Tissue Typing Laboratory, 1996: 405–415.

Curtis JJ, Luke RG, Jones P, et al. Hypertension in cyclosporine-treated renal transplant recipients is sodium dependent. *Am J Med* 1989;85:134–138.

Dennis VW, Robinson K. Homocysteinemia and vascular disease in end-stage renal disease. *Kidney Int* 1996;50(Suppl. 57):S11–S17.

Edwards MS, Doster S. Renal transplant diet recommendations: results of a survey of renal dietitians in the United States. *J Am Diet Assoc* 1990;90:843–846.

El Haggan W, Vendrely B, Chauveau P, et al. Early evolution of nutritional status and body composition after kidney transplantation. *Am J Kidney Dis* 2002;40:629–637.

Ellis CN, Gorsulowsky DC, Hamilton TA, et al. Cyclosporine improves psoriasis in a double blind study. *JAMA* 1981;256:3110–3116.

Feehally J, Harris KP, Bennett SE, et al. Is chronic renal transplant rejection a non-immunological phenomenon? *Lancet* 1986;2: 486–488.

Friedman AN, Miskulin DC, Rosenberg IH, et al. Demographics and trends in overweight and obesity in patients at time of kidney transplantation. *Am J Kidney Dis* 2003;41:480–487.

Gonzalez MT, Gonzalez C, Grino JM, et al. Long-term evolution of renal osteodystrophy after kidney transplantation: comparative study between intact PTH levels and bone biopsy. *Transplant Proc* 1990;22:1407–1411.

Hodgson SF. Corticoid-induced osteoporosis. *Endocrinol Metab Clin North Am* 1990;19:95–111.

Horber FF, Hoppeler H, Herren D, et al. Altered skeletal muscle ultrastructure in renal transplant patients on prednisone. *Kidney Int* 1986;30:411–416.

Horber FF, Scheidegger JR, Gruing BE, et al. Evidence that prednisone-induced myopathy is reversed by physical training. *J Clin Endocrinol Metab* 1985;61:83–88.

Hoy WE, Sargent JA, Hall D, et al. Protein catabolism during the postoperative course after renal transplantation. *Am J Kidney Dis* 1985;5:186–190.

Hricik DE, Mayes JT, Schulak JA. Independent effects of cyclosporine and prednisone on posttransplant hypercholesterolemia. *Am J Kidney Dis* 1991;17:353–358.

Hricik DE, Whalen CC, Lautman J, et al. Withdrawal of steroids after renal transplantation: clinical predictors of outcome. *Trans plantation* 1992;53:41–45.

Jindal RM, Zawada ET. Obesity and kidney transplantation. *Am J Kidney Dis* 2004;43:943–952.

Johnson CP, Gallagher-Lepak S, Zhu Y-R, et al. Factors influencing weight gain after renal transplantation. *Transplantation* 1993; 56:822–827.

Julian BA, Laskow DA, Dubousky J, et al. Rapid loss of vertebral mineral density after renal transplantation. *N Engl J Med* 1991;325: 544–550.

Kamel K, Ethier JH, Quaggin S, et al. Studies to determine the basis for hyperkalemia in recipients of a renal transplant who are treated with cyclosporine. *J Am Soc Nephrol* 1991;2:1279–1284.

Kasiske BL, Cosio FG, Beto J, et al, National Kidney Foundation Working Group. Clinical practice guidelines for managing dyslipidemias in kidney transplant recipients: a report from the Managing Dyslipidemias in Chronic Kidney Disease Work Group of the National Kidney Foundation Kidney Disease Outcomes Quality Initiative. *Am J Transplant* 2004;4(Suppl. 7):13–53.

Kasiske BL, Umen AJ. Persistent hyperlipidemia in renal transplant patients. *Medicine* 1987;66:309–316.

Kasiske BL, Vazquez M, Harmon WE, et al. Recommendations for outpatient surveillance of renal transplant recipients. *J Am Soc Nephrol* 2000;11(Suppl. 15):S1–S86.

Kelleher J, Humphrey CS, Homer D, et al. Vitamin A and its transport protein in patients with chronic renal failure receiving maintenance hemodialysis and after renal transplantation. *Clin Sci* 1983;65:619–626.

Laskow DA, Curtis JJ. Posttransplant hypertension. *Am J Hypertens* 1990;3:721–725.

Markell M. New-onset diabetes in transplant patients: pathogenesis, complications and management. *Am J Kidney Dis* 2004;43: 953–965.

Merion RM, Twork AM, Rosenberg L, et al. Obesity and renal transplantation. *Surg Gynecol Obstet* 1991;172:367–376.

Milman N, Larsen L. Iron absorption after renal transplantation. *Acta Med Scand* 1976;200:25–30.

Moore RA, Callahan MF, Cody M, et al. The effect of the American Heart Association step one diet on hyperlipidemia following renal transplantation. *Transplantation* 1990;49:60–62.

Mor E, Facklam D, Hasse J, et al. Weight gain and lipid profile changes in liver transplant recipients: long-term results of the American FK506 multicenter study. *Transplant Proc* 1995;27:1126.

Nehme D, Rondeau E, Pollard F, et al. Aseptic necrosis of bone following renal transplantation: relationship with hyperparathyroidism. *Nephrol Dial Transplant* 1989;4:123–128.

Nuti R, Vattimo A, Turchetti V, et al. 25-hydroxy cholecalciferol as an agonist of adverse corticosteroid effects on phosphate and calcium metabolism in man. *J Endocrinol Invest* 1984;7:445–448.

Painter PL, Topp KS, Krasnoff JB, et al. Health-related fitness and quality of life following steroid withdrawal in renal transplant recipients. *Kidney Int* 2003;63:2309–2316.

Pei Y, Richardson R, Greenwood C, et al. Extrarenal effect of cyclosporin A on potassium homeostasis in renal transplant recipients. *Am J Kidney Dis* 1993;22:314–319.

Pirsch JD, Armbrust MJ, Knechtle SJ, et al. Obesity as a risk factor following renal transplantation. *Transplantation* 1995;59:631–647.

Pirsch JD, Miller J, Deierhoi MH, et al. A comparison of tacrolimus (FK506) and cyclosporine for immunosuppression after cadaveric renal transplantation. *Transplantation* 1997;63:977–983.

Prummel MF, Weirsinga WM, Lips P, et al. The course of biochemical parameters of bone turnover during treatment with corticosteroids. *J Clin Endocrinol Metab* 1991;72:382–386.

Rosenberg ME, Salahudeen AK, Hostetter TH. Dietary protein and the renin-angiotensin system in chronic renal allograft rejection. *Kidney Int* 1995;48(Suppl. 52):S102–S106.

Salahudeen AK, Hostetter TH, Raatz SK, et al. Effects of dietary protein in patients with chronic renal transplant rejection. *Kidney Int* 1992;41:183–190.

Sambrook P, Birmingham J, Kelly P, et al. Prevention of corticosteroid osteoporosis: a comparison of calcium, calcitriol, and calcitonin. *N Engl J Med* 1993;328:1747–1752.

Shen SY, Lukens CW, Alongi SU, et al. Patient profile and effect of dietary therapy on post-transplant hyperlipidemia. *Kidney Int* 1983;16:S147–S152.

Shihab FS. Metabolic complications. In: Norman DJ, Turka LA, eds. *Primer on transplantation*, 2nd ed. Mt. Laurel, NJ: American Society of Transplantation, 2001:247–256.

Short CD, Durrington PN. Hyperlipidemia and renal disease. *Baillieres Clin Endocrinol Metab* 1992;4:777–806.

Sinclair NR, Canadian Muticentre Transplant Study Group. Low-dose steroid therapy in cyclosporine-treated renal transplant recipients with well-functioning grafts. *Can Med Assoc J* 1992; 147:645–657.

Slatopolsky E, Martin K. Glucocorticoids and renal transplant osteonecrosis. *Adv Exp Med Biol* 1984;171:353–359.

Stern L, Iqbal N, Seshadri P, et al. The effects of low-carbohydrate versus conventional weight loss diet in severely obese adults: one-year follow-up of a randomized trial. *Ann Intern Med* 2004;140:778–785.

Suzuki Y, Ichikawa Y, Saito E, et al. Importance of increased urinary calcium excretion in the development of secondary hyperparathyroidism of patients under glucocorticoid therapy. *Metabolism* 1983; 32:151–156.

Terasaki PI, Koyama H, Cecka JM, et al. The hyperfiltration hypothesis in human renal transplantation. *Transplantation* 1994; 57:1450–1454.

The U.S. Multicenter FK506 Liver Study Group. A comparison of tacrolimus (FK506) and cyclosporine for immunosuppression in liver transplantation. *N Engl J Med* 1994;331:1110–1115.

Tonstad S, Holdaas H, Gorbitz C, et al. Is dietary intervention effective in post-transplant hyperlipidemia? *Nephrol Dial Transplant* 1995;10:82–85.

Toole JF, Malinow MR, Chambless LE, et al. Lowering homocysteine in patients with ischemic stroke to prevent recurrent stroke, myocardial infarction, and Death. The Vitamin Intervention for Stroke Preventions (VISP) randomized controlled trial. *JAMA* 2004;291:565–575.

Torres A, Machado M, Concepcion MT, et al. Influence of vitamin D receptor genotype on bone mass changes after renal transplantation. *Kidney Int* 1996;50:1726–1733.

Vathsala A, Wienberg RB, Schoenberg L, et al. Lipid abnormalities in cyclosporine-prednisone-treated renal transplant recipients. *Transplantation* 1989;48:37–43.

Whittier FC, Evans DH, Dutton S. Nutrition in renal transplantation. *Am J Kidney Dis* 1985;6:405–411.

Windus DW, Lacson S, Delmez JA. The short-term effects of a low-protein diet in stable renal transplant recipients. *Am J Kidney Dis* 1986;17:693–699.

Yancy WS, Olsen MK, Guyton JR, et al. A low-carbohydrate, ketogenic diet versus a low-fat diet to treat obesity and hyperlipidemia. A randomized controlled trial. *Ann Intern Med* 2004;140:769–777.

Nutrition Intervention for Chronic Renal Diseases

Jordi Goldstein-Fuchs

Nutrition therapy for kidney diseases is an integral component of medical care for the patient with progressive or end-stage renal disease, as well as for the patient who has undergone a renal transplant. Nutritional management is multifaceted and includes not only diet education but also nutrition assessment, development of individualized interventions, monitoring for changes, treating comorbid conditions, and documenting patient outcomes. Other chapters in this handbook address the science of nutrition assessment and malnutrition. This chapter provides applicable clinical information concerning the diet for different stages of kidney disease, for the common comorbid conditions associated with kidney disease, and for recipients of kidney transplants.

The traditional primary objectives of diet therapy for patients with progressive and end-stage kidney disease were to control uremic symptoms, potentially to forestall the progression of kidney disease, and to maintain an adequate nutritional status. Although these objectives are still valid, nutrition intervention goals now additionally include methods to improve overall patient outcomes and comorbid conditions, such as anemia, bone disease, and cardiovascular disease (CVD).

Nutrition therapy for patients with kidney disease is based on an extensive and continually expanding scientific literature. Empirical interventions that are observation-based are discouraged unless studied in a systematic manner. Although the relation of many components of nutrition manipulations to outcomes is even more controversial than the use of low-protein diets to slow progression, or is inconclusive, as in the role of homocysteine-causing CVD, the importance of adequate protein and calorie intake to avoid malnutrition is an established fact. Malnourished patients have a higher risk than others for morbidity and mortality. Specific nutrition recommendations have not been as consistently verified.

In an effort to provide evidence-based clinical guidelines, the National Kidney Foundation (NKF) launched the NKF Kidney Disease Outcomes Quality Initiatives (NKF-K/DOQI) in March 1995 [American Journal of Kidney Diseases (AJKD), 1995]. The guidelines have been completed for key issues in renal disease, including nutrition (NKF-K/DOQI, 2000). The American Dietetic Association (ADA) has compiled clinical protocols of care for the Medical Nutrition Therapy (MNT) program, which is legislation that provides for the reimbursement of nutrition intervention for the patient with progressive kidney disease (ADA, 2002). These primer publications provide a framework for evidence-based clinical work and enable the Registered Dietitian (RD) and renal care team to provide patients with nutritional care within a medical mode.

DIET THERAPY FOR PROGRESSIVE KIDNEY DISEASE

Protein

Chronic kidney disease (CKD) is defined by the level of kidney function and the evidence of kidney damage. The NKF-K/DOQI Clinical Practice Guidelines for CKD (NKF-K/DOQI, 2002) identified five stages of kidney disease, defined by the glomerular filtration rate (GFR) (see Table 14-1). These guidelines include specific nutrition recommendations for protein and calories for patients with stage 4 CKD.

For individuals with a GFR less than 25 mL per minute who are not undergoing maintenance dialysis, a low protein diet that provides 0.60 g protein/kg b.w./d should be considered. However, if the individual cannot tolerate such a diet or is unable to maintain an adequate intake (AI) of calories, then the individual should eat up to 0.75 g protein/kg b.w./d (see Chapter 6).

Regarding total energy intake: For individuals with a GFR less than 25 mL per minute who are not undergoing maintenance dialysis, the recommended intake is 35 kilocalories (kcal)/kg b.w./d for those younger than 60 years and 30 to 35 kcal per kg for individuals who are 60 years and older.

Although the K/DOQI guideline primarily addresses GFR less than 25, application of dietary protein restriction varies widely among practitioners. No real standard of practice exists, because of the controversial nature of the scientific literature. For a stable, well-nourished patient who has an established progressive kidney disease (CKD stages 1 to 4), a daily protein intake equivalent to the Recommended Dietary Allowance (RDA)—0.8 g protein/kg b.w./d—is reasonable. For a patient who is obese or underweight, the amount of protein should be based on an appropriately defined body weight. Alternatively, the NKF-K/DOQI Clinical Practice Guidelines on Hypertension and Antihypertensive Agents in CKD include a recommendation based on kidney disease stage of 1.4 g of protein/kg b.w./d for stages 1 to 2 and 0.6 to 0.8 g of protein/kg b.w./d for stages 3 to 4 (NKF-K/DOQI, 2004).

Table 14-1.   Stages of chronic kidney disease

Stage	Description	GFR (mL/min/1.73m^2)
1	Kidney damage with normal GFR	>90
2	Kidney damage with mild decrease in GFR	60–90
3	Moderate decrease GFR	30–60
4	Severe decrease GFR	15–30
5	Kidney failure	<15

GFR, glomerular filtration rate.
From NKF-K/DOQI. Clinical practice guidelines for chronic kidney disease: Evaluation, classification, and stratification. *Am J Kidney Dis* 2002;39(Suppl 1):S1–S46, with permission.

Calories

Calorie needs depend upon equations derived from direct and indirect calorimetry. A calorie needs assessment for a patient with stage 1 to 4 CKD would include calculations in the range of 28 kcal per kg of actual body weight to 35 kcal per kg b.w., based upon the appropriateness of weight for height. The Body Mass Index (BMI) could be used to identify the appropriateness of weight for height. Total calorie needs can then be adjusted for weight goals (i.e., gain, loss, or maintenance), metabolic status (anabolic or catabolic), and activity level. Table 14-2 lists clinical approaches to determine calorie requirements. These determinations are best made by an experienced renal RD, because the RD has extensive training and education in clinical nutrition and diet therapy. New technologies may soon enable individual calorie expenditure measurements; for example, a handheld portable device called the *Medgem* (Health-e-tech, Inc.) can measure resting energy expenditure (REE) within 10 minutes. Studies are currently

Table 14-2. Clinical approaches to determining calorie requirements of patients with chronic kidney disease (CKD) stages 1–4

No one ideal methodology is yet available to estimate energy needs. Therefore, calculating a range of needs may be the best approach until a more accurate technique is available:

1. Obtain food recall and weight history from patient. Estimate kcal intake factoring in weight history: loss, gain, maintenance; weight goal: loss, gain, maintenance.
2. To determine BEE
    a.   Harris–Benedict Equation:

Male (kcal) = 66 + (13.7 × b.w.^{a}) + (5.0 × height^b) − (6.8 × age^c)

Female (kcal) = 655 + (9.6 × b.w.^{a}) + (1.8 × height^b) − (4.7 × age^c)^d

    b.   Multiply BEE × activity factor as follows: sedentary, 1.2; moderate, 1.3
    c.   Additionally, multiply by stress factor when indicated
    d.   If the patient requires weight gain, add 500–1,000 kcal/d to identify approximated calorie needs for weight gain
    e.   If the patient requires weight loss, deduct 500–1,000 kcal/d to identify approximate calorie needs for weight loss
III. Use 28–35 kcal/kg b.w., depending on weight goal and patient reported activity level.
IV. Compare results from above methods and provide range of kcal needs.

CKD, chronic kidney disease; BEE, basal energy expenditure.
^{a} Actual body weight (b.w.) in kilograms.
^{b} Height in centimeters.
^{c} Age in years.
^{d} Currently, a validated equation to adjust for obesity is not available; therefore, empirical adjustment continues to be necessary.
From Harris JA, Benedict FG. *A biometric study of metabolism in man.* Washington, DC: Carnegie Institution, 1919:1–266, with permission.

being done with this tool to determine its accuracy and utility in patients with chronic CKD.

Carbohydrate

Several organizations including the American Heart Association, the American Diabetes Association, and the American Institute for Cancer Research have recently published new or updated dietary guidelines referred to as Therapeutic Lifestyle Changes (TLC) in response to growing evidence that suggests that nutrition has a positive role to play in preventing disease. Although different organizations have proposed a variety of recommendations, some common guidelines include increased consumption of fresh fruits and vegetables and whole grains and a reduced intake of total fat, saturated fatty acids, and cholesterol. Applying these guidelines translates into recommendations that carbohydrates provide 50% to 60% of calories and fats provide 25% to 30% of total calories.

These recommendations should be considered for patients with CKD, because of the high incidence of CVD in this patient group. In addition, with obesity as a risk factor for CVD and type 2 diabetes as the main cause of CKD, Lifestyle changes might offer some benefit to patient outcomes. This potential benefit needs to be explored with more research. The Lifestyle or TLC guidelines are compatible with CKD diets, because the recommendations include reduced intake of red meat. A challenge for some patients with Stages 1 to 4 CKD might be the high potassium intake. This challenge is discussed in the section called "Potassium."

Fat

Although total fat intake as a percentage of calories is important, the fatty acid composition of the fat also plays a role in CVD prevention. Saturated and transfatty acids are known to modify serum lipoprotein patterns toward a pattern that is associated with CVD risk. Therefore, fatty acid recommendations have been to keep saturated fatty acid intake at less than 10% of total calories and linoleic acid (n-6 polyunsaturated fatty acids) as 5% to 10% of total calories.

ω-3 Fatty Acids

In response to the growing body of evidence that indicates that ω-3 fatty acids have a beneficial role in preventing CVD, the American Heart Association revised its dietary intake recommendations in November 2002 to include an ω-3 fatty acid guideline for patients without or with documented CVD and for individuals who have elevated triglyceride levels (see Table 14-3).

The Institute of Medicine (IOM) recently published Acceptable Macronutrient Distribution Ranges (AMDRs) that include n-3 fatty acids. The AMDRs are based on the results of epidemiologic studies and a literature review that evaluated associations between diet intake and risk of chronic disease. The AMDR for fat is 20% to 35% of calories, 5% to 10% of calories for linoleic acid (n-6 polyunsaturated fatty acids, PUFAs) and 0.6% to 1.2% of energy for α-linolenic acid (ω-3 PUFAs). Up to 10% of the AMDR for ω-3 fatty acids can be consumed as eicosapentaenoic acid (EPA), docosahexaenoic acid (DHA), or both, equaling 0.06% to 0.12% of energy.

**Table 14-3.   American Heart
Association guidelines for ω-3 fatty acids**

Patients without documented CHD:
Eat a variety of (preferably oily) fish at least twice per week.
  Include oils and foods rich in α-linolenic acid (flaxseed, canola,
  and soybean oils; flaxseed and walnuts).
Patients with documented CHD:
Consume approximately 1 g EPA + DHA/d, preferably from oily
  fish. EPA + DHA supplements could be considered in
  consultation with the physician.
Patients who need triglyceride lowering: 2–4 g of EPA + DHA/d
  provided as capsules under a physicians care.

CHD, coronary heart disease; EPA, eicosapentaenoic acid; DHA, docosahexaenoic
acid.
From Kris-Etherton P, William H, Appel L. Fish consumption, fish oil,
omega-3 fatty acids, and cardiovascular disease. *Circulation* 2002;106:
2747–2757, with permission.

The IOM also introduced a new reference value: AI for the general population. AI is defined as the recommended average daily intake level based on observed or experimentally determined approximations or estimates of nutrient intake by a group (or groups) of apparently healthy people who are assumed to have an AI when an RDA cannot be determined.

The AI for α-linolenic acid is 1.6 and 1.1 g for men and women, respectively. Up to 10% can be consumed as EPA, DHA, or both. This amount of ω-3 fatty acid can be obtained by eating at least two servings of fatty fish per week or by taking supplements. For linoleic acid, the AI is 17 g per day for adult men and 12 g for adult women (National Academies Press, 2002).

Although no specific guidelines are currently available for patients with CKD, applying these fatty acid recommendations to stable, well-nourished patients in order to potentially lower CVD risk is reasonable. Little evidence exists to indicate that clinical problems related to bleeding occur with intakes less than 3 g per day. The US Food and Drug Administration (FDA) has identified 3 g per day of ω-3 fatty acids as the amount Generally Recognized as Safe (GRAS). This guideline can be applied to the CKD diet by adding cold-water fish, a main dietary source of ω-3 fatty acids, twice a week in lieu of red meat or poultry; this diet would provide an AI of EPA and DHA. A 3 oz portion of fatty cold-water fish can provide 0.13 to 1.7 g of EPA and DHA, depending upon the fish selected. Individuals who dislike fish can consider low-dose supplements of ω-3 fatty acids, but they should be monitored medically. Nonmarine sources of ω-3 fatty acids are available that are enriched in α-linolenic acid, the precursor to the elongated 20:5 EPA and the 22:5 DHA. These sources include soybean, olive, canola, and linseed oils. Aside from the oils, whole food sources of α-linolenic acid tend to be rich in potassium and phosphorus and cannot be readily included into the diet of a patient with CKD, because these patients need to restrict those minerals. Table 14-4 identifies the ω-3 fatty acid content of selected foods.

Table 14-4. ω-3 fatty acid content of selected foods

A. Sources of α-Linolenic Acid	g/tbls
Canola oil	1.3
Soybean oil	0.9
Flaxseed (linseed) oil	8.5 g fatty acids/100 g food
Walnut, English	6.8
Bean, common	0.6
Broccoli	0.1
Soybean	2.1
Spinach	0.9
B. Sources of EPA + DHA	**g/3 oz serving of fish**
Tuna, light, canned in water, drained	0.26
Sardines	0.98–1.70
Herring, Pacific	1.81
Flounder/Sole	0.42
Salmon, Pink	1.09

EPA, eicosapentaenoic acid; DHA, docosahexaenoic acid.
Modified from Simopoulos AP, Robinson J. *The Omega diet: the lifesaving nutritional program based on the diet of the island of Crete.* New York: Harper Collins, 1999 and Kris-Etherton P, William H, Appel L. Fish consumption, fish oil, omega-3 fatty acids, and cardiovascular disease. *Circulation* 2002;106:2747–2757.

Sodium

Because of the complex interactions between dietary sodium, hypertension, CVD, and CKD, the NKF-K/DOQI Clinical Practice Guidelines on Hypertension and Antihypertensive Agents (2004) recommends a dietary sodium intake of less than 2.4 g per day for most patients with CKD. Individualized modification is needed if the patient has a sodium-wasting disease or is prescribed medications that cause sodium loss. Figure 14-1 is an example of a patient handout that can be used as part of diet education to help patients with CKD lower sodium intake.

Potassium

Dietary intake of potassium is not restricted in patients with CKD unless potassium retention, the need to prescribe potassium-retaining medications, or both are evident. Individual metabolic abnormalities related to hormonal imbalances or glucose metabolism could also result in hyperkalemia. The TLC recommendations for CVD prevention include a diet that is rich in fruits, vegetables, and whole grains. This diet results in a daily potassium intake that is, on average, greater than 6 g. This intake can result in hyperkalemia. The NKF-K/DOQI Guidelines for Hypertension (2004) suggest a potassium intake greater than 4 g per day for stages 1 to 2 and ranging between 2 and 4 g of potassium per day for CKD stages 3 to 4. Table 14-5 identifies the potassium content of selected fruits, vegetables, and miscellaneous foods.

Phosphorus and Calcium

Early intervention for managing alterations in vitamin D metabolism and hyperparathyroidism is being strongly recommended by the nephrology community. As a result, dietary intake of phosphorus and calcium should be evaluated earlier in the course of CKD than has previously been recommended. The NKF-K/DOQI Clinical Practice Guidelines for Bone Metabolism and Disease (2003) recommend restricting dietary phosphorus to 800 to 1,000 mg per day (adjusted for dietary protein needs) when the serum phosphorus level is more than 4.6 mg per dL (1.49 mmol per L),

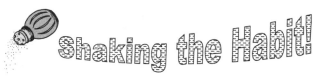

Here are some tips to reduce the amount of salt (sodium) in your diet:

✓ Limit salty snack foods such as chips, salty crackers or pretzels, and salted popcorn.

✓ Watch canned or frozen vegetables—many have added sodium.

✓ Processed foods have more sodium—buy fresh, natural foods more often.

✓ Limit the times you eat at fast food restaurants as their food is usually higher in sodium.

✓ Use seasoning blends like Mrs. Dash.

✓ Season with herbs and spices, most of which are sodium-free.

> **Put the saltshaker in the cupboard and use sparingly**
>
> ¼ tsp. salt = 575 mg sodium
>
> ½ tsp. salt = 1,150 mg sodium
>
> 1 tsp. salt = 2,300 mg sodium

Foods that are high in sodium

✓ Cured meats: ham, bacon, sausage, luncheon meat (bologna, salami, etc.)
✓ Fish, canned in oil or brine
✓ Canned shellfish
✓ Salted nuts, seeds, and snack mixes
✓ Soy protein products
✓ Pizza
✓ Lasagna
✓ Frozen dinners
✓ Dehydrated and canned soups
✓ Cheeses
✓ Buttermilk
✓ Instant cocoa mixes
✓ Bouillon cubes
✓ Olives, pickles, pickle relish
✓ Meat tenderizers
✓ Seasoning salts

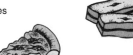

Figure 14-1. A sodium education handout designed to help patients undergoing dialysis to control salt and fluid intake. (DaVita, Inc., with permission).

Read the Labels!

Here are key words that indicate that a food may be high in sodium or have ingredients that contain sodium.

★ salt ★ sodium ★ monosodium glutamate (MSG) ★ baking powder ★ baking soda ★ disodium phosphate ★ sodium benzoate ★ sodium hydroxide ★ sodium nitrite ★ sodium propionate ★ sodium sulfite

Herb it UP!

Herbs are a great way to add flavor to your meals without adding salt. Here is a list of herbs and the foods they compliment.

Herbs	Vegetables
Anise	Green salads, vegetable soup
Basil	Green salads, pasta salad
Chervil	Green salads, vegetable soup
Chives	Use instead of onion for milder flavor
Sweet marjoram	String beans
Mint	Green peas
Parsley	Green salads, vegetable soup

Try any of these herbs to compliment these foods:

Herbs	Vegetables
Caraway seed, marjoram	Cauliflower
Basil, caraway seed, dill, Marjoram, nutmeg, savory	Green Beans
Basil, curry, marjoram, mint, Rosemary	Peas
Basil, celery seed, dill, paprika, Tarragon	Green salad
Basil, dill, garlic, parsley	Fish
Lovage, marjoram, sage, Tarragon	Poultry
Basil, dill, garlic, parsley	Fish

Figure 14-1. *Continued.*

when the plasma levels of parathyroid hormone (PTH) are elevated (see target ranges, Table 14-6), or when both levels are elevated.

Serum levels of phosphorus are controlled by diet modification and medication. Prescribing phosphate binders to patients with CKD who have elevated phosphorus levels is routine; phosphorus binders are usually prescribed to be taken during a meal or within 15 minutes of eating (either before or after). Most of the phosphorus binders that are available for use are calcium-based. Only one product currently on the market is a noncalcium binding resin (sevelamer); see Table 14-7. Side effects include excessive gas production, nausea, and bloating. There are now two calcium-free binders available. Sevelamer is a nonabsorbable-phosphate binder. A lanthanum carbonate product is now available.

Total dietary intake of calcium has become a concern because of the evidence that an excessive calcium intake can exacerbate

Buying Fresh Herbs

Most of these herbs are commonly found in markets: bay leaf, mint, oregano, parsley, rosemary, sage, thyme, and basil. Choose herbs that are clean, fresh, and fragrant, without signs of wilting or browning. They can be stored in the refrigerator in a plastic bag for up to five days.

Seasoning Strength

Strong herbs: bay leaves, cardamom, curry, ginger, hot peppers, mustard, pepper, rosemary, and sage—Use 1 teaspoon for 6 servings.
Medium herbs: basil, celery seed, cumin, dill, fennel, garlic, marjoram, mint, oregano, savory, thyme, and turmeric—Use 1 teaspoon for 6 servings.
Delicate herbs: burnet, chervil chives, parsley—Use as desired.

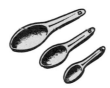

Figure 14-1. *Continued.*

vascular and other extraskeletal calcifications. The amount of dietary calcium that can be labeled as excessive in the population of patients with CKD has not to date been defined by any research. Maintaining total calcium intake within the RDA of calcium for adults is a reasonable goal until new evidence suggests otherwise. The RDA for calcium is 1,200 mg (for both men and women aged 19 to 75 years).

DIET FOR DIALYSIS

The diet therapy for patients who require renal replacement therapy addresses the same nutrients as those for earlier CKD stages, except that fluid intake is restricted. Individualizing each patient's nutrition plan is imperative, based on current nutritional status, nutrition history, food preferences, pertinent serum laboratory values, medical status, and the treatment method.

Protein

Protein intake must meet nutritional needs and compensate for any losses. Excessive intake simply enhances the production of nitrogenous toxins, whereas an inadequate intake can promote protein malnutrition. Amino acid and protein losses occur with dialysis, requiring a higher intake than that needed for healthy adults. During hemodialysis (HD), free amino acid losses average 4.5 to 7.7 g, and bound amino acid losses average 3.7 g per

Table 14-5. Potassium content of selected fruits, vegetables, and miscellaneous foods

Food	Serving Size	Amount of Potassium (mg)	Potassium Classification (considered low, medium, or high potassium content)
Apples	$^1/_2$ cup peeled, sliced	62	Low
Banana	1 medium	451	High
Blueberries, raw	$^1/_2$ cup	65	Low
Nectarine	1 medium	288	High
Strawberries, raw	$^1/_2$ cup	124	Low
Cauliflower, frozen, cooked	$^1/_2$ cup	125	Low
Chickpeas, cooked	$^1/_2$ cup	239	High
Green beans, cooked from raw	$^1/_2$ cup	185	Medium
Bread, white	1 slice	28	Low
Bread, whole wheat	1 slice	71	Low
Chocolate Kisses	1.4 oz (8 pieces)	152	Medium
Peanuts, dry roasted	1.0 oz	180	Medium
Jelly beans	1.0 oz	10	Low
Ice cream, chocolate	$^1/_2$ cup	164	Medium
Tomato sauce	$^1/_2$ cup	453	High

Created from Pennington, J. *Bowes & Church's food values of portions commonly used,* 17th ed. Philadelphia: Lippincott Williams & Wilkins, 1998.

treatment, depending upon the type of dialyzer. With peritoneal dialysis (PD), both amino acids and albumin are lost across the peritoneal capillary membranes. Of the 4 to 15 g lost daily, 50% to 80% is lost as albumin. Current protein recommendations for patients receiving HD or PD therapy are 1.2 g protein/kg b.w./d (NKF-K/DOQI, 2000a).

The quality of protein needed to meet essential amino acid (EAA) requirements is also important. Two thirds of protein should be from high biologic value (HBV) sources to ensure that minimal EAA requirements are met. A strict vegan (plant products only) vegetarian diet can be difficult when planning to meet these guidelines. Combinations of legumes, soy products, and limited amounts of nuts and seeds may be adequate for some patients.

Table 14-6. Target range of intact plasma parathyroid hormone (PTH) by stage of chronic kidney disease (CKD)

CKD Stage	GFR Range (mL/min/1.73 m^2)	Target "Intact" PTH [pg/mL (pmol/L)]
3	30–59	35–70 (3.85–7.7 pmol/L) (opinion)
4	15–29	70–110 (7.7–12.1 pmol/L) (opinion)
5	<15 or dialysis	150–300 (16.5–33.0 pmol/L) (evidence)

CKD, chronic kidney disease; GFR, glomerular filtration rate; PTH, parathyroid hormone.
From NKF-K/DOQI. Clinical practice guidelines for bone metabolism and disease in chronic kidney disease. *Am J Kidney Dis* 2003;42(Suppl. 3):S1–S202, with permission.

Calorically dense nondairy nutritional supplements are available to enhance vegan diets and provide a source of EAAs.

Energy

Energy requirements for patients receiving HD therapy is important for maintaining weight, and the requirements to avoid weight loss is an area of nutrition that needs further research. Studies that have actually measured energy expenditure in this patient population are limited in number and were conducted in small numbers of patients. Recent studies by Ikizler et al. (1996, 2002, 2003) suggest that REE in patients receiving HD therapy is greater than in control subjects, greater during dialysis than before and after dialysis, and greater during dialysis days than during nondialysis days. These investigators' most recent report also concluded that energy expenditure is greater in patients receiving HD therapy than in patients with CKD stages 1 to 4.

Until new data indicates otherwise, current energy recommendations for this patient population are based on an integration of data from studies that evaluated energy intake, energy measurements, and nitrogen balance. The NKF-K/DOQI Clinical Practice Guidelines for Nutrition in Chronic Renal Failure state that "The recommended daily energy intake for maintenance hemodialysis or chronic peritoneal dialysis patients is 35 kcal/kg body weight per day for those who are less than 60 years of age and 30–35 kcal/kg body weight per day for individuals 60 years or older." This guideline statement is based on both evidence and opinion. The rationale has been summarized as follows: (a) studies evaluating calorie intake in patients receiving HD therapy have documented low energy intakes, averaging about 24 to 27 kcal per kg; (b) REE studies have reported that patients receiving HD therapy have the same or slightly increased REE measurements compared to controls undergoing mild physical activity; and (c) nitrogen balance studies have indicated that at a calorie intake of 35 kcal per kg,

**Table 14-7.   Foods that count as
fluids and methods to control thirst**

1. Foods considered to be fluids

   Any food that is liquid at room temperature:
   Jello ices of any type
   Ice cream
   Popsicles
   Soups
   Thin stews
   Sorbets
   Ice chips and cubes
   Watermelons
   Any fluid that you drink, including nutritional supplements,
      alcohol, coffee, tea, water for medications

2. Methods to control thirst

   Avoid salty foods
   Keep mouth moist with mouth rinses (do not swallow)
   Brush teeth often
   Chewing gum (regular or sugar)
   Hard candy (regular or sugar)
   Frozen lemon slices
   Frozen blueberries
   Frozen grapes
   Products specific to help dry mouth and lips:
      Laclede, Inc., products, for example
   Use a humidifier in dry rooms or put a bowl
      of water by a heating vent.

neutral nitrogen balance is achieved, and serum albumin and anthropometric measures normalize.

For patients receiving PD therapy, energy requirements are complicated by the use of dextrose as an osmotic agent in dialysate. Total energy intake recommended should include both the oral and the dialysate content. Grodstein et al. (1981) proposed the following formula to calculate calories from absorbed dextrose:

$$Y = [(11.3\ X) - 10.9] \times L\ dialysate \times 3.7\ kcal/g\ glucose$$

where Y is the grams glucose absorbed per liter of dialysate and X is the concentration of glucose (g per L). As much as 60% to 80% (100 to 250 g) of the dialysate dextrose can be absorbed and may account for more than one third of the patient's daily caloric needs. This extra energy was initially thought to aid nutritionally compromised patients. However, a spontaneous decrease in patients' intake seems to occur in response to the dextrose load, so desired weight gains or reversal of signs of malnutrition are not achieved. Conversely, restricting calories for weight reduction or weight maintenance in patients who are prone to obesity is complicated by the high protein requirements. In such patients, the use of protein supplements can help replace protein losses. The entire renal team can work together to encourage increased physical activity to prevent or help treat undesired weight gain.

Dietary Potassium

The kidney is the primary route for excretion of potassium. Therefore, once a patient's urine output decreases to less than 600 mL per day, GFR less than 10 mL per minute, or both, a potassium restriction is usually required to maintain normal serum potassium levels. Hyperkalemia, defined as a serum potassium level 6 mEq per mL or greater, can result in death. Whereas dialysis therapy removes potassium from the serum, dietary potassium intake determines how much potassium accumulates between treatments. The usual dietary potassium prescription for patients receiving HD therapy is 2 g per day. Patients receiving PD therapy are treated with greater frequency and are therefore allowed a more liberal prescription, typically in the range of 4 g daily. Individualization of these guidelines should take several factors into consideration: residual renal function; body size; the presence of anabolism, catabolism, or infection; and the potassium content of the dialysate. The food groups that typically require special selection for adequate potassium intake are fruits and vegetables. Dairy products are also concentrated sources of potassium. Miscellaneous high-potassium foods include nuts and seeds, chocolate, and whole grain breads. Although diet indiscretion is most often the primary cause of hyperkalemia, other conditions could also result in hyperkalemia, including medications, acidemia, inadequate dialysis, and abnormal glucose metabolism. All these potential conditions, in addition to diet, must be considered when determining intervention for high potassium levels. Table 14-5 lists the potassium content of selected foods.

Sodium and Fluid

Dietary intake of sodium and fluid are interrelated. Both factors play a role in maintaining sodium and fluid balance but also in producing edema, hypertension, and cardiac problems such as congestive heart failure. The recommended sodium intake for patients receiving HD therapy is usually 2 g per day. This intake complements the fluid restriction required for patients with anuria (500 mL or more of urine per day) of 1,000 mL per 24 hours. A high sodium intake not only contributes to thirst but also causes fluid retention. Patients receiving HD therapy who retain fluid and sodium experience intradialytic hypotension, pre- and postdialysis hypertension, cramping, and overall malaise because of the need to remove excess amounts of fluid during a short dialysis period. This sodium and fluid prescription facilitates minimizing interdialytic weight gains, of which the goal is 2 kg or 0.3% to 0.5% of estimated dry weight. Table 14-7 identifies foods that count as liquids, which should be considered when monitoring daily fluid intake. Maintaining a fluid intake of 1,000 mL per day is one of the most challenging and difficult components of the dialysis diet for most patients.

Because of the continual nature of PD therapy and the osmotic nature of the glucose-containing dialysate solutes, sodium and fluid losses occur. Therefore, restricting sodium (less than 3 g per day) and fluid is typically unnecessary. Patients learn to monitor for both dehydration and overhydration and to make the appropriate adjustments in their dialysis regimen.

Phosphorus, Calcium, and Vitamin D

As GFR decreases, the generation of active vitamin D hormone (1,25-dihydroxycholecalciferol) is decreased, intestinal calcium absorption declines, and phosphate is retained, resulting in overstimulation of PTH. Hyperparathyroidism can lead to cardiovascular and extraskeletal calcification of soft tissues such as blood vessels, lungs, and joints; bone disease; and increased mortality.

Phosphorus and Phosphate Binders

As in the earlier stages of CKD, serum phosphorus levels for patients with stage 5 CKD can be controlled with diet, phosphate binders, vitamin D therapy, and newer pharmaceuticals that modulate PTH function. The NKF-K/DOQI guidelines for bone disease management recommend that patients receiving dialysis replacement therapy maintain serum phosphorus levels no greater than 5.5 mg per dL. Clinical recommendations for the patient with stage 5 CKD are very specific in regard to total calcium intake. The K/DOQI recommendations specify that the total dose of elemental calcium resulting from the use of calcium-based phosphate binders should not exceed 1,500 mg per day and that the total calcium intake, from dietary sources and phosphate binders combined, should not exceed 2,000 mg per day. Calcium-containing phosphate binders are not recommended for patients undergoing dialysis who are hypercalcemic, defined as corrected serum calcium greater than 10.2 mg per dL.

The recommended dietary phosphorus intake is 800 to 1,000 mg per day. Restricting dietary phosphate, prescribing phosphate binders, and ensuring adequate dialysis are all necessary to maintain serum phosphorus levels between 2.5 and 5.5 mg per dL. The main food group that is rich in phosphorus is the dairy products, followed by animal protein. Whole grains, nuts, and dried beans and peas are foods rich in dietary phosphate. Table 14-8 identifies the phosphate content of selected foods. Patients who are used to eating 1 to 4 servings of dairy protein and large amounts of animal protein find it difficult to adhere to phosphate-restricted diets. Adhering to phosphate binder therapy is also a major challenge for many patients.

Several different types of phosphate binders are available (see Table 14-9). Calcium carbonate, calcium acetate, and calcium citrate are the typical calcium-containing phosphate binders used. All three binders allow for at least 20% absorption of calcium. Magnesium carbonate is less commonly used as a phosphate binder. Magnesium carbonate can lead to hypermagnesemia and may a play a role in adynamic bone disease. Aluminum hydroxide is a powerful phosphate-binding agent but can lead to osteomalacia, encephalopathy, and aluminum toxicity. Although aluminum hydroxide was widely used before the 1990s, this class of phosphate binder is now reserved for "rescue therapy," an intervention for hyperphosphatemia that is accompanied by highly elevated PTH and serum calcium levels. In response to concerns regarding elemental calcium intake, a noncalcium-based

Table 14-8. Phosphate content of selected foods

Food	Measure	Phosphorus (mg)
Beans, black	1 cup	251
Brown rice	$^1/_2$ cup	81
White rice	$^1/_2$ cup	12
Tofu, firm	100g	76
Cheese, cream	1 tbsp	15
Custard	$^1/_2$ cup	142
Milk, 2%	1 cup	232
Yogurt, lowfat	4 oz	162
Salmon	3 oz	282
Shrimp	3 oz	116
Peanuts, roasted	1 oz	147
Chocolate, semi sweet	1 oz	37
Bread, wheat bran	1 slice	67
Caramel	1 package (2.5 oz)	81
Peanut butter	2 tbsp	118
Eggnog	1 cup	277

Created from Pennington J. *Bowes & Church's food values of portions commonly used*, 17th ed. Philadelphia: Lippincott Williams & Wilkins, 1998 and *Nutritionist five* [computer program]. Version 1.6. San Bruno, CA: First Data Bank Inc., 1998.

binder has become available: sevelamer hydrochloride (Renagel) (Genzyme, Inc., MA). Sevelamer is a cationic polymer that is not absorbed but is excreted in the feces. Renagel has been shown to be as effective at binding phosphorus as calcium carbonate and offers the additional benefit of lowering LDL cholesterol. A main advantage of sevelamer hydrochloride over the calcium-based binders is that it can bind dietary phosphate without contributing to a positive calcium balance or resulting in hypercalcemia. A phosphate binder containing lanthanum carbonate is now available for clinical use (Fosrenol Shire).

Intravenous Vitamin D

Hyperparathyroidism is controlled in the patient with stage 5 CKD by administering active metabolites of vitamin D. Intravenous (IV) calcitriol and paricalcitol administered during dialysis suppress PTH. However, both IV treatments increase intestinal calcium and phosphorus absorption and boost calcium mobilization from the bone. Therefore, serum calcium, serum phosphorus, and the calcium × phosphorus product require frequent (biweekly or monthly) monitoring to avoid unrecognized consequences. Cinacalcet (Sensipar, Amgen, CA), a calcimimetic that suppresses PTH, was recently approved by the FDA. This compound binds to the PTH calcium-sensing receptor and lowers serum PTH, calcium, and phosphorus (see Chapter 3). Cinacalcet is indicated for patients who become hypercalcemic with IV vitamin D,

Table 14-9.   Identification of phosphate binders

Type	Brand Name	% Ca	Dose	Elemental Calcium	Potential Side Effects
Sevelamer hydrochloride · Given *with* meals (and snacks, if prescribed) as a calcium-free phosphate binder · Difficult to provide adequate dosage with reasonable number of pills per meal without using 800 mg version	Renagel	0%	800 mg hard tablet 400 mg hard tablet 403 mg soft capsule	Contains no calcium	Diarrhea, nausea, constipation, flatulence, dyspepsia, ↓ Chol, ↓ LDL
Calcium acetate · Given *with* meals (and snacks, if prescribed) as phosphate binder	PhosLo	25%	667 mg gel cap or tablet	167 mg	Constipation, nausea, hypercalcemia, metastatic calcification
Lanthanum carbonate	Fosrenol	0%	250 mg or 500 mg	Contains no calcium	Nausea, vomiting

Calcium carbonate • Given *with* meals (and snacks, if prescribed) as phosphate binder • Given between meals as Ca supplement • Tums and Calcichew are chewable • CalciMix can be swallowed or opened and mixed with food • Oscal 500 and Nephrocalci are swallowed	Tums regular Tums EX Tums ultra Tums 500 Calcichew Calcimix Oscal 500 (oyster shell should not be used for patients with renal disease — increase risk of lead) Nephrocalci	40%	500 mg 750 mg 1,000 mg 1,250 mg 1,250 mg 1,250 mg 1,250 mg 1,500 mg	200 mg 300 mg 400 mg 500 mg 500 mg 500 mg 500 mg 600 mg	Constipation, hypercalcemia, metastatic, calcification
Calcium citrate • Not recommended because it enhances aluminum absorption, especially when combined with Al-based phosphate binders	Citracal	22%	950 mg	209 mg	Enhances aluminum absorption, hypercalcemia, metastatic, calcification

continued

Table 14-9. Continued.

Type	Brand Name	% Ca	Dose	Elemental Calcium	Potential Side Effects
Magnesium carbonate in combination with calcium carbonate • Use with caution—may cause increased magnesium levels • Serum magnesium levels need to be monitored	Magnebind 200	25%	200 mg MgCO$_3$ 400 mg Ca^{2+}CO$_3$	160 mg Ca^{2+} 100 mg Ca^{2+}	Diarrhea, ↑ magnesium
	Magnebind 300		300 mg MgCO$_3$ 250 mg Ca^{2+}CO$_3$	80 mg Ca^{2+}	
	Magnebind 400 Rx		400 mg MgCO$_3$ 200 mg Ca^{2+}CO$_3$ 1 mg Folic acid		
Aluminum hydroxide • Use with caution on short-term basis only • Serum aluminum levels need to be monitored	Alu-cap Alu-tab AlternaGel Amphojel	0%	1 capsule 1 tablet 5 mL 5 mL	175 mg Al 175 mg Al 208 mg Al 111 mg Al Contains no calcium	Aluminum bone disease, dementia

Chol, cholesterol; LDL, low-density lipoprotein.
DaVita, Inc. An internal DaVita patient education piece (in press) used with permission.

demonstrate PTH resistance in the presence of vitamin D infusion, or both.

Other Vitamins and Minerals for Chronic Kidney Disease, Stages 1 to 5

Patients with renal disease are at increased risk for deficiencies of water-soluble vitamins, particularly vitamin C, folate, and pyridoxine (B_6). Causes include altered intake of foods, drug-nutrient interactions, changes in retention and excretion patterns, interference in metabolism by uremic toxins, and losses to the dialysate. High doses of vitamin C may result in elevated plasma levels of oxalate. Supplementation should not exceed 75 to 90 mg per day. Supplementation with fat-soluble vitamin A is not recommended. Studies have shown that patients develop hypervitaminosis A and may develop bone resorption. Requirements for fat-soluble vitamins E and K are thought to be similar to those of the general population (see Chapter 10). Patients need to have an explanation of why they should take a special vitamin rather than the multivitamin preparations that contain vitamin A or the standard form of vitamin D.

Vitamin formulations containing high-dose folic acid have become available for the patient undergoing dialysis in response to the literature suggesting that hyperhomocysteinemia is linked to CVD and poor outcome in this patient population (see Table 14-10). The literature about this issue is controversial; until the results of clinical trials currently in process are completed, supplements in the range of 1 to 5 mg folate per day may be prudent. In addition, vitamin supplements containing vitamin E, selenium, and zinc have also become available. Whether the higher cost of these supplements results in a cardioprotective effect is not known. The potential for toxicity in each individual patient must be considered when selecting a vitamin supplement (Chapter 10).

Iron and Anemia

Iron metabolism plays an essential role in the anemia of chronic renal failure. Factors that contribute to anemia include failure of the kidney to secrete erythropoietin, blood loss of two to five liters per year from HD treatments, and possible binding of iron to the dialysis membrane. If left untreated, anemia can result in cardiac enlargement, ventricular hypertrophy, angina, heart failure, and malnutrition. Supplementation with recombinant human erythropoietin (rhEPO), as a replacement for the natural hormone, dramatically decreases the incidence and severity of anemia. The K/DOQI-recommended hematocrit and hemoglobin target levels are 33% to 36% and 11 to 12 g per dL, respectively (NKF-K/DOQI, 2000). The general dose required for adult patients is 80 to 120 U rhEPO/kg b.w./wk in two to three doses, if administered subcutaneously. If the IV route is used, the general dosing is 120 to 180 U/kg b.w./wk, given over three dialysis sessions. The absolute dose depends on patient response.

As a result of rhEPO administration, most patients receiving dialysis replacement therapy will require iron replacement therapy. This requirement is evaluated by monitoring serum ferritin and transferrin levels. Patients with iron deficiencies may not respond to erythropoietin. Patients can be prescribed oral iron

Table 14-10.   Sample of vitamin formulations available for chronic kidney disease (CKD)

Ingredient	Nephrocaps (Fleming Labs)	Renal Tab (Rena Lab)	Dialy-vite 800 with Zinc (Hill-estad)	Diatx (Pamlab)	Renax (Everett Labs)
Vitamin C (mg)	100	125	60	60	50
Thiamine (mg)	1.5	12.5	1.5	1.5	3.0
Riboflavin (mg)	1.7	7.5	1.7	1.5	2.0
Niacin (mg)	20.0	50.0	20.0	20.0	20.0
Pyridoxine (mg)	10.0	20.0	10.0	50.0	15.0
Folic acid (mg)	1.0	1.0	0.8	5.0	2.5
B12 (μg)	6.0	12.5	6.0	1000	12.0
Biotin (μg)	150.0	300	300.0	300	300
Pantothenic acid (mg)	5.0	30.0	10.0	10.0	10
Zinc (mg)	—	15	50.0	—	20
Selenium (μg)	—	—	—	—	70
Vitamin E (IU)	—	15.0	—	—	35
Manganese (mg)	—	7.5	—	—	—
Chromium (μg)	—	150	—	—	—
Molybdenum (μg)	—	50.0	—	—	—
Glutamic acid HCL (mg)	—	150	—	—	—
Lipase (mg)	—	100.0	—	—	—

supplements of 250 to 500 mg ferrous sulfate or the equivalent ferrous fumerate or glutamate. However, IV iron administration has been observed to be more effective in treating iron deficiency anemia. An example of a recipe incorporating TLC diet guidelines for a patient with CKD who does not require potassium restriction is shown in Table 14-11. Table 14-12 provides an example of a 1-week menu that is appropriate for a patient receiving HD therapy.

Table 14-11. Sample recipe suitable for a patient with chronic kidney disease (CKD) who does not require a potassium restriction

Wild rice with vegan sausage

10 oz of a 15-1/2 oz. can black-eyed peas, drained
2 tbsp plus 2 tsp all-purpose flour
3 tbsp fresh button mushrooms, finely chopped
1/2 tsp onion powder
2 tsp fennel seed
2 dashes crushed red pepper flakes
2 tsp basil
4 sprigs of parsley, chopped
Pinch ground black pepper
2 tsp crushed rosemary
2 tsp sage
1 tbsp olive oil
1/2 onion, diced (4 oz)
1 carrot, diced (2 oz)
1 clove garlic, minced
3 Granny Smith apples, diced (15 oz)

3 tbsp fresh thyme
1/4 tsp marjoram
4 oz Mori-Nu tofu, soft
1 tbsp lemon juice
1/8 tsp garlic powder
1/8 tsp onion powder
3 drops of Tabasco sauce
3 cups cooked wild rice

Nutritional information
Servings per recipe: 6
Amount per serving: 1-1/2 cups
Calories: 222
Total fat: 4 g
Saturated fat: 0.5 g
Monounsaturated fat: 2 g
Polyunsaturated fat: 1 g
Cholesterol: 0 mg
Sodium: 166 mg
Phosphorus: 157 mg
Potassium: 445 mg
Total carbohydrates: 41 g
Dietary fiber: 6 g
Protein: 8 g

Mash black-eyed peas; add flour, mushrooms, 1/2 teaspoon of onion powder together. Form into 6 small very flat patties. Blend these spices together: fennel, red pepper flakes, basil, parsley, black pepper, rosemary, and sage. Coat the black-eyed pea/mushroom patties with the spice mixture. Save leftover spice mixture. Spray patties with olive oil and fry the patties on medium heat in a nonstick pan until golden brown. Gently turn over and brown the other side. Layer these patties in the bottom of an 8 × 8 inch baking dish. Sauté on medium heat 1-1/2 teaspoons olive oil, carrots, and onions until onions start turning brown; add apples, garlic, fresh thyme, and marjoram and cook for 2 more minutes. Mix tofu with lemon juice, garlic powder, onion powder, and Tabasco sauce. Mix wild rice, tofu, and apple mixture and 1-1/2 teaspoons of sausage spices together; pour wild rice mixture over tops of the black-eyed patties in the baking dish. Bake in a preheated 350°F oven for 30 minutes.

NUTRITION FOR THE RECIPIENT OF A KIDNEY TRANSPLANT

The overall goal of the posttransplant diet is to promote blood pressure control, prevent weight gain, normalize electrolyte imbalances, maximize bone density, control blood glucose levels, and promote overall good nutritional status. Although renal transplantation restores near-normal kidney function, many metabolic challenges occur, both in the acute posttransplant stage and during

Table 14-12.   Seven-day menu for a patient undergoing hemodialysis using recipes from a cookbook for patients with chronic renal disease

1ST MENU

First Meal
1/4 cup scrambled
    egg substitute
2 slices white toast
    with margarine
1/2 cup fruit cocktail
1 cup coffee with nondairy
    creamer and sugar

Second Meal
Deluxe tuna salad mold
One lettuce leaf
8 pieces white melba toast
1/2 cup sauteed zucchini
1 tangerine

Snack
2 oatmeal cookies

Third Meal
1 lemon pork chop
1/2 cup noodles with parsley
    and margarine
1/2 cup sunshine carrots
1/2 cup applesauce
1 dinner roll with margarine
Apple crisp

Snack
1 slice angel food cake
1 cup cranberry juice

Calories 2,070
Carbohydrate .... 286 g
Protein .... 63 g
Fat .... 64 g
Sodium .... 1,740 mg
Potassium .... 1,863 mg
Phosphorus .... 760 mg

2ND MENU

First Meal
1/2 cup cream of rice with sugar
1/2 cup light (1%) milk
1/2 cup red raspberries
1, 2 oz bagel
2 tablespoons lite cream cheese
1 cup coffee with nondairy
    creamer and sugar

Second Meal
Egg salad sandwich on light
    rye bread
Fresh medium peach
Vanilla wafers

Snack
Graham cracker snacks
Cup lemonade

Third meal
7 petite meat balls with mustard
    sauce
1/2 cup parsley potatoes with
    margarine
1/2 cup waxed beans
1/2 cup apricot halves
1 cup tea with sugar

Snack
3 cups popcorn

Calories 1,850
Protein .... 63 g
Fat .... 77 g
Sodium .... 1,467 mg
Potassium .... 2,008 mg
Phosphorus .... 893 mg

3RD MENU

First Meal
3, 4-inch pancakes with
    margarine and maple syrup
1/2 cup canned peaches
1 cup coffee with nondairy
    creamer and sugar

Second Meal
Fresh fruit salad:
    1/2 medium apple
    1/2 small orange
    10 grapes
    1 slice pineapple

Table 14-12. *Continued.*

1/2 cup cottage cheese
10 saltines with unsalted tops
1 cup lemonade

Snack
1/2 cup light (1%) milk
12 animal crackers

Third Meal
1 baked best chicken breast
1/4 cup cranberry sauce
1/2 cup boiled rice with
   margarine

1/2 cup asparagus
Corn bread (2 oz piece)
   with margarine
1 cup tea with sugar

Snack
1 piece chocolate chip cake

Calories 1,988
Carbohydrate .... 303 g
Fat .... 54 g
Sodium .... 2,180 mg
Potassium .... 1,865 mg
Phosphorus .... 1,080 mg

4TH MENU

First Meal
English muffin with
   margarine and jelly
1-1/4 cup Rice Krispies
1/2 cup light (1%) milk
1 cup coffee with nondairy
   creamer and sugar

Second Meal
3 oz meatloaf sandwich on
   white bread
Angel food cake with 1/2 cup
   frozen strawberries and
   whipped topping
1 cup lemonade

Third Meal
Sole parmesan

1/2 cup savory stuffing
1/2 cup frozen corn niblets
1 cup tossed salad with olive oil
   and vinegar dressing
Cheesecake puff
1 cup tea with sugar

Snack
Hard unsalted pretzels (1 oz)
1 cup ginger ale

Calories 2,093
Carbohydrate .... 324 g
Protein .... 76 g
Fat .... 60 g
Sodium .... 2,284 mg
Potassium .... 2,389 mg
Phosphorus .... 1,100 mg

5TH MENU

First Meal
1 cup corn flakes
1/2 cup light (1%) milk
1/2 cup blueberries
Apple muffin with margarine
1 cup coffee with nondairy
   creamer and sugar

Second Meal
1/2 cup chicken salad
   with lettuce in a pita pocket
2 small plums

10 vanilla wafers
1 cup lemonade

Third Meal
Filet of sole with lemon and
   chive sauce
1/2 cup broccoli
Dinner roll with margarine
1/2 cup peaches
1 slice orange chiffon cake
1 cup tea with sugar

continued

Table 14-12. *Continued.*

Calories 1,914
Carbohydrate .... 292 g
Protein .... 63 g
Fat .... 66 g

Sodium .... 1,925 mg
Potassium .... 1,885 mg
Phosphorus .... 964 mg

6TH MENU

First Meal
2 slices french toast made with
  1/2 cup egg substitute
Maple syrup and margarine
1/2 cup applesauce
1 cup coffee with nondairy
  creamer and sugar

Second Meal
Turkey sandwich with berry
  cream cheese
1 medium, fresh pear
3 graham crackers
1/2 cup gingerale

Third Meal
Clam chowder
Crepes St. Jacques
Broccoli Italianne
Butterscotch pudding
1 cup tea with sugar

Calories 2,165
Carbohydrate .... 280 g
Protein .... 58 g
Fat .... 82 g
Sodium .... 2,170 mg
Potassium .... 2,165 mg
Phosphorus .... 940 mg

7TH MENU

First Meal
Apple pancakes with
  margarine
1/2 cup grapefruit
1 cup coffee with nondairy
  creamer and sugar

Second Meal
Ham sandwich with 2 slices of
  lower salt ham on white
  bread with mayonnaise
15 grapes
2 nutty meringue cookies
  1 cup lemonade

Third Meal
Chicken marsala
1 cup angel hair pasta with

margarine
1 slice Italian bread with
  margarine
1/2 cup peas and onions
1/2 cup pineapple sherbet with
  1/2 cup crushed pineapple

Snack
Rich cranberry shake

Calories 2,212
Carbohydrate .... 314 g
Protein .... 71 g
Fat .... 84 g
Sodium .... 1,775 mg
Potassium .... 2,284 mg
Phosphorus .... 900 mg

From *Now you're cooking... A resource for people with kidney disease.* National
Kidney Foundation/Council on Renal Nutrition of New England, 1999, with
permission.

long-term maintenance, from side effects of antirejection medication and often require special nutrition intervention.

During the acute posttransplant state, electrolyte imbalances may develop, including hypophosphatemia, which can aggravate the decrease in bone density. Serum electrolytes should be closely monitored, with appropriate intervention as indicated. Table 14-13 identifies nutrition recommendations for the posttransplant recovery phase.

Long-term metabolic abnormalities occur during the long-term maintenance posttransplant phase. For example, 60% of recipients develop hyperlipidemia, and approximately 40% of posttransplant mortality is attributed to cardiovascular death. Glucose intolerance is common and is associated with a high risk for infection and decreased survival. Excessive weight gain exacerbates the hyperlipidemia and glucose intolerance and can

**Table 14-13. Nutrition recommendations
for the immediate posttransplant recovery phase**

Goals	1. Promote wound healing
	2. Promote anabolism
	3. Prevent infection
	4. Minimize side effects of medications
Nutrient requirements	**Recommendations**
Calories	• 1.3–1.5 (BEE or 30–35 kcal/kg dry wt or wt, adjusted for obesity)
Protein	• 1.3–2.0 g/kg dry wt or wt, adjusted for obesity
Carbohydrate	• 50%–70% nonprotein kcal; diabetic diet as appropriate
Fat	• 30%–50% nonprotein kcal
Fluid	• Ad lib or 1.0 mL/kg dry wt; increase intake to equal output unless diuresis is goal
Vitamins	• RDA; supplementation usually not necessary
Minerals	• Sodium: 4.0 g/d or no added salt; unrestricted if HTN/edema absent
	• Potassium: unrestricted unless necessary
	• Calcium: 1,000–1,500 mg/d; supplement if necessary
	• Phosphorus: supplementation may be necessary
	• Magnesium: supplementation may be necessary

BEE, basal energy expenditure; RDA, recommended dietary allowance; HTN, hypertension.
© 2002, American Dietetic Association, used with permission.

contribute to a metabolic syndrome, increasing the risk of graft rejection. Diet interventions recommended to avoid dyslipidemia and to control body weight include exercise and a low-fat diet. Table 14-14 details the long-term posttransplant nutrition therapy recommended for adults who are recipients of kidney transplants.

Nutrition Assessment

Evaluating and monitoring nutritional status is a fundamental component of providing nutrition care to patients with renal disease. The nutritional assessment procedure includes methods to detect, diagnose, characterize, and classify deficiencies and to predict outcome. Mechanisms to monitor patient response to therapeutic intervention are also necessary parts of a comprehensive assessment protocol. Traditionally, nutritional compromise has been viewed as a secondary phenomenon that resolves spontaneously when the primary disorder is corrected. Loss of protein stores is now recognized as a disease entity that requires diagnosis and treatment.

Table 14-14.   Long-term nutritional therapy for the recipient of a kidney transplant

Goals	1. Achieve or maintain desirable weight 2. Maintain acceptable blood glucose levels 3. Maintain cholesterol levels ≤200 mg/dL 4. Maintain normal blood pressure 5. Maintain optimal bone density 6. Minimize side effects of medications 7. Maintain healthy lifestyle
Nutrient Requirements	**Recommendations**
Calories	• 1.2–1.3 3 × BEE or adequate to maintain desirable weight
Protein	• 0.8–1.0 g/kg b.w.
Carbohydrate	• 45%–50% total calories, 25–30 g dietary fiber/d
Fat	• ≤30% total kcal • ≤10% polyunsaturated • 10%–15% monounsaturated • 7%–10% saturated • <300 mg cholesterol/d
Fluid	• Ad lib
Vitamins	• RDA; supplement as needed
Minerals	• RDA; supplement or restrict as needed

BEE, Basal Energy Expenditure; RDA, Recommended Dietary Allowance.
© 2002, American Dietetic Association, used with permission.

The global objective of nutritional assessment is to ascertain a patient's nutritional status and to use the information to determine the specific intervention(s) required to maintain or obtain optimal nutrition and overall health. Loss of protein stores causes substantial morbidity and mortality beyond that associated with the primary disease and can prevent patient recovery from infection, injury, and surgery. These and other adverse consequences of poor nutrition have been most comprehensively studied in hospitalized patients. The importance of routine nutritional assessment for the patient receiving renal replacement therapy has been scientifically documented by several studies and demonstrates a direct relation between nutritional indices and morbidity and mortality in this patient population. These observations have resulted in renewed interest in identifying specific and reliable methods to assess the nutritional status of the patient with chronic and end-stage renal disease.

The optimal protocol to use in a predictive, reliable, and sensitive manner for patients with kidney disease has not been identified, in part because of a variety of metabolic, anthropometric, and biochemical abnormalities that accompany the uremic state and characterize patients receiving renal replacement therapy. The nutritional assessment procedure should detect subclinical abnormalities; diagnose loss of protein stores; identify macronutrient, micronutrient, and substrate deficiencies; ascertain the risk for the development of poor nutrition; and rate the overall nutritional status of each patient. No single measurement can accomplish all of these goals. Therefore, an array of indices, each representing a specific data category, are measured independently and then evaluated collectively to ascertain the nutritional status of the patient with renal disease. Table 14-15 lists the components that must be evaluated in the clinical setting when completing a nutrition assessment.

Serum Albumin as a Nutrition Assessment Parameter

Serum albumin has been relied upon as a marker of visceral stores for more than 20 years. Nutrition assessment protocols have depended heavily on serum albumin as a parameter by which to determine nutrition intervention. For example, a patient with hypoalbuminemia who loses weight has traditionally been encouraged to increase dietary intake of both calories and HBV protein. Patients with hypoalbuminemia who have adequate and stable body weight have been instructed to increase animal protein intake to restore albumin and presumably improve nutritional status. However, nutrition interventions that provide an increased intake of protein calories, either through food intake or the use of supplements, do not result in uniform improvement. The obvious hypothesis regarding hypoalbuminemia is that the serum albumin concentration is affected by nonnutritional factors, and the available information indicates that this hypothesis is true.

For example, recent reports have determined that patients undergoing dialysis who have low serum albumin values have evidence of systemic inflammation. This inflammation is manifested through elevations in serum levels of proinflammatory cytokines, such as tumor necrosis factor, interleukin-1, and

Table 14-15. Components of nutrition assessment for patients with chronic kidney disease (CKD)

Clinical	Food and Diet Intake	Biochemical	Body Weight	Body Composition
Physical examination	Diet history, food record or food frequency questionnaire	Visceral protein stores	History	Adipose stores
Nutrition assessment scoring/screening	Appetite assessment	Static protein reserves	Actual	Lean body mass (skeletal muscle)
Medical history	Quantitative food intake	Immune competence	Compared to standards, BMI	
Psychosocial history	Qualitative food intake	Vitamins, minerals, and trace elements		
Demographics	Food habits and patterns	Fluid, electrolyte, and acid-base balance	Weight change over time	
Physical activity level	Fluid intake/balance	Anemia labs		
Current medical/surgical issues	Lifestyle issues: physical activity	Cardiovascular disease: Lipid status, cardiac calcification		Goal weight
Prescribed medications; nutrient/drug interactions		Evidence of systemic inflammation		
		Bone disease labs		

BMI, body mass index.

interleukin-6. These cytokines can also be associated with anorexia, muscle wasting, and fat wasting and generate an overall catabolic state of metabolism. Similarly, metabolic acidosis results in low serum albumin, fatigue, loss of muscle protein, anorexia, and so on. Hepatic synthesis of acute phase protein decreases serum albumin levels, whereas metabolic acidosis suppresses albumin synthesis. In short, hypoalbuminemia is principally a manifestation of systemic inflammation or acidosis, rather than a consequence of inadequate protein and energy intakes. From this perspective, it is clear why aggressive diet and nutrition support does not correct the catabolic effects of systemic inflammation, acidosis, or insulin resistance.

Which factors trigger systemic inflammation is currently not clear. Hypotheses include the dialysis procedure itself, bioincompatible dialysis membranes, oxidative stress, or CVD. CVD is a main cause of mortality in patients receiving HD therapy. A complex interplay between CVD and systemic inflammation is thought to affect nutritional status. The additive effects of systemic inflammation and potential catabolism, which result in weight loss, visceral muscle wasting, and poor outcome, emphasize the need to maintain strict and persistent nutritional assessment, monitoring, and interventions.

PROTOCOLS TO PROVIDE NUTRITION CARE

Although nutrition assessment methodology is not definitive, and optimal nutrient intakes are individualized, standardized protocols are available for nutrition assessment, monitoring, and nutritional counseling for patients with CKD. Examples are listed in Table 14-16 for CKD stages 1 to 4 and Table 14-17 for the patient receiving renal replacement therapy.

Costs for nutrition care provided by an RD formerly were covered by Medicare, but only for patients with stage 5 CKD. In January 2002, Medicare implemented the MNT program, which provides reimbursement for nutrition care provided by RDs to Medicare patients who have a diagnosis of chronic renal insufficiency or diabetes. This coverage is not sufficient and is an area in which the ADA is currently working to improve patient access to nutrition care provided by an RD.

PATIENT EDUCATION, MOTIVATION, AND ADHERENCE TO RECOMMENDATIONS

The diet for patients with CKD, particularly for patients with stage 5 CKD, frequently requires lifestyle changes in specific food selection, culinary methods, and social eating. Restricting total fluid, intake of seasonal fruits and vegetables, and minimizing intake of dairy products can be difficult to adjust to and maintain.

Geographical and social challenges exist as well. For example, patients living in desert regions are used to drinking large quantities of water. Phosphate binders are large pills that not only require fluid for swallowing but can also cause nausea, bloating, and excessive gas production. Binders have to be taken at work, at social events, and when eating out. How does the renal care team motivate patients to adhere to all these multiple components of care?

Table 14-16.   A protocol for the nutritional management of chronic kidney disease (CKD) stages 1-4

Initial Nutrition Assessment
Session: Initial Length, *60–90 minutes*; Time, *Within 1 month of referral*

Factor	Assessments
Clinical data	1. Review minimum baseline data table.
	2. Obtain current height, weight, and BMI.
	3. Obtain weight history, recent weight changes, and weight goals.
	4. Determine IBW and/or UBW adjusted for amputation or obesity and percentage IBW and/or percentage UBW (see Appendix B).
	5. Assess muscle and fat stores, presence of edema.
	6. Assess for physical signs of nutrient deficiencies/excesses or increased needs (e.g., decubiti, poor wound healing, thinning hair, pale conjunctiva, cheilosis).
	7. Determine nitrogen balance using urea kinetics, if appropriate (see Appendix D).
	8. Assess blood pressure control.
Dietary evaluation	1. Determine previous dietary instruction and practices.
	2. Determine usual food intake and pattern of intake.
	3. Assess appetite, GI issues, tolerance of oral intake, and food allergies/intolerances.
	4. Assess feeding issues (e.g., chewing, swallowing).
	5. Determine use of vitamin/mineral, herbal, or other nutrition supplements.
	6. Determine alcohol/drug/tobacco use and history.
	7. Assess intake of calories, protein, sodium, and other nutrients as indicated (e.g., carbohydrates, fats, potassium, phosphorus, calcium, and fluids).
	8. Assess diet order, tube feeding order, and/or parenteral nutrition order for appropriateness.
Functional ability/exercise	1. Determine level of functional ability and recent changes.
	2. Assess ability to feed self and needs for assistance.

continued

Table 14-16. *Continued.*

Factor	Assessments
	3. Determine activity level and exercise habits
	4. Determine physical or motivational limitations to exercise.
Psychosocial and economic issues	1. Assess living situation, cooking facilities, finances, educational background, employment, literacy, and other factors that may affect availability of food.
	2. Assess ethnic or religious belief considerations.
	3. Assess availability of support systems.
	4. Determine whether other relevant psychosocial or economic issues exist.
Knowledge, skill level, attitudes, and motivation	1. Assess basic knowledge level of dietary guidelines for renal insufficiency
	2. Assess basic knowledge level of impact of renal insufficiency on nutrition.
	3. Assess attitudes toward nutrition and health.
	4. Determine patient's willingness and ability to learn and make appropriate changes.

BMI, body mass index; IBW, ideal body weight; UBW, usual body weight; GI, gastrointestinal.
From Wiggins Kerry L, Renal Dietitians Dietetic Practice Group. *Guidelines for nutrition care of renal patients.* Chicago: American Dietetic Association, 2002, with permission.

Studies have been completed that investigate demographics and rationale for nonadherence to diet and medication. Barriers that have been identified to have a role in nonadherence include behavioral, socioeconomic, medical, or some combination of these factors. Behavioral issues include high hostility levels towards components of their new lifestyle and frequent travel. Medical barriers are related to the presence of comorbid conditions, physical limitations, or depression. Financial difficulties imposed by the need to purchase multiple medications (on average 14 to 15 doses of five to six medications daily) can result in a patient's decision to disregard a prescription drug regimen.

Components of care that have been identified to help foster adherence to recommendations in patients receiving dialysis therapy, as described by Morton de Souza (2001), include the following:

Table 14-17. A protocol that identifies expected outcomes from nutritional therapy for adult patients receiving hemodialysis therapy

Expected Outcomes of Medical Nutrition Therapy

Outcome Assessment Factors	Expected Outcome of Therapy	Ideal/Goal Value
Clinical outcomes		
• Biochemical parameters	Measure <30 days prior to nutrition session	
–BUN, creatinine	BUN and creatinine levels stabilized	BUN and creatinine levels stabilized
–Albumin	Albumin increasing to ≥4.0	Albumin ≥4.0 g/dL
–Potassium	Potassium maintained within goal range	Potassium 3.5–5.5 mEq/L
–Phosphorus	Phosphorus and calcium levels progressing toward goal ranges	Phosphorus 4.0–6.0 mg/dL
–Calcium		Calcium 8.5–10.5 mg/dL
–Serum glucose (casual)	Blood sugar levels maintained within goal range	Serum glucose 80–200 mg/dL
–HbA1c (diabetes)		HbA1c <7%
–Cholesterol	Cholesterol levels progressing toward goal range	Cholesterol 150–250 mg/dL
–PTH (intact)	PTH maintained within goal range	PTH 100–300 pg/mL
• Hematologic parameters		
–Hematocrit/hemoglobin	Adequate erythropoiesis maintained	Hematocrit 33%–36%, hemoglobin 11.0–12.0 g/dL
–Ferritin	Adequate iron stores maintained for erythropoiesis	Ferritin 100–800 ng/mL
–Transferrin saturation		Transferrin saturation 20%–50%
• Dialysis adequacy		
–Kt/V (URR)	Kt/V (URR) maintained at or above target goal	Kt/V ≥1.2 or URR 65 (hemodialysis)
		Weekly Kt/V ≥2.0, creatinine clearance ≥60 L/wk/1.73 m² (CAPD)
–nPNA (stable state)	nPNA maintained at or above goal	nPNA ≥0.8

		MNT goals
Anthropometrics –Dry weight –Interdialytic fluid gains (hemodialysis)	Reasonable weight achieved/maintained Fluid gains achieved/maintained at goal	Within reasonable b.w. weight (BMI 20–25) Fluid gains 2%–5% b.w.
Clinical signs and symptoms	Adequate body mass maintained	Adequate muscle/fat stores Optimum functional ability
	Level of functional ability maintained Good appetite maintained	Minimum GI symptoms Food intake >80% recommended intake Blood pressure within appropriate limits
	Appropriate blood pressure control maintained	
Patient/caregiver behavioral outcomes		1. Makes appropriate food choices and takes medications as prescribed
Food selection/meal planning	Exhibits positive changes in food selection and amounts If diabetic, times meals and snacks appropriately	2. Maintains adequate protein intake 3. Maintains lab values within acceptable limits
Nutrient needs	Identifies foods high in protein, sodium, potassium, and phosphorus content Identifies fluid sources and limits	4. If diabetic, maintains stable glucose levels through appropriate dietary practices 5. If no medical limitations, maintenance of an exercise program
Potential food/drug interactions	Verbalizes potential food/drug interactions	
Exercise	If no medical limitations, gradually increases or continues physical activity level	

BUN, blood, urea, nitrogen; PTH, parathyroid hormone; URR, urea reduction ratio; CAPD, continuous ambulatory peritoneal dialysis; BMI, body mass index; GI, gastrointestinal; MNT, Medical Nutrition Therapy.

From Wiggins Kerry L, Renal Dietitians Dietetic Practice Group. *Guidelines for nutrition care of renal patients.* Chicago: American Dietetic Association, 2002, with permission.

- Patient-centered care—a model in which the patient sets his or her own health goals with support and assistance from the renal care team.
- Positive patient–staff interaction—receiving extra attention and multiple interactions improves adherence, as does a positive patient–doctor interaction.
- Ongoing accessibility of staff—all members of the healthcare team have a role to play in improving patient adherence to guidelines. Consistent and frequent feedback from the dietitian has been demonstrated to improve patient adherence to diet guidelines. The social worker can identify barriers to adherence. Nurses, who have the most contact with the patient, are in a position to identify or notice problems, changes, or new developments in following medical and nutritional advice.

Compliment patients for positive efforts—continuous positive reinforcement and acknowledgment of improved behaviors are inherent to the success of a model geared toward improving adherence. Noting an improved weight gain or a lower potassium level can make a difference in a patient's behavior over time.

A large variety of materials are available to assist patients in adhering to diet guidelines, particularly for phosphate, fluid, and potassium. Although standardized monthly nutrition care of patients is critical, innovative approaches, such as Phosphorus Buddy programs, unit contests, and games, are becoming increasingly popular. An example of one of these innovative type materials is reproduced in Figure 14-2.

SUMMARY

Diet is an integral component of the overall treatment of patients with kidney disease. The diet is complex, and the challenge of caring for these patients continues to grow with advances in research and technology. Results from research in the areas of nutrition assessment methods, metabolism, systemic inflammation, and CVD will continue to challenge renal care practitioners to use nutrition intervention optimally to improve patient outcomes. In the meantime, nutrition assessment, monitoring, patient education with continual reinforcement, and individualized diet application are among the best clinical approaches the nephrology team can offer.

Name of Game or Contest	Nutri-Bowling Game
Individual or Team	Individual Patient Game
Length of Time to Play	One or More Months
Parameters Measured	Phosphorus, Calcium, Potassium, Albumin, Fluid Gains & Treatment Attendance
Objective of the Game	To knock down as many "bowling pins" as possible
How to Play Nutri-Bowling	The patient knocks down a specific number of "bowling pins" based on his or her lab results and average monthly fluid gains. If all five of the above parameters are within the acceptable range, the patient receives a "STRIKE" (10 pins). If only four parameters are met, 8 pins are knocked down. If only three parameters are met, 6 pins are knocked down. If only two parameters are met, 4 pins are knocked down. A "Gutter Ball" is bowled if only one or none of the parameters are met. "**BONUS PINS**" (1 pin for each) can be added to the total score if the patient 1.) Attended all treatments 2.) Stay for entire treatment each time.
What to Give Patients	Nutri-Bowling Game handout (included)
How to Keep score STRIKE!	As you prepare each patient's lab "report card," count the number of "pins" the patient knocked down. Use stats from the previous month (from the date of last month's lab draw) for average fluid gains and treatment attendance records. Your unit's secretary may be able to assist you in keeping track of patients who were a "No Show" (don't count hospitalization) and who left treatments early (AMA) *Against Medical Advice*. Write the patient's "bowling score" on his or her lab report card, give it to the patient and keep a copy for your records. Place the names of the patients in the appropriate raffle container for 1st, 2nd, or 3rd place winners.
Clinic Display	Attach the bowling pin visuals (included) to a bulletin board or walls and doors in the clinic. Provide educational information regarding each parameter along side the bowling pins. Use additional bowling visuals such as bowling balls, score cards, bowling shoes and shirts, etc.
Rewards Certificate of Achievement	Hold raffles for 1st place: 10 or more pins, 2nd place for 8 pins & 3rd place for 6 pins. You may choose to hold a monthly raffle or wait until three months. Prizes may include t-shirts, bowling alley gift certificates (if patients are able to use their nonaccess arm to bowl—best to check with physician), key chains containing a bowling ball, etc. Be sure to award all the first place "bowlers" with a small prize or recognition. You may post their names or initials. Give each one a certificate of achievement or an award ribbon.

Figure 14-2. Example of an innovative intervention to improve patient adherence. From Morton de Souza D. *Handbook of creative approaches to patient compliance. A guide to assist renal dietitians working with dialysis patients.* **South Florida, Professional Nutrition Services, 2001, with permission.**

NUTR◯ - BOWL◯NG GAME

Your Bowling Game Is Scored as Follows:

Two "PINS" for *each* within the desirable range:

Phosphorus = 3.5–5.5   Calcium = 8.4–10.2

Albumin: ↑3.5   Potassium: 3.5–5.5

Fluid gains: 2.0 kg average

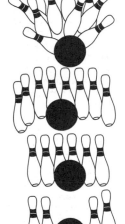

STRIKE (10 Pins)

If all five of the values listed above are within the desirable range

(8 Pins)

If four out of the five values listed above are within the desirable range

(6 Pins)

If three out of the five values listed above are within the desirable range

(4 Pins)

If two out of the five values listed above are within the desirable range

GUTTER BALL (☹ Pins)

If only one or *none* of the values listed above are within the desirable range

BONUS PINS (1 pin for each)

-If you attended all treatments in the month

-If you stayed for your complete treatment each time

Raffle Drawings for 1st place (10 + pins), 2nd place (8 pins), and 3rd place (6 pins)

Go for the STRIKE!!!

Figure 14-2. *Continued.*

SELECTED READINGS

American Dietetic Association. *Medical nutrition therapy evidence based guides for practice. chronic kidney disease (non-dialysis) medical nutrition therapy protocol.* Chicago: American Dietetic Association, 2002.

Blue L. Adult kidney transplantation. In: Hasse J, Blue L, eds. *Comprehensive guide to transplant nutrition.* Chicago: American Dietetic Association, 2002:44–57.

Chertow GM. Slowing the progression of vascular calcification in hemodialysis. *J Am Soc Nephrol* 2003;14:S310–S314.

Ford J, Pope JF, Hunt AE, et al. The effect of diet education on the laboratory values and knowledge of hemodialysis patients with hyperphosphatemia. *J Renal Nutr* 2004;14(1):36–44.

Grodstein GP, Blumenkrantz MJ, Kopple JD, et al. Glucose absorption during continuous ambulatory peritoneal dialysis. *Kidney Int* 1981;19(4):564–567.

Ikizler TA, Pupim LB, Brouillette JR, et al. Hemodialysis stimulates muscle and whole body protein loss and alters substrate oxidation. *Am J Endocrinol Metab* 2002;282:E107–E116.

Ikizler TA, Wingard R, Sun M, et al. Increased energy expenditure in hemodialysis patients. *J Am Soc Nephrol* 1996;7:2646–2653.

Karalis M. Ways to increase protein intake. *J Renal Nutr* 2002; 12(2):136–138.

Kaysen G. Role of inflammation and its treatment in ESRD patients. *Blood Purif* 2002;20:70.

Kris-Etherton P, William H, Appel L. Fish consumption, fish oil, omega-3 fatty acids, and cardiovascular disease. *Circulation* 2002;106:2747–2757.

Martin C, Reams R. The renal dietitian's role in managing hyperphosphatemia and secondary hyperparathyroidism in dialysis patients: a national survey. *J Renal Nutr* 2003;13(2):133–136.

Morton de Souza D. *Handbook of creative approaches to patient compliance. A guide to assist renal dietitians working with dialysis patients.* Florida: Professional Nutrition Services, 2001.

National Academy of Sciences, Institute of Medicine. *Dietary reference intakes for energy, carbohydrates, fiber, fat, fatty acids, cholesterol, protein and amino acids (macronutrients),* Chapter 8. Washington, DC: The National Academies Press, 2002.

Neyra R, Chen KY, Un M, et al. Increased resting energy expenditure in patients with end-stage renal disease. *J Parenter Enteral Nutr* 2003;27:36–42.

NKF-K/DOQI. Clinical practice guidelines for nutrition in chronic renal failure. *Am J Kidney Dis* 2000a;35(Suppl. 2):S1–S140.

NKF-K/DOQI. Clinical practice guidelines for the treatment of anemia of chronic kidney disease. *Am J Kidney Dis* 2000b;37(Suppl. 1):S182–S238.

NKF-K/DOQI. Clinical Practice Guidelines for Chronic Kidney Disease: Evaluation, Classification, and Stratification. (2002). *Am J Kidney Dis* 2002;39(Suppl. 1):S1–S46.

NKF-K/DOQI. Clinical practice guidelines for bone metabolism and disease in chronic kidney disease. *Am J Kidney Dis* 2003;42(Suppl. 3):S1–S202.

NKF-K/DOQI. Clinical practice guidelines on hypertension and antihypertensive agents in chronic kidney disease. *Am J Kidney Dis* 2004;43(Suppl. 1):S1–S290.

Paret CL. Calcium containing phosphate binder use associated with accelerated atherosclerotic coronary calcification. *J Ren Nutr* 2003;13(4):1–8.

Stenvinkel P, Heimbürger O, Lindholm B, et al. Are there two types of malnutrition in chronic renal failure? Evidence for relationships between malnutrition, inflammation and atherosclerosis (MIA syndrome). *Nephrol Dial Transplant* 2000;15(7):953–960.

Wiggins Kerry L, Renal Dietitians Dietetic Practice Group. *Guidelines for nutrition care of renal patients.* Chicago, Ill: American Dietetic Association, 2002.

Williams M, Chianchiano JD. Medicare medical nutrition therapy: Legislative process and product. *J Renal Nutr* 2002;12(1):1–7.

Subject Index

Figures are indicated by page numbers followed by *f*; tables are indicated by page numbers followed by *t*